T0127869

Vascular Surgery

Editors

RAVI VEERASWAMY
DAWN M. COLEMAN

SURGICAL CLINICS
OF NORTH AMERICA

www.surgical.theclinics.com

Consulting Editor
RONALD F. MARTIN

August 2023 • Volume 103 • Number 4

ELSEVIER

1600 John F. Kennedy Boulevard • Suite 1800 • Philadelphia, Pennsylvania, 19103-2899

http://www.surgical.theclinics.com

SURGICAL CLINICS OF NORTH AMERICA Volume 103, Number 4
August 2023 ISSN 0039–6109, ISBN-13: 978-0-323-93935-5

Editor: John Vassallo (j.vassallo@elsevier.com)

Developmental Editor: Anita Chamoli

Surgical Clinics of North America (ISSN 0039–6109) is published bimonthly by Elsevier Inc., 360 Park Avenue South, New York, NY 10010-1710. Months of publication are February, April, June, August, October, and December. Business and Editorial Offices: 1600 John F. Kennedy Blvd., Suite 1800, Philadelphia, PA 19103-2899. Periodicals postage paid at New York, NY and additional mailing offices. Subscription prices are $479.00 per year for US individuals, $1045.00 per year for US institutions, $100.00 per year for US & Canadian students and residents, $575.00 per year for Canadian individuals, $1327.00 per year for Canadian institutions, $580.00 for international individuals, $1327.00 per year for international institutions and $250.00 per year for foreign students/residents. To receive student/resident rate, orders must be accompanied by name of affiliated institution, date of term, and the *signature* of program/residency coordinator on institution letterhead. Orders will be billed at individual rate until proof of status is received. Foreign air speed delivery is included in all *Clinics* subscription prices. All prices are subject to change without notice. POSTMASTER: Send address changes to *Surgical Clinics*, Elsevier Health Sciences Division, Subscription Customer Service, 3251 Riverport Lane, Maryland Heights, MO 63043. **Customer Service (orders, claims, online, change of address): Telephone: 1-800-654-2452 (U.S. and Canada); 314-447-8871 (outside U.S. and Canada). Fax: 314-447-8029. E-mail: journalscustomerservice-usa@elsevier.com (for print support); journalsonlinesupport-usa@elsevier.com (for online support).**

Reprints. For copies of 100 or more, of articles in this publication, please contact the Commercial Reprints Department, Elsevier Inc., 360 Park Avenue South, New York, New York 10010-1710. Tel. 212-633-3874, Fax: 212-633-3820, E-mail: reprints@elsevier.com.

Surgical Clinics of North America is also published in Spanish by McGraw-Hill Interamericana Editores S.A., P.O. Box 5-237 06500 Mexico D.F. Mexico; and in Portuguese by Interlivros Edicoes Ltda., Rua Comandante Coelho 1085, CEP 21250, Rio de Janeiro, Brazil; and in Greek by Paschalidis Medical Publications, Athens Greece.

Surgical Clinics of North America is covered in *MEDLINE/PubMed (Index Medicus), EMBASE/Excerpta Medica, Current Contents/Clinical Medicine, Current Contents/Life Sciences, Science Citation Index,* and *ISI/BIOMED.*

Contributors

CONSULTING EDITOR

RONALD F. MARTIN, MD, FACS
Colonel (Retired), United States Army Reserve, Department of General Surgery, Pullman Regional Hospital and Clinic Network, Pullman, Washington, USA

EDITORS

RAVI VEERASWAMY, MD
The Elliot-Robison Endowed Professor of Surgery; Chief of Vascular Surgery and Associate Chief Medical Officer, Medical University of South Carolina, MUSC Health Ashley River Tower, Charleston, South Carolina, USA

DAWN M. COLEMAN, MD
Formerly, Marion and David Handleman Research Professor of Vascular Surgery, University of Michigan, Vascular Surgery, Ann Arbor, Michigan, USA; Currently, Professor of Surgery, Division Chief, Vascular and Endovascular Surgery, Duke University, Duke University Medical Center, Durham, North Carolina, USA

AUTHORS

AJIBOLA GEORGE AKINGBA, MD, PhD
Vascular Surgeon, DC VAMC, Adjunct Associate Professor, Uniformed Services University of Health Sciences, Washington, DC, USA

CHARLES ADAM BANKS, MD
Division of Vascular Surgery and Endovascular Therapy, The University of Alabama at Birmingham, Birmingham, Alabama, USA

ROBERT J. BEAULIEU, MD, MSE
Assistant Professor, Vascular Surgery, Department of Surgery, University of Michigan, Ann Arbor, Michigan, USA

WARREN BRYAN CHOW, MD, MS
Assistant Professor of Surgery, Division of Vascular Surgery and Endovascular Therapy, David Geffen School of Medicine at UCLA, Los Angeles, California, USA

VENITA R. CHANDRA, MD
Clinical Professor of Surgery (Vascular), Stanford School of Medicine, Program Director of Stanford Vascular Surgery Residency and Fellowship, Co-Medical Director of Stanford Wound Care Center; Division of Vascular and Endovascular Surgery, Department of Surgery, Stanford University, Stanford, California, USA

DAWN M. COLEMAN, MD
Formerly, Marlon and David Handleman Research Professor of Vascular Surgery, University of Michigan, Vascular Surgery, Ann Arbor, Michigan, USA; Currently, Professor

of Surgery, Division Chief, Vascular and Endovascular Surgery, Duke University, Duke University Medical Center, Durham, North Carolina, USA

NICOLE D'AMBROSIO, MD
Department of Vascular Surgery, Georgetown University Hospital, MedStar Health, Washington, DC, USA

JESSIE DALMAN
University of Michigan, Ann Arbor, Michigan, USA

SIMON DE FREITAS, MD
Department of Vascular Surgery, Georgetown University Hospital, MedStar Health, Washington, DC, USA

AUDRA A. DUNCAN, MD, FACS, FRCSC
Professor, Chair/Chief, Division of Vascular and Endovascular Surgery, Western University, London, Ontario, Canada

YOUNG ERBEN, MD
Associate Professor, Division of Vascular and Endovascular Surgery, Mayo Clinic, Jacksonville, Florida, USA

YANA ETKIN, MD
Associate Professor of Surgery, Division of Vascular and Endovascular Surgery, Department of Surgery, Zucker School of Medicine at Hofstra/Northwell, Hempstead, New York, USA

JAVAIRIAH FATIMA, MD, FACS, RPVI, DFSVS
Associate Professor, Department of Vascular Surgery, Georgetown University Hospital, MedStar Health, Washington, DC, USA

ARASH FEREYDOONI, MD, MS, MHS
Division of Vascular and Endovascular Surgery, Department of Surgery, Stanford University, Stanford, California, USA

ANA FUENTES
Division of Vascular and Endovascular Surgery, Mayo Clinic, Jacksonville, Florida, USA

KARAN GARG, MD
Associate Professor of Surgery, Division of Vascular Surgery, NYU Langone Medical Center, New York, New York, USA

RYAN GEDNEY, MD
Vascular Surgery Resident, Medical University of South Carolina, Charleston, South Carolina, USA

LONDON GUIDRY, MD
Clinical Associate Professor of Surgery, Division of Vascular and Endovascular Surgery, Department of Surgery, Louisiana State University Health and Science Center, New Orleans, Louisiana, USA

JOHN IGUIDBASHIAN, MD
Department of Surgery, University of Colorado Anschutz School of Medicine, Aurora, Colorado, USA

RABBIA IMRAN, MS
University of Colorado Anschutz School of Medicine, Aurora, Colorado, USA

ALLISON LEARNED, BS, NP
Department of Surgery, Division of Vascular Surgery, University of Massachusetts Chan Medical School, Worcester, Massachusetts, USA

TAMMY T. NGUYEN, MD, PhD
Assistant Professor, Department of Surgery, Division of Vascular Surgery, University of Massachusetts Chan Medical School; University of Massachusetts Diabetes Center of Excellence, Worcester, Massachusetts, USA

BENJAMIN J. PEARCE, MD, FACS
Associate Professor, Division of Vascular Surgery and Endovascular Therapy, The University of Alabama at Birmingham, Birmingham, Alabama, USA

SUDIE-ANN ROBINSON, MD
Department of Surgery, Division of Vascular Surgery, University of Massachusetts Chan Medical School, Worcester, Massachusetts, USA

CARON B. ROCKMAN, MD
Florence and Joseph Ritorto Professor of Surgery, Division of Vascular Surgery, NYU Langone Medical Center, NYU Grossman School of Medicine, New York, New York, USA

VINCENT LOPEZ ROWE, MD
Professor and Chief, Division of Vascular Surgery and Endovascular Therapy, David Geffen School of Medicine at UCLA, Los Angeles, California, USA

OONAGH H. SCALLAN, MD, FRCSC
Assistant Professor, Division of Vascular and Endovascular Surgery, Western University, London, Ontario, Canada

NITEN SINGH, MD
Professor of Surgery, Division of Vascular Surgery, Department of Surgery, University of Washington, Seattle, Washington, USA

NICOLAS A. STAFFORINI, MD
Division of Vascular Surgery, Department of Surgery, University of Washington, Seattle, Washington, USA

KYLE STEIGER, MD
Mayo Clinic Alix School of Medicine, Mayo Clinic, Scottsdale, Arizona, USA

KAREN WOO, MD, PhD
Professor of Surgery, Division of Vascular Surgery, Department of Surgery, David Geffen School of Medicine at UCLA, Los Angeles, California, USA

MATHEW WOOSTER, MD, MBA
Associate Professor of Surgery, Director of Aortic Surgery, Division of Vascular Surgery, Medical University of South Carolina, Charleston, South Carolina, USA

JENIANN A. YI, MD, MS
Assistant Professor, Department of Surgery, University of Colorado Anschutz School of Medicine, Aurora, Colorado, USA

Contents

> We offer an overview of lipid lowering, antiplatelet, antihypertensive, and glucose-lowering therapies for vascular surgeons and their respective medical teams. Further reviews should offer additional guidance on smoking cessation, exercise therapy, and nutritional optimization.

> Patients with vascular disease represent a particularly high-risk surgical population. Many of the comorbidities that contribute to their vascular presentation impact a number of vascular beds or other organ systems. As a result, these patients have the highest rates of cardiac and pulmonary complications among patients with noncardiac surgery. The vascular surgeon is in a unique position to help evaluate and treat many of these conditions to not only reduce the perioperative risk but also to improve the patient's overall health. This article presents a comprehensive review of the common preoperative evaluations that have a high impact on patients with vascular disease.

> Abdominal aortic aneurysms are found in up to 6% of men and 1.7% of women over the age of 65 years and are usually asymptomatic. The natural history of aortic aneurysms is continued dilation leading to rupture, which is associated with an overall 80% mortality. Of the patients with ruptured aneurysms that undergo intervention, half will not survive their hospitalization. Reduction in aneurysm mortality is therefore achieved by prophylactic repair during the asymptomatic period. On a population-based level, this is supported by abdominal aortic aneurysm screening programs. Approximately 60% of abdominal aortic aneurysms are confined to the infrarenal portion of the aorta and are amenable to repair with off-the-shelf endovascular devices. Endovascular techniques have now replaced open surgery as the primary modality for aneurysm repair.

Aortic arch and descending thoracic pathology have historically remained in the realm of open surgical repair. Technology is quickly pushing to bring these under the endovascular umbrella, with lower morbidity repairs proving safe in their early experience. Much work remains particularly for acute aortic syndromes, however, to understand who is best treated medically, surgically, endovascularly, or with hybrid approaches.

Stroke is a persistent leading cause of morbidity and mortality, and carotid artery atherosclerosis remains a treatable cause of future stroke. Although most patients with asymptomatic carotid artery disease may be at a relatively low risk for future stroke, most completed strokes are unheralded; thus, the identification and appropriate treatment of patients with asymptomatic carotid artery disease remains a critical part of overall stroke prevention. Select patients with asymptomatic carotid artery stenosis with an increased risk of future stroke based on the degree of stenosis and other imaging or patient-related characteristics are appropriate to consider for carotid artery intervention.

Atherosclerotic carotid artery disease has been well studied over the last half-century by multiple randomized controlled trials attempting to elucidate the appropriate modality of therapy for this disease process. Surgical techniques have evolved from carotid artery endarterectomy and transfemoral carotid artery stenting to the development of hybrid techniques in transcarotid artery revascularization. In this article, the authors provide a review of the available literature regarding operative and medical management of carotid artery disease.

End-stage kidney disease (ESKD) affects nearly 800,000 patients in the United States. The choice of peritoneal dialysis (PD) versus hemodialysis (HD) should be patient centric. An ESKD Life-Plan is crucial with the goal of creating the right access, for the right patient, at the right time, for the right reason. Complex access should be considered when straightforward access options have been exhausted. Evolving techniques such as percutaneous access for HD and PD should be further investigated. Shared decision-making and palliative care is an essential part of the care of patients with CKD and ESKD..

Many end-stage kidney failure patients require hemodialysis as a life-sustaining treatment. Hemodialysis access via arteriovenous fistula or graft creation is preferred over long-term dialysis catheters, but intervention to maintain patency and prevent access failure is common. Endovascular and open surgical techniques are both utilized to address the underlying etiology of failure. Endovascular options include balloon angioplasty, angioplasty with stenting, and drug-eluting stents. Open revision is commonly needed for recurrent stenosis, aneurysmal or pseudoaneurysmal change, hemodialysis access-induced distal ischemia, and infection. Treatment plans should be guided by patient's individualized goals of care and require a multidisciplinary approach to the management of this complex disease.

Current Approaches for Mesenteric Ischemia and Visceral Aneurysms   703

Oonagh H. Scallan and Audra A. Duncan

This article provides an overview of acute mesenteric ischemia, chronic mesenteric ischemia, and visceral aneurysms, with a focus on treatment. Acute mesenteric ischemia can be a challenging diagnosis. Early recognition and adequate revascularization are key to patient outcomes. Chronic mesenteric ischemia is a more insidious process, typically caused by atherosclerosis. Various options for revascularization exist, which must be tailored to each patient. Visceral aneurysms are rare and the natural history is not well defined. However, given the risk of rupture and high mortality, treatment may be complex.

Nonatherosclerotic Renovascular Hypertension   733

Jessie Dalman and Dawn M. Coleman

Renovascular hypertension (RVH) is a secondary form of high blood pressure resulting from impaired blood flow to the kidneys with subsequent activation of the renin-angiotensin-aldosterone system. Often, this occurs due to abnormally small, narrowed, or blocked blood vessels supplying one or both kidneys (ie: renal artery occlusive disease) and is correctable. Juxtaglomerular cells release renin in response to decreased pressure, which in turn catalyzes the cleavage of circulating angiotensinogen synthesized by the liver to the decapeptide angiotensin I. Angiotensin-converting enzyme then cleaves angiotensin I to form the octapeptide angiotensin II, a potent vasopressor and the primary effector of renin-induced hypertension. The effects of angiotensin II are mediated by signaling downstream of its receptors. Angiotensin receptor type 1 is a G-protein-coupled receptor that activates vasoconstrictor and mitogenic signaling pathways resulting in peripheral arteriolar vasoconstriction and increased renal tubular reabsorption of sodium and water which promotes intravascular volume expansion. Angiotensin II stimulates the adrenal cortical release of aldosterone, which promotes renal tubular sodium reabsorption, resulting in volume expansion. Angiotensin II acts on glial cells and regions of the brain responsible for blood pressure regulation increasing renal sympathetic activation. Angiotensin II simulates the release of vasopressin from the pituitary which stimulates thirst and water reabsorption from the kidney to expand the intravascular volume and cause peripheral vasoconstriction (increased sympathetic tone). All of these mechanisms coalesce to increase arterial pressure by way of arteriolar constriction, enhanced cardiac output, and the retention of sodium and water.

SURGICAL CLINICS
OF NORTH AMERICA

SERIES OF RELATED INTEREST

Advances in Surgery
https://www.advancessurgery.com/
Surgical Oncology Clinics
https://www.surgonc.theclinics.com/
Thoracic Surgery Clinics
https://www.thoracic.theclinics.com/

THE CLINICS ARE AVAILABLE ONLINE!
Access your subscription at:
www.theclinics.com

Foreword

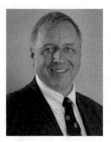

Ronald F. Martin, MD, FACS
Consulting Editor

It has been said no one thinks about oxygen when one has plenty of it, but when one does not have enough oxygen, it is the only thing one thinks about. I submit the same can be said for time. At the beginning of my career, it seemed like it would be forever until I had practiced enough to be comfortable. Now, very much toward the latter part of my career, I wonder where all the time went. During my time in training, we were all frequently taught that change was the only constant. And if we forgot it, someone with gray hair (or no hair) would be quick to remind us. The bitter irony though was despite our mentors constantly telling us change was coming, almost none could say how things would change. Even after the change had happened, most of them would say, "I didn't see that coming."

Vascular surgery is one of the best areas of surgical interest that typifies the above. The worlds of vascular surgery from the 1970s and 1980s are completely unrecognizable from the vascular surgery world of 2023 plus. The basic principles we relied on then and rely on now are not too different. The critical care trinity of air goes in and out, blood goes round and round, and oxygen is good, still pretty much holds up (looked at from a respectable distance). As far as the "blood-going-round-and-round" piece, cardiac output still pretty much equals cardiac return. The aphorism about revascularization being dependent on inflow, outflow, and conduit still holds. And the big arterial problems of blood leaking out, blood not getting through (clots, emboli, plaques), and arteries getting overly stretchy still make up the mainstay of troubles.

After that, though, just about everything in vascular is no longer the same.

This issue of the *Surgical Clinics*, expertly compiled by Drs Veeraswamy and Coleman along with their fellow contributors, is a phenomenal compendium to explain where we have landed on this journey. There is also plenty to outline the map of how we got here and where we might be going. Detailed descriptions of how the prevention of some disorders is as, if not more, important than the treatment—particularly when considering aneurysms—refocus our center of effort. The paradigm shift regarding open surgical procedures: originally open surgery was the only way to get arterial problems set to right, then endovascular procedures should only be done in specialized centers, to the more contemporary view that endovascular procedures can be

Surg Clin N Am 103 (2023) xiii–xiv
https://doi.org/10.1016/j.suc.2023.06.001
0039-6109/23/© 2023 Published by Elsevier Inc.

performed more widely, and major open procedures should only be done at specialized centers. (Parenthetically, that circle of logic applies to many general surgical operations as well.)

Of course, the advancement of diagnostic capability, technical capability, and engineering of devices have all led to huge improvements in care for patients with vascular disorders using far less morbid treatment plans. Yet, as with all other advances, it creates a new set of issues (eg, endoleaks) that require new tools and plans to manage and, preferably, prevent.

It should be clear now that vascular surgery has become almost completely dissociated from its progenitor, general surgery. For decades, many of us lived through the squabbles about that division from the heights of "Big Surgery" to the medical staff meetings. In retrospect, I respect the arguments that were made for and against the separation, but history has been clear on who was correct—our Vascular surgical colleagues. Whether by excellent foresight or self-fulfilling prophecy, the metamorphosis of the discipline into something that had historical links to general surgery but is clearly fundamentally separate and distinct is complete.

What general surgery and vascular surgery do have still in common, which it is hoped will never change, is that need to care for the whole patient to expect good results. After all, we all frequently are operating on focal aspects of systemic problems. In vascular surgery, one is almost always treating a focal manifestation of a systemic disease. In order to get the best results for our patients and our communities, we must all speak a common medical language and realize where our subspecialty fits into the larger picture. This issue of the *Surgical Clinics* should help anyone, from the beginning resident to the more seasoned surgeon, achieve those lofty goals. We are deeply indebted to our contributors for sharing their keen insights.

Ronald F. Martin, MD, FACS
Colonel (retired), United States Army Reserve
Department of General Surgery
Pullman Surgical Associates
Pullman Regional Hospital and Clinic Network
825 Southeast Bishop Boulevard, Suite 130
Pullman, WA 99163, USA

E-mail address:
rfmcescna@gmail.com

Preface

An Overview of Current Treatment Algorithms and Upcoming Opportunities in Vascular Surgery

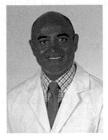
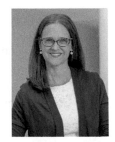

Ravi Veeraswamy, MD   Dawn M. Coleman, MD

Editors

Vascular surgery is an incredibly dynamic and innovative field in medicine. Our specialty has evolved and the landscape of comprehensive vascular care that we offer our patients is vast, as the endovascular revolution has altered the landscape for vascular interventions. New technology and techniques have been rapidly assimilated, accelerated by "cross-pollination" from other specialties.

In this issue, we review the current state of common vascular pathologies, treatments, and interventions across a variety of arterial beds. We emphasize broad concepts, with an algorithmic approach to treating aneurysmal and occlusive arterial disease. This issue is not intended to be comprehensive, nor a technical procedural guide. Rather, it is an attempt to provide those outside, or new to, the specialty with a general layout of the clinical problems that vascular surgeons manage and what solutions they might offer.

In addition to open surgical and percutaneous interventions, vascular surgeons continue to provide medical care that mitigates disease progression and promotes optimal results before and after interventions. This is an often-undervalued aspect of comprehensive vascular care, and, as appropriate, is highlighted throughout the articles. Finally, there are previews into the upcoming direction of the field with a focus on novel devices and the expansion of patients who can be helped via the advances in vascular surgery.

When we embarked on this project, our goal was to provide a succinct, yet thorough educational text, which would allow others to understand the breadth of the field and the multitude of creative approaches that the vascular surgeon can provide to treat a wide variety of arterial problems. We hope this will be of value to the medical field at

Surg Clin N Am 103 (2023) xv–xvi
https://doi.org/10.1016/j.suc.2023.05.008
0039-6109/23/© 2023 Published by Elsevier Inc.

large and are grateful for the opportunity to share our excitement about vascular surgery with others.

Ravi Veeraswamy, MD
Medical University of South Carolina
MUSC Health Ashley River Tower
25 Courtenay Drive
Charleston, SC 29425, USA

Dawn M. Coleman, MD
University of Michigan
Vascular Surgery
1500 East Medical Center Drive 5867 CC
Ann Arbor, MI 48109-5867, USA

E-mail addresses:
veeraswa@musc.edu (R. Veeraswamy)
dawn.coleman@duke.edu (D.M. Coleman)

Medical Management of Cardiovascular Disease

Kyle Steiger, MD[a], Ana Fuentes[b], Young Erben, MD[b],*

KEYWORDS

- Medical management • Hypertension • Diabetes mellitus • Hyperlipidemia
- Cardiovascular disease • Non surgical management

BACKGROUND

Medical management is critical in the treatment of all patients with cardiovascular disease. However, patients with peripheral vasculopathy are known to be medically undertreated by comparison to those with cardiac disease despite wide agreement that peripheral vascular disease is a broad indicator cerebrovascular and cardiovascular risk and current guidelines urging medical optimization of these patients.[1–4] This has been cited as a possible reason for worse outcomes in patients with peripheral arterial disease (PAD) as compared with those with coronary artery disease.[5] We provide an overview of consensus recommendations and evidence base regarding best medical therapy in patients typically seen by vascular surgeons with an emphasis on lipid-lowering and antiplatelet medications as well as blood pressure (BP) and glycemic control. Smoking cessation, exercise therapy, and nutritional optimization are important pieces of overall best medical management that we do not address.

LIPID REDUCTION

Patients achieving low levels of low-density lipoprotein-cholesterol (LDL-C) have fewer major cardiovascular events.[6] For patients with PAD, the Heart Protection Study was the first randomized controlled trial to illustrate that those with PAD treated with statins have a 25% reduction in rate of first major vascular event and 17% reduction in peripheral vascular events.[7] Patients with carotid disease have experienced similar reductions in randomized controlled trials.[8] Observational studies have further demonstrated statins decrease mortality and risk of amputation with increasing benefit linked to greater statin intensity and decreasing levels of LDL-C.[9,10] Consequently, the 2018 American College of Cardiology (ACC) and American Heart Association (AHA) guideline on management of blood cholesterol recommends high-intensity statin therapy or maximally tolerated statin therapy in all patients with clinically significant

[a] Department of Internal Medicine, Mayo Clinic, Rochester, Minnesota, USA; [b] Division of Vascular and Endovascular Surgery, Mayo Clinic, Jacksonville, FL, USA
* Corresponding author. Division of Vascular and Endovascular Surgery, Mayo Clinic Florida, 4500 San Pablo Road, Jacksonville, FL 32224.
E-mail address: erben.young@mayo.edu

Surg Clin N Am 103 (2023) 565–575
https://doi.org/10.1016/j.suc.2023.04.019
0039-6109/23/© 2023 Elsevier Inc. All rights reserved.
surgical.theclinics.com

atherosclerotic cardiovascular disease (ASCVD) including aortic aneurysm, even in those with normal LDL levels with a goal to reduce LDL-C levels by 50% or greater.[11] They further suggest higher risk patients with ASCVD, defined as those who have had an additional ASCVD event or more than one high-risk condition should achieve an LDL level of less than 70 mg/dL.[11] In these high-risk patients, ezetimibe or proprotein convertase subtilisin/kexin type 9 (PCSK9) inhibitor adjuvant therapy is to be considered in those who are unable to achieve this goal with statins alone.[11,12] In 2022, the ACC encouraged more aggressive treatment of lipids with statin and nonstatin therapies suggesting high-risk patients should achieve a goal of both a 50% or greater reduction in LDL-C and an LDL-C level of less than 55 mg/dL for a non-HDL-C of less than 85 mg/dL. They further state patients unable to achieve this goal should be referred to a lipid specialist.[13]

PCSK9 inhibitor therapy is supported by the FOURIER trial (Further Cardiovascular Outcomes Research With PCSK9 Inhibition in Subjects With Elevated Risk), which showed a 3.5% absolute reduction in cardiovascular events as well as a 42% reduction in major adverse limb events in patients with PAD treated with evolocumab.[12,14] Long-term follow-up of both arms of the FOURIER trial has shown persistently low rates of adverse events at 8 years with further reductions in cardiovascular events in those receiving treatment longest compared with those originally randomized into the placebo arm.[15] The greatest challenge with this medication is cost effectiveness (>US$150,000 per quality-adjusted life year according to the 2018 guideline).[11] Ezetimibe therapy has not been well studied in patients with PAD, with the body of evidence relying on the IMPROVE-IT trial (Improved Reduction of Outcomes: Vytorin Efficacy International Trial), which showed the greatest reduction in cardiovascular events among those with greatest Thrombolysis in Myocardial Infarction score; however, no studies have evaluated meaningful outcomes specifically in patients with PAD.[16] Nonetheless, the presumed benefit in patients with atherosclerosis coupled with its cost-effectiveness makes this the nonstatin drug of choice in most high-risk patients. Despite the growing body of evidence detailing improved outcome in patients with noncardiac vasculopathy treated with lipid-lowering medications and society guidelines encouraging their use in this population, prescribing rates of lipid lowering therapies remain low among those with noncoronary atherosclerosis.[17]

ANTIPLATELET AND ANTICOAGULATION MEDICATIONS

For the vascular surgeon, atherosclerosis with or without stenting is the primary indication for antiplatelet therapies. For patients with intermittent claudication from PAD, a large meta-analysis showed antiplatelet agents reduce all cause (RR 0.76) and cardiovascular (RR 0.54) mortality and decrease the need for revascularization (RR 0.65).[18] Regarding the use of single antiplatelet therapies, aspirin alone has been compared with P2Y12 inhibitors in clinically significant atherosclerotic disease. A large meta-analysis of 9 clinical trials comparing the 2 generally in patients with significant atherosclerosis found those who received P2Y12 inhibitors had borderline reduction in the risk of myocardial infarction (NNT 244) but that there were no differences in overall mortality, vascular mortality, or stroke incidence.[19] However, only one of these trials included patients with PAD: the CAPRIE trial (Clopidogrel Versus Aspirin in Patients at Risk for Ischemic Events). Importantly, this trial demonstrated the superiority of clopidogrel in patients with PAD via an 8.7% decrease in major adverse cardiovascular events by comparison without a significant difference in bleeding risk.[20] Other trials have shown no superiority of other antiplatelet agents to clopidogrel.[21] Nonetheless, the American guidelines (ACC/AHA) recommend either aspirin or clopidogrel monotherapy for all patients with PAD, whereas European guidelines favor clopidogrel, citing the CAPRIE trial.[22] Similarly, antiplatelet monotherapy is recommended in patients with asymptomatic and symptomatic carotid artery stenosis.[23,24]

The story of dual antiplatelet therapy (DAPT) is less straightforward. Regarding PAD as the sole indication for DAPT, large meta-analyses have shown varied clinical benefit and bleeding risk, culminating in a call for greater investigation.[25,26] The data on DAPT cannot be presented without considering patients who have experienced percutaneous intervention, bypass, or endarterectomy. Most of the data regarding DAPT and stenting is derived from the coronary literature resulting in the 2016 ACC/AHA consensus recommending that it should be continued for at least 1 month and sometimes indefinitely after coronary artery stenting.[27] A very-small, randomized, controlled clinical trial did examine DAPT after lower extremity stenting, which resulted in much lower rates of lesion revascularization at 6 months (5% vs 20%); however, these outcomes did not persist at 1 year when the intervention was stopped at 6 months.[28] Nonetheless, global vascular guidelines recommend that DAPT be considered for 1 to 6 months after endovascular revascularization.[29,30] With respect to bypass, DAPT is not superior to monotherapy in patients with native infrainguinal bypasses; however, it may confer benefit in patients receiving prosthetic grafts via reduction in composite occlusion, revascularization, amputation, or death (HR 0.65) with the tradeoff of doubled risk of mild/moderate bleeding without significantly increasing major bleeding.[31] Global vascular guidelines encourage consideration of DAPT for 6 to 24 months in these patients.[29] Considering carotid disease, clinical trials and metanalyses suggest DAPT reduces risk of TIA in the perioperative period in patients undergoing carotid artery stenting.[32–34] Although there is no consensus as to how long it should be continued, a survey of vascular surgeons participating in ACST-2, showed 82% used it preoperatively and 86% postoperatively for an average of 3 months after intervention (range 1–12 months).[35] It is important to note those undergoing carotid endarterectomy are thought to receive no increased benefit from DAPT.[36]

Although antiplatelet therapies have been considered a mainstay in the treatment of atherosclerosis, clinicians often ponder whether patients on full anticoagulation for another indication need antiplatelet therapy or if it unnecessarily increases bleeding risk without benefit. The ACC has provided guidelines for these situations in 2020.[37] Aside from those situations, anticoagulants are being considered more relevant to the field as newer therapies with less frequent surveillance and lower bleeding risk are developed. Rivaroxaban with aspirin has been the subject of investigation in patients with vascular disease in several recent clinical trials, namely COMPASS (Cardiovascular Outcomes for People Using Anticoagulation Strategies) and VOYAGER PAD (Vascular Outcomes Study of ASA Along With Rivaroxaban in Endovascular or Surgical Limb Revascularization for Peripheral Artery Disease). The COMPASS trial evaluated the effect of rivaroxaban with aspirin compared with aspirin monotherapy, finding that those treated with rivaroxaban had decreased composite of cardiovascular death, stroke, myocardial infarction, fatal bleeding, or symptomatic bleeding (HR 0.8) with the best reduction of risk in those patients with polyvascular disease, heart failure, renal dysfunction, and/or diabetes mellitus (DM).[38] VOYAGER PAD evaluated rivaroxaban plus aspirin versus aspirin and placebo in patients undergoing peripheral stenting and demonstrated decreased composite acute limb ischemia, major amputation, MI, stroke, or death from cardiovascular cause (HR 0.85) at the cost of increased risk of major bleeding (HR 1.42).[39] These studies and more will likely be discussed in future guidelines.

BLOOD PRESSURE CONTROL

For every 10 mm Hg increase in BP there is a 30% to 45% increase in the risk of stroke.[40] Effective long-term BP management is a mainstay in the prevention of morbimortality in patients with vascular disease.[41] The AHA's 2017 BP guideline is the most recent at the time of this writing and suggests all patients with clinical ASCVD be initiated on both BP-lowering medication and lifestyle modification for BPs 130/80 or greater averaged on 2 or more BP readings with monthly follow-up to ensure goal achievement.[42] Furthermore, the 2022 ACC/AHA guideline on aortic disease agrees with this BP goal, even in patients with thoracic aortic aneurysms; however, it vitally decreases the goal for patients with acute aortic syndromes (<120 mm Hg systolic and heart rate of 60 to 80 mm Hg) and acknowledges select patients deferring asymptomatic aneurysm repair may benefit from a lower goal.[43] Both the BP and aortic disease guidelines acknowledge contemporary studies demonstrating decreased mortality in those with a more intensive BP goal (systolic <120 mm Hg); however, note the BP readings obtained in typical clinical practice are inflated by comparison to those obtained by trialists.[44] There is also some thought that patients with PAD may suffer from decreased limb perfusion at lower BP goals due to a j-shaped curve of mortality and BP in a post hoc analysis of the INVEST trial (International Verapamil-SR/Trandolapril Study); however, this theory has only affected guidelines in Europe where these patients have a goal blood pressure of 140/90.[45,46]

It is important to recognize antihypertensives are not generally thought to alter the course of limb-threatening ischemia or aortic aneurysms; however, they improve overall survival.[47–50] Marfan syndrome is an exception to this rule, where beta-blockers and angiotensin receptor blockers (ARBs) are known to decrease the progression of aortic dilatation in these patients.[51] Consequently, beta-blockers and ARBs are first-line and second-line antihypertensives, respectively, in all patients with aneurysmal disease.[43] With respect to antihypertensive choice for other comorbid conditions, the AHA blood pressure guidelines provide an overview of best practices where the data are most robust, for example, guideline-directed medical therapy in those with heart failure with reduced ejection fraction.[42]

Of course, consideration of BP in the preoperative and perioperative periods is important for vascular surgeons. In those with mild-to-moderate hypertension without other metabolic or cardiovascular abnormalities, there is no evidence to suggest delaying surgery is beneficial.[52] If BP is greater than 180/110 mm Hg, benefits of surgery should be compared with benefits of BP optimization with antihypertensive medicine.[52] Continuation of the medical therapy that the patient is already on is generally considered the best course of action unless there is a contraindication.[53] Initiating a beta-blocker before noncardiac surgery is not recommended because of its association with higher risk of stroke, as well as all-cause mortality.[52,54,55] However, continuing therapy with beta-blocker, if the patient was already on such a drug is recommended.[52,54,55] In cases where initiation of betablockade is necessary before the surgery, it is recommended that the drug is started well in advanced, at least 1 day before the surgery, to assess tolerability and safety.[55] The recommended heart rate for patients with BB therapy is 60 to 70 beats per minute.[56] In the past, some have omitted angiotensin-converting enzyme inhibitors and ARBs 24 hours before noncardiac surgery due to periprocedural hypotension; however, current evidence is not strong enough to make this suggestion. In patients with current hypertension or heart failure, it is adequate to continue the drug with continuous periprocedural monitoring of the BP.[57] In those stopping an ACE or ARB, reinitiating therapy as soon as possible after surgery is vital because nonreinitiation has been associated with higher 30-day mortality.[58] Finally, it is not recommended to drastically reduce BP in patients in the hyperacute period of stroke because it can reduce cerebral perfusion and should rather be managed according to respective guidelines for hemorrhagic (2022) and ischemic (2019) situations.[59,60] Patients beyond this timeframe can be managed per standard AHA/ACC guidelines.[40]

GLYCEMIC CONTROL

DM is the most frequent comorbidity in patients with cardiac disease and is a significant risk factor for cardiovascular and cerebrovascular events.[40,52] Many studies have evaluated to what degree glucose control is associated with optimal reduction in morbimortality, with current guidelines targeting hemoglobin A1C of less than 7% to reduce diabetic microvascular and macrovascular complications. However, this is without impact on stroke risk.[29,40] Furthermore, contemporary advancement in pharmacologic strategies with cardiorenal and weight control benefits have shifted diabetes management toward pharmacologic individualization. The American Diabetes Association's 2023 guideline on pharmacologic approaches to glycemic treatment details guidance on cardiorenal risk reduction in patients with ASCVD, heart failure, and chronic kidney disease (CKD).[61] They favor the use of SGLT2 inhibitors in patients with heart failure, CKD, and ASCVD. They note GLP-1 receptor agonists can be chosen as first line in those with ASCVD as well and may also be chosen in patients with CKD for whom SGLT2 inhibitors are not tolerated or in whom they are contraindicated. Metformin monotherapy is still recognized as the best initial therapeutic agent in patients with type II DM who do not have other risk factors.[61]

With respect to the hospitalized patient, it is considered acceptable to maintain higher levels of plasma glucose especially to avoid associated risk with hypoglycemia.[62] In these situations, the plasma glucose goal should be between 140 and 180 mg/dL in most patients because moderate glucose control has corresponded to decreased mortality and stroke as compared with higher glycemic targets and without increased benefit in those achieving tighter control in clinical trials and metaanalyses.[63] Preoperatively, the A1C target should be less than 8% for elective operations. SGLT2 inhibitors should be discontinued 3 to 4 days before surgery to avoid ketoacidosis and urinary tract infections. Metformin and all oral glucose-lowering agents should be held on the day of surgery to avoid lactic acidosis and hypoglycemia, respectively. Preoperatively, patients should be administered half of their neutral protamine Hagedorn (NPH) insulin or 75% to 80% doses of long-acting analog or insulin pump basal insulin. Blood glucose should be monitored at least every 2 to 4 hours while the individual takes nothing by mouth and should be dosed with short-acting or rapid-acting insulin as needed. The ADA does not provide guidance on the use of glucagon-like peptide 1 (GLP1)-receptor agonists or ultra-long-acting insulin analogs during the perioperative period.[62]

Although the risk of contrast-induced AKI has been overstated, the risk for lactic acidosis from metformin use is elevated in patients who develop an AKI.[64] Because creatinine elevations are delayed after kidney injury, the FDA recommends continuing to hold metformin for 2 days after contrast exposure while monitoring for AKI "in patients with eGFR between 30 and 60 mL/min/1.73 m^2; in patients with a history of liver disease, alcoholism, or heart failure; or in patients who will be administered intra-arterial iodinated contrast."[65] If kidney function is stable at 48 hours after contrast exposure, metformin can be restarted. Metformin should be avoided in patients with eGFR less than 30 altogether.[65]

SUMMARY

Effective medical management decreases mortality and morbidity in patients with cardiovascular disease in the long term; however, patients with noncardiac vascular disease are undertreated especially with respect to statin usage.[1] Furthermore, special attention to perioperative medical management is key to patient safety.[52] Every vascular surgery practice should implement a mechanism to guarantee each patient presenting for vascular surgery is offered the very best perioperative and long-term medical therapy whether through self-reliance or well-versed coordination with vascular medicine, advanced practice providers, primary care colleagues, or other specialists.[66]

CLINICS CARE POINTS

- All patients with clinically significant atherosclerosis should be offered highest tolerated statin therapy, with those at high risk being offered adjuvant lipid lowering therapies as necessary.
- All patients with clinically significant atherosclerosis should be offered single antiplatelet therapy. Those with PAD may benefit more from clopidogrel.
- DAPT is indicated in peripheral artery stenting, carotid artery stenting, and may be offered in those with prosthetic peripheral bypasses.
- All patients with clinically significant ASCVD should achieve a long-term BP goal of 130/80 mm Hg or lesser.
- Glycemic control has moved toward an individualized approach with SGLT2 inhibitors being favored in patients with heart failure, ASCVD, and CKD with a goal to reduce A1C of less than 7%. GLP1 receptor agonists are also considered first line in those with ASCVD.
- SGLT2 inhibitors should be stopped 3 to 4 days before surgery and all other noninsulin glucose-lowering medications should be stopped on the day of surgery.
- Metformin should be held immediately before contrast exposure and should often be held for 48 hours after contrast exposure pending stable renal function.
- Insulin is the preferable glucose-lowering medication in the hospitalized patient with a glucose goal being 140 to 180 mg/dL in most patients.

DISCLOSURE

The authors have nothing to disclose.

REFERENCES

1. Berger JS, Ladapo JA. Underuse of prevention and lifestyle counseling in patients with peripheral artery disease. J Am Coll Cardiol 2017;69(18):2293–300.
2. Gerhard-Herman MD, Gornik HL, Barrett C, et al. 2016 AHA/ACC guideline on the management of patients with lower extremity peripheral artery disease: executive summary: a report of the american college of cardiology/American heart association task force on clinical practice guidelines. Circulation 2017;135(12): e686–725.

3. Criqui MH, Langer RD, Fronek A, et al. Mortality over a period of 10 years in patients with peripheral arterial disease. N Engl J Med 1992;326(6):381–6.
4. Agnelli G, Belch JJF, Baumgartner I, et al. Morbidity and mortality associated with atherosclerotic peripheral artery disease: a systematic review. Atherosclerosis 2020;293:94–100.
5. Pereg D, Elis A, Neuman Y, et al. Comparison of mortality in patients with coronary or peripheral artery disease following the first vascular intervention. Coron Artery Dis 2014;25(1):79–82.
6. Boekholdt SM, Hovingh GK, Mora S, et al. Very low levels of atherogenic lipoproteins and the risk for cardiovascular events: a meta-analysis of statin trials. J Am Coll Cardiol 2014;64(5):485–94.
7. Randomized trial of the effects of cholesterol-lowering with simvastatin on peripheral vascular and other major vascular outcomes in 20,536 people with peripheral arterial disease and other high-risk conditions. J Vasc Surg 2007;45(4):645–54 [discussion: 53-4].
8. Sillesen H, Amarenco P, Hennerici MG, et al. Atorvastatin reduces the risk of cardiovascular events in patients with carotid atherosclerosis: a secondary analysis of the Stroke Prevention by Aggressive Reduction in Cholesterol Levels (SPARCL) trial. Stroke 2008;39(12):3297–302.
9. Feringa HH, Karagiannis SE, van Waning VH, et al. The effect of intensified lipid-lowering therapy on long-term prognosis in patients with peripheral arterial disease. J Vasc Surg 2007;45(5):936–43.
10. Arya S, Khakharia A, Binney ZO, et al. Association of statin dose with amputation and survival in patients with peripheral artery disease. Circulation 2018;137(14): 1435–46.
11. Grundy SM, Stone NJ, Bailey AL, et al. 2018 AHA/ACC/AACVPR/AAPA/ABC/ACPM/ADA/AGS/APhA/ASPC/NLA/PCNa guideline on the management of blood cholesterol: a report of the American college of cardiology/American heart association task force on clinical practice guidelines. Circulation 2019;139(25): e1082–143.
12. Sabatine MS, Giugliano RP, Keech AC, et al. Evolocumab and clinical outcomes in patients with cardiovascular disease. N Engl J Med 2017;376(18):1713–22.
13. Lloyd-Jones DM, Morris PB, Ballantyne CM, et al. 2022 ACC expert consensus decision pathway on the role of nonstatin therapies for LDL-cholesterol lowering in the management of atherosclerotic cardiovascular disease risk. J Am Coll Cardiol 2022;80(14):1366–418.
14. Bonaca MP, Nault P, Giugliano RP, et al. Low-density lipoprotein cholesterol lowering with evolocumab and outcomes in patients with peripheral artery disease: insights from the FOURIER trial (Further cardiovascular outcomes research with PCSK9 inhibition in subjects with elevated risk). Circulation 2018;137(4): 338–50.
15. O'Donoghue ML, Giugliano RP, Wiviott SD, et al. Long-term evolocumab in patients with established atherosclerotic cardiovascular disease. Circulation 2022; 146(15):1109–19.
16. Cannon CP, Blazing MA, Giugliano RP, et al. Ezetimibe added to statin therapy after acute coronary syndromes. N Engl J Med 2015;372(25):2387–97.
17. Nastasi DR, Smith JR, Moxon JV, et al. Prescription of pharmacotherapy and the incidence of stroke in patients with symptoms of peripheral artery disease. Stroke 2018;49(12):2953–60.
18. Wong PF, Chong LY, Mikhailidis DP, et al. Antiplatelet agents for intermittent claudication. Cochrane Database Syst Rev 2011;11:Cd001272.

19. Chiarito M, Sanz-Sánchez J, Cannata F, et al. Monotherapy with a P2Y(12) inhibitor or aspirin for secondary prevention in patients with established atherosclerosis: a systematic review and meta-analysis. Lancet 2020;395(10235):1487–95.

20. A randomised, blinded, trial of clopidogrel versus aspirin in patients at risk of ischaemic events (CAPRIE). Lancet 1996;348(9038):1329–39.

21. Jones WS, Baumgartner I, Hiatt WR, et al. Ticagrelor compared with clopidogrel in patients with prior lower extremity revascularization for peripheral artery disease. Circulation 2017;135(3):241–50.

22. Kithcart AP, Beckman JA. ACC/AHA versus esc guidelines for diagnosis and management of peripheral artery Disease: JACC guideline comparison. J Am Coll Cardiol 2018;72(22):2789–801.

23. Brott TG, Halperin JL, Abbara S, et al. 2011 ASA/ACCF/AHA/AANN/AANS/ACR/ ASNR/CNS/SAIP/SCAI/SIR/SNIS/SVM/SVS guideline on the management of patients with extracranial carotid and vertebral artery disease: executive summary. A report of the American College of Cardiology Foundation/American Heart Association Task Force on Practice Guidelines, and the American Stroke Association, American Association of Neuroscience Nurses, American Association of Neurological Surgeons, American College of Radiology, American Society of Neuroradiology, Congress of Neurological Surgeons, Society of Atherosclerosis Imaging and Prevention, Society for Cardiovascular Angiography and Interventions, Society of Interventional Radiology, Society of NeuroInterventional Surgery, Society for Vascular Medicine, and Society for Vascular Surgery. Circulation 2011;124(4): 489–532.

24. Aboyans V, Bauersachs R, Mazzolai L, et al. Antithrombotic therapies in aortic and peripheral arterial diseases in 2021: a consensus document from the ESC working group on aorta and peripheral vascular diseases, the ESC working group on thrombosis, and the ESC working group on cardiovascular pharmacotherapy. Eur Heart J 2021;42(39):4013–24.

25. Navarese EP, Wernly B, Lichtenauer M, et al. Dual vs single antiplatelet therapy in patients with lower extremity peripheral artery disease - A meta-analysis. Int J Cardiol 2018;269:292–7.

26. Savarese G, Reiner MF, Uijl A, et al. Antithrombotic therapy and major adverse limb events in patients with chronic lower extremity arterial disease: systematic review and meta-analysis from the European Society of Cardiology Working Group on Cardiovascular Pharmacotherapy in Collaboration with the European Society of Cardiology Working Group on Aorta and Peripheral Vascular Diseases. Eur Heart J Cardiovasc Pharmacother 2020;6(2):86–93.

27. Levine GN, Bates ER, Bittl JA, et al. 2016 ACC/AHa guideline focused update on duration of dual antiplatelet therapy in patients with coronary artery disease: a report of the American College of Cardiology/American Heart Association task force on clinical practice guidelines: an update of the 2011 ACCF/AHA/SCAI guideline for percutaneous coronary intervention, 2011 ACCF/AHA guideline for coronary artery bypass graft surgery, 2012 ACC/AHA/ACP/AATS/PCNA/SCAI/ STS guideline for the diagnosis and management of patients with stable ischemic heart disease, 2013 ACCF/AHA guideline for the management of ST-elevation myocardial infarction, 2014 AHA/ACC guideline for the management of patients with non-ST-elevation acute coronary syndromes, and 2014 ACC/AHA guideline on perioperative cardiovascular evaluation and management of patients undergoing noncardiac surgery. Circulation 2016;134(10):e123–55.

28. Strobl FF, Brechtel K, Schmehl J, et al. Twelve-month results of a randomized trial comparing mono with dual antiplatelet therapy in endovascularly treated patients with peripheral artery disease. J Endovasc Ther 2013;20(5):699–706.

29. Conte MS, Bradbury AW, Kolh P, et al. Global vascular guidelines on the management of chronic limb-threatening ischemia. J Vasc Surg 2019;69(6S): 3S–125S.e40.

30. Hussain MA, Al-Omran M, Creager MA, et al. Antithrombotic therapy for peripheral artery disease: recent advances. J Am Coll Cardiol 2018;71(21):2450–67.

31. Belch JJF, Dormandy J. Results of the randomized, placebo-controlled clopidogrel and acetylsalicylic acid in bypass surgery for peripheral arterial disease (CASPAR) trial. J Vasc Surg 2010;52(4):825–33.e2.

32. Barkat M, Hajibandeh S, Hajibandeh S, et al. Systematic review and meta-analysis of dual versus single antiplatelet therapy in carotid interventions. Eur J Vasc Endovasc Surg 2017;53(1):53–67.

33. McKevitt FM, Randall MS, Cleveland TJ, et al. The benefits of combined antiplatelet treatment in carotid artery stenting. Eur J Vasc Endovasc Surg 2005; 29(5):522–7.

34. Dalainas I, Nano G, Bianchi P, et al. Dual antiplatelet regime versus acetyl-acetic acid for carotid artery stenting. Cardiovasc Intervent Radiol 2006;29(4):519–21.

35. Huibers A, Halliday A, Bulbulia R, et al. Antiplatelet therapy in carotid artery stenting and carotid endarterectomy in the asymptomatic carotid surgery trial-2. Eur J Vasc Endovasc Surg 2016;51(3):336–42.

36. Ku JC, Taslimi S, Zuccato J, et al. Editor's choice - peri-operative outcomes of carotid endarterectomy are not improved on dual antiplatelet therapy vs. aspirin monotherapy: a systematic review and meta-analysis. Eur J Vasc Endovasc Surg 2022;63(4):546–55.

37. Kumbhani DJ, Cannon CP, Beavers CJ, et al. 2020 ACC expert consensus decision pathway for anticoagulant and antiplatelet therapy in patients with atrial fibrillation or venous thromboembolism undergoing percutaneous coronary intervention or with atherosclerotic cardiovascular disease. J Am Coll Cardiol 2021;77(5):629–58.

38. Steffel J, Eikelboom JW, Anand SS, et al. The COMPASS trial: net clinical benefit of low-dose rivaroxaban plus aspirin as compared with aspirin in patients with chronic vascular disease. Circulation 2020;142(1):40–8.

39. Bonaca MP, Bauersachs RM, Anand SS, et al. Rivaroxaban in peripheral artery disease after revascularization. N Engl J Med 2020;382(21):1994–2004.

40. Ricotta JJ, Aburahma A, Ascher E, et al. Updated Society for Vascular Surgery guidelines for management of extracranial carotid disease. J Vasc Surg 2011; 54(3):e1–31.

41. Kolls BJ, Sapp S, Rockhold FW, et al. Stroke in patients with peripheral artery disease. Stroke 2019;50(6):1356–63.

42. Whelton PK, Carey RM, Aronow WS, et al. 2017 ACC/AHA/AAPA/ABC/ACPM/ AGS/APhA/ASH/ASPC/NMA/PCNA guideline for the prevention, detection, evaluation, and management of high blood pressure in adults: executive summary: a report of the American college of cardiology/American heart association task force on clinical practice guidelines. Hypertension 2018;71(6):1269–324.

43. Isselbacher EM, Preventza O, Black JH, et al. 2022 ACC/AHA guideline for the diagnosis and management of aortic disease: a report of the American heart association/American college of cardiology joint committee on clinical practice guidelines. Circulation 2022;146(24):e334–482.

44. A randomized trial of intensive versus standard blood-pressure control. N Engl J Med 2015;373(22):2103–16.

45. Bavry AA, Anderson RD, Gong Y, et al. Outcomes among hypertensive patients with concomitant peripheral and coronary artery disease: findings from the INternational VErapamil-SR/Trandolapril STudy. Hypertension 2010;55(1):48–53.

46. Aboyans V, Ricco J-B, Bartelink M-LEL, et al. 2017 ESC guidelines on the diagnosis and treatment of peripheral arterial diseases, in collaboration with the european society for vascular surgery (ESVS): document covering atherosclerotic disease of extracranial carotid and vertebral, mesenteric, renal, upper and lower extremity arteriesEndorsed by: the European Stroke Organization (ESO)The Task Force for the Diagnosis and Treatment of Peripheral Arterial Diseases of the European Society of Cardiology (ESC) and of the European Society for Vascular Surgery (ESVS). Eur Heart J 2017;39(9):763–816.

47. Brewster DC, Cronenwett JL, Hallett JW, et al. Guidelines for the treatment of abdominal aortic aneurysms. Report of a subcommittee of the Joint Council of the American Association for Vascular Surgery and Society for Vascular Surgery. J Vasc Surg 2003;37(5):1106–17.

48. Bergqvist D. Pharmacological interventions to attenuate the expansion of abdominal aortic aneurysm (AAA) - a systematic review. Eur J Vasc Endovasc Surg 2011;41(5):663–7.

49. Lederle FA, Noorbaloochi S, Nugent S, et al. Multicentre study of abdominal aortic aneurysm measurement and enlargement. Br J Surg 2015;102(12):1480–7.

50. Bahia SS, Vidal-Diez A, Seshasai SR, et al. Cardiovascular risk prevention and all-cause mortality in primary care patients with an abdominal aortic aneurysm. Br J Surg 2016;103(12):1626–33.

51. Pitcher A, Spata E, Emberson J, et al. Angiotensin receptor blockers and β blockers in Marfan syndrome: an individual patient data meta-analysis of randomised trials. Lancet 2022;400(10355):822–31.

52. Fleisher LA, Beckman JA, Brown KA, et al. ACC/AHA 2007 guidelines on perioperative cardiovascular evaluation and care for noncardiac surgery: a report of the American College of Cardiology/American Heart Association Task Force on Practice Guidelines (Writing Committee to Revise the 2002 Guidelines on Perioperative Cardiovascular Evaluation for Noncardiac Surgery) developed in collaboration with the American Society of Echocardiography, American Society of Nuclear Cardiology, Heart Rhythm Society, Society of Cardiovascular Anesthesiologists, Society for Cardiovascular Angiography and Interventions, Society for Vascular Medicine and Biology, and Society for Vascular Surgery. J Am Coll Cardiol 2007;50(17):e159–241.

53. Auerbach AD, Goldman L. beta-Blockers and reduction of cardiac events in noncardiac surgery: scientific review. JAMA 2002;287(11):1435–44.

54. Chaikof EL, Dalman RL, Eskandari MK, et al. The Society for Vascular Surgery practice guidelines on the care of patients with an abdominal aortic aneurysm. J Vasc Surg 2018;67(1):2–77.e2.

55. Fleisher LA, Beckman JA, Brown KA, et al. 2009 ACCF/AHA focused update on perioperative beta blockade incorporated into the ACC/AHA 2007 guidelines on perioperative cardiovascular evaluation and care for noncardiac surgery. J Am Coll Cardiol 2009;54(22):e13–118.

56. Feringa HH, Bax JJ, Boersma E, et al. High-dose beta-blockers and tight heart rate control reduce myocardial ischemia and troponin T release in vascular surgery patients. Circulation 2006;114(1 Suppl):I344–9.

57. Roshanov PS, Rochwerg B, Patel A, et al. Withholding versus continuing angiotensin-converting enzyme inhibitors or angiotensin II receptor blockers before noncardiac surgery: an analysis of the vascular events in noncardiac surgery patients cOhort evaluatioN prospective cohort. Anesthesiology 2017;126(1): 16–27.

58. Lee SM, Takemoto S, Wallace AW. Association between withholding angiotensin receptor blockers in the early postoperative period and 30-day mortality: a cohort study of the veterans affairs healthcare system. Anesthesiology 2015;123(2): 288–306.

59. Powers WJ, Rabinstein AA, Ackerson T, et al. Guidelines for the early management of patients with acute ischemic stroke: 2019 update to the 2018 guidelines for the early management of acute ischemic stroke: a guideline for healthcare professionals from the American Heart Association/American Stroke Association. Stroke 2019;50(12):e344–418.

60. Greenberg SM, Ziai WC, Cordonnier C, et al. 2022 Guideline for the Management of Patients With Spontaneous Intracerebral Hemorrhage: A Guideline From the American Heart Association/American Stroke Association. Stroke 2022;53(7): e282–361.

61. ElSayed NA, Aleppo G, Aroda VR, et al. 9. Pharmacologic approaches to glycemic treatment: standards of care in diabetes-2023. Diabetes Care 2023;46(Suppl 1). S140-s57.

62. ElSayed NA, Aleppo G, Aroda VR, et al. 16. Diabetes care in the hospital: standards of care in diabetes-2023. Diabetes Care 2023;46(Suppl 1). S267-s78.

63. Sathya B, Davis R, Taveira T, et al. Intensity of peri-operative glycemic control and postoperative outcomes in patients with diabetes: a meta-analysis. Diabetes Res Clin Pract 2013;102(1):8–15.

64. Davenport MS, Perazella MA, Yee J, et al. Use of intravenous iodinated contrast media in patients with kidney disease: consensus statements from the American College of Radiology and the National Kidney Foundation. Radiology 2020; 294(3):660–8.

65. FDA revises warnings regarding use of the diabetes medicine metformin in certain patients with reduced kidney function. In: Administration USFaD, editor. Available at: https://www.fda.gov/drugs/drug-safety-and-availability/fda-drug-safety-communication-fda-revises-warnings-regarding-use-diabetes-medicine-metformin-certain#:~:text=The%20current%20drug%20labeling%20strongly,builds%20up%20in%20the%20blood. Accessed January 01, 2023.

66. Weissler EH, Jones WS. Who will own the responsibility to prescribe statins? Tragedy of the commons. JAMA Netw Open 2021;4(12):e2137605.

Preoperative Assessment of Patients with Vascular Disease

Robert J. Beaulieu, MD, MSE

KEYWORDS

- Vascular surgery • Cardiac risk • Pulmonary risk

KEY POINTS

- Cardiac complications occur more frequently among vascular surgery patients than any other non-cardiac surgery and preoperative medical maximization may be the best strategy to reduce these risks.
- Active tobacco abuse increases the risk of pulmonary complications 5 fold following vascular surgery but cessation 6-12 months in advance reduces these risks back to the level of the general population.
- Frailty is an evolving concept in vascular surgery and represents an independent risk from other comorbid conditions including CAD, DM, COPD and CKD.

INTRODUCTION

Patients with vascular disease often have a complex list of comorbid conditions that affect both their presentation and treatment. Highly prevalent conditions such as atherosclerosis and diabetes have both vascular-specific and systemic manifestations. Even acute presentations of isolated vascular insults can exacerbate underlying chronic conditions. Further, the acuity of many vascular surgery presentations may preclude a more elective referral to a specific preoperative evaluation clinic. As such, it has become increasingly important for the practicing vascular surgeon to rapidly and effectively triage a wide array of conditions that affect the patient's perioperative risks. Many of these are intuitive, linked by the common bond of vessels affected by atherosclerosis, such as with coronary artery disease. Others involve risk factors that potentiate both vascular disease and additional organ involvement, such as the risk of tobacco abuse to both vessels and pulmonary function. More recently, novel measures of "fitness" for surgery, such as frailty, are becoming increasingly important predictors of patient outcomes. This article will aim to present

Department of Surgery, University of Michigan, 1500 E. Medical Center Drive, Ann Arbor, MI, USA
E-mail address: robeauli@med.umich.edu

Surg Clin N Am 103 (2023) 577–594
https://doi.org/10.1016/j.suc.2023.05.005
0039-6109/23/© 2023 Elsevier Inc. All rights reserved.

a concise summary of preoperative risk evaluation and management, as well as highlight new areas for estimating patient risk prior to vascular surgery.

Cardiac Evaluation

Cardiac complications are more common among patients undergoing vascular surgery than any other type of noncoronary surgery.[1,2] Not surprisingly, with a mixture of endovascular and open operation types, there is further stratification within this cohort. Cardiac risk is highest among open aortic operations and open infrainguinal bypass as compared with endovascular procedures and carotid endarterectomy.[3] In some instances, this distinction drives the choice of operative type. This trend has become apparent with an evaluation of vascular registry data showing a migration of high-risk patients from open aortic repair to endovascular over the past 2 decades.[4] Interestingly, this has been associated with an increasing rate of cardiac complications being seen among patients with EVAR, perhaps emphasizing the high-risk nature of all vascular procedures.[4] However, an improved appreciation of this fact combined with increased adherence to best medical management may be driving an overall decreasing trend in cardiac risk with vascular surgery (**Fig. 1**).[5] An accurate assessment of cardiac risk for patients undergoing vascular surgery is of paramount importance to help ensure the patient gets the highest efficacy operation with the lowest possible cardiac risk.

There are several factors that contribute to the high rates of postoperative cardiac complications among vascular patients. First, many of the risk factors that predispose patients to atherosclerotic vascular disease, such as smoking, hypertension, hyperlipidemia, and diabetes, are known to contribute to coronary artery disease as well. Secondly, large volume shifts occur frequently in major vascular surgery and are predictors of major complications following surgery.[6] And the impact of these shifts is not limited to the patient's time in the operating room. Patients that require a blood transfusion in the postoperative setting, or in both the postoperative and intraoperative setting, as compared with just during the operation, are at higher risk for postoperative myocardial infarction (POMI).[7] Finally, the physiologic stress response is pronounced during vascular surgery, resulting in significantly elevated levels of circulating

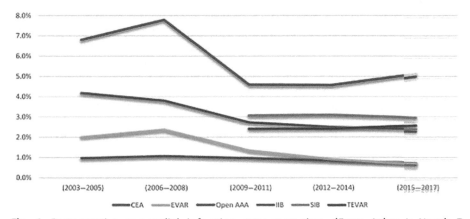

Fig. 1. Postoperative myocardial infarction rates over time. (*From* Axley J, Novak Z, Blakeslee-Carter J, et al. Long-Term Trends in Preoperative Cardiac Evaluation and Myocardial Infarction after Elective Vascular Procedures. Ann Vasc Surg. 2021;71:19-28; with permission.)

catecholamines both during the operation and in the perioperative period.[8] Increased circulating catecholamines have been linked with elevated troponins after noncardiac surgery, a sensitive marker for myocardial ischemia.[9] It is likely a combination of these factors, rather than any single factor, which contributes to the high risk of cardiac complication during vascular surgery. For instance, while endovascular aortic repair blunts the rise in cortisol response to surgery compared with open repair, rates of MI after EVAR still approach 5%.[10,11]

A thorough examination of the patient's current medication regimen is a good initial first step and can often yield important clues to the cardiac risk of a procedure. Antiplatelet and statin therapy have become the cornerstone of medical management for most vascular patients, owing largely to the reduction in cardiovascular events among this high-risk group.[12,13] However, evidence suggests that a disappointingly low percentage of vascular patients are being offered this best medical therapy.[14] This neglect has implications on both preoperative cardiac event rates and, more pertinent to this report, postoperative cardiac event rates. High-intensity statin therapy has been shown to reduce the postoperative cardiac event rate by two-thirds (8% vs 26%, $P = .031$).[15] Recognition of an absence of maximal medial therapy before may allow for prompt risk reduction through starting therapy. The introduction of statins in the immediate preoperative period reduces the risk of postoperative cardiac events.[16]

Beyond aspirin and statin therapy, many vascular surgery patients are on targeted therapies for hypertension or heart failure that may impact their perioperative cardiac risk. Angiotensin-converting enzyme (ACE) inhibitor therapy is increasingly prescribed in vascular surgery patients to reduce both cardiovascular and cerebrovascular risks.[17] A distinction should be made about the indication for ACE inhibitor therapy, both to understand cardiac risks but also to help guide perioperative management. For instance, patients on ACE inhibitor for the purposes of hypertension alone should likely have their ACE inhibitor held for 24 hours prior to an operation to reduce the risk of hypotension whereas those on it for left ventricular dysfunction may be better served by keeping therapy in place.[1] Dihydropyridines are a type of calcium channel blockers that include nifedipine and amlodipine and have indications for both hypertension and angina. However, it should be noted that their use has also been found to be independently associated with an increased perioperative mortality risk, primarily driven by higher postoperative MI rates, in patients undergoing open aortic repair.[18] These examples show the value in a thorough review of current medications both as a clue to underlying cardiac conditions and to quickly identify medication changes that will impact the patient's perioperative cardiac risk.

Medical management alone may not be an effective strategy to reduce postoperative cardiac risk. Even with adherence to an aggressive medical therapy regimen with antiplatelet and high-intensity statin, the risk of postoperative myocardial ischemia remains high.[19] This appears to be especially true of patients with Metabolic Syndrome who had a 66% increased risk of POMI after infrainguinal bypass by multivariate analysis, an increase that did not some blunted by adherence to statin, aspirin and beta blockade.[20] Patients who suffer a POMI have a 1-year mortality significantly higher than patients who undergo the operation but do not have a cardiac event.[19] Absence of combined statin and antiplatelet therapy afterward predicts even worse outcomes.[21]

Presumably, an exhaustive cardiac workup on all vascular patients prior to surgery would minimize the cardiac risk. However, this has not borne out to be true. Routine stress testing before vascular surgery does not reduce perioperative cardiac risk and may unnecessarily delay vascular surgery.[22] Among patients undergoing open aortic aneurysm repair or suprainguinal bypass, a negative preoperative stress test was associated with a *higher* risk of postoperative cardiac event.[23] Further, in some patients with stable CAD undergoing major vascular surgery, even operative revascularization of "at risk" lesions does not reduce the risk of postoperative ischemia.[24] In a study of patients undergoing open thoracabdominal aortic aneurysm repair or aortoiliac occlusive disease treatment, patients with coronary revascularization history had an *increased* cardiac risk compared to nonrevascularized patients, possibly due to the need to antiplatelet therapy in the perioperative setting.[25] This suggests there is a no "one size fits all" approach for cardiac risk calculation/management for patients undergoing vascular surgery. Rather, the aim should be to perform the right workup, in the right patient, at the right time before surgery.

Cardiac risk calculators have been developed to help address this concern. Initial iterations of these calculators were based on those derived for all patients undergoing surgery and were agnostic to specific risks associated with vascular patients, with the most notable being the Revised Cardiac Risk Index (RCRI). While well-validated on general surgery patients, the RCRI significantly underestimates the risk of adverse cardiac outcomes among vascular surgery patients.[26] The widespread use of the Vascular Quality Initiative (VQI) and the granularity of the information entered helped inform the development of a new, vascular-specific risk index with the Vascular Quality Initiative Cardiac Risk Index (VQI-CRI) with the aim to address this disparity.[3] Despite the increasing detail available for inclusion in risk calculators, even vascular specific calculators still appear to underestimate the cardiac risk following vascular surgery.[27] This helps to appropriately frame the challenge in predicting postoperative cardiac risks despite an incomplete understanding of the pathophysiology that underlies the problem. Despite the scope of this problem, there are meaningful evaluations that can be completed both in the office and in the lab In preparation for vascular surgery.

Functional capacity
Assessment of the patient's functional status is often used as a quick way to estimate a patient's risk of cardiac complication. Traditionally, this has been accomplished by asking a patient about their ability to climb a flight of stairs or run a short distance (4 METs or greater activity). When combined with a risk calculator, a reduced self-reported functional capacity was associated with improved predictive capability.[28] However, these data may be more related to a patient's pulmonary status than cardiovascular status. Among patients undergoing noncardiac surgery, functional capacity reporting alone has limited capability to predict cardiac complications or mortality.[29] Additionally, many vascular patients are limited in both walking distance and climbing capabilities because of underlying peripheral ischemia. It seems that the use of functional capacity assessment may be best used in conjunction with a risk calculator and as an initial guide for those who need additional workup.

Electrocardiography
Electrocardiography (ECG) is frequently performed in patients with or without a history of ischemic heart disease in the anticipation of vascular surgery. The American Heart Association/American College of Cardiology recommendations consider obtaining an ECG as "reasonable" in all patients undergoing vascular surgery and recommend it for patients undergoing vascular surgery who have at least one risk factor for heart disease (Level of Evidence: B).[30] Evidence suggests that for TEVAR, the determination of cardiac symptomatology and resting ECG alone may be enough to evaluate cardiac risk.[31] Pathologic q-waves on resting ECG are of specific interest. These may occur

even in the absence of patient reporting symptoms and have been associated with increased cardiac risk for patients undergoing noncardiac surgery.[32] As such, a resting ECG is often a useful initial step to help identify "at risk" patients.

Echocardiography and stress testing
The use of transthoracic echocardiography (TTE) can help to evaluate left ventricular (LV) function, mitral regurgitation, and aortic valve gradients among patient's undergoing high-risk surgery. The routine use of TTE in all patients, however, does not appear to help inform risk, especially in otherwise low-risk patients.[33] It should be considered in patients with dyspnea, especially those with a history of heart failure.[34] Additionally, patients with known aortic valvular disease of moderate or greater degree who have not had recent imaging (within the last year) should be evaluated.[35] In many patients, an evaluation of myocardial perfusion with stress is pursued to replicate the stress of surgery and predict postoperative cardiac events. Chemical stress testing with dobutamine stress echocardiography (DSE) can be performed in patients unable to complete the exercise needed for standard myocardial perfusion imaging (MPI). In this case, the degree of inducible ischemia appears to be important. Patients with ischemia induced in less than 20% of the LV myocardium do not have a higher likelihood of perioperative cardiac risk.[36] Fixed defects as well as angina during the testing have been identified as independent predictors of cardiac risk after vascular surgery as well.[37] Ideally, preoperative stress testing should only be performed in high-risk patients with low exercise tolerance in whom an abnormal finding will prompt a change in therapy.

Biomarkers
Preoperative biomarker testing to determine surgical risk should be considered distinctly from perioperative testing to evaluate symptoms following surgery. In the latter, even small increases in cardiac troponins may likely correspond with myocardial injury and worse cardiac outcomes.[38] There is some evidence that trending troponins postoperatively can be indicative of cardiac risk, with the peak values even elevated above 0.02 ng/mL reflect an increased risk.[39] The role of preoperative troponin values is less certain.[40] Moderate elevation of high sensitivity troponins above 12 ng/L have been shown to have an increased risk of 30-day mortality, though even a mild elevation is associated with an increased risk of myocardial injury after noncardiac surgery (MINS).[41] Preoperative brain natriuretic peptide (BNP) has become an increasingly important predictor of cardiovascular risk as well. Pooled data from multiple studies, though not exclusively vascular surgery patients have shown that elevated BNP is strongly associated with increased risk of cardiac death or MI (OR 19.3, 95% CI 8.5–43.7).[42] While there are no current guideline recommendations for obtaining these markers in preoperative vascular surgery patients, they are becoming an increasingly popular tool to risk stratify these patients.

Preoperative revascularization
As stated previously, preoperative coronary revascularization for patients undergoing vascular surgery remains a controversial topic. The Coronary Artery Revascularization Prophylaxis (CARP) trial failed to demonstrate a reduction in long-term cardiac outcomes or perioperative MI rates among patients with stable coronary disease undergoing preoperative coronary revascularization.[24] The current recommendations from the ACC/AHA recommend coronary revascularization only if it would be otherwise indicated in the nonoperative setting.[35] Despite being seemingly less invasive, percutaneous coronary intervention should be reserved for patients with the left main disease who cannot tolerate a bypass or those with unstable coronary disease who

would be appropriate candidates for urgent or emergent revascularization.[43] The potential delay in subsequent vascular surgery should be strongly considered in this group. Currently, nonemergent noncardiac surgery should be performed no earlier than 30 days after bare metal stenting and ideally 365 days after drug-eluting stent (DES) implantation (Class 1 Recommendation, Level of Evidence B).[35]

Pulmonary Evaluation

Patients undergoing vascular surgery warrant special consideration of potential pulmonary complications. Many will have risk factors that have contributed to both vascular disease and decreased pulmonary function, such as tobacco abuse, chronic obstructive pulmonary disease (COPD), and age greater than 65.[44–46] Additionally, the extent of the operation (open abdominal aortic or thoracoabdominal exposures), as well as the duration of the operation (greater than 2.5 hours), will have increased pulmonary risk.[44,47] Pulmonary complications with endovascular versus open aortic repair are significantly reduced with an odds ratio of 0.14 (CI, 0.04–0.47).[48] Identification and management of these risk factors is especially important as the occurrence of postoperative pulmonary complication is associated with a significantly higher rate of postoperative mortality.[47] Therefore, a complete workup of preoperative pulmonary risk factors, particularly among this high-risk population, can both help guide method of surgical management as well as improve postoperative outcomes.

A thorough history and physical exam is a sensitive initial tool for evaluating the pulmonary risk in vascular patients. Factors such as tobacco abuse, known COPD (including if supplemental oxygen is required), congestive heart failure, and functional capacity should all be explored. As discussed earlier, limitations in functional capacity can often be driven by pulmonary, rather than cardiovascular, status. Therefore, it should be clearly elucidated if the patient's reduced capacity is due to shortness of breath, chest pain, or claudication. Many vascular patients are elderly and sedentary, a combination which is highly associated with respiratory impairment and dyspnea.[49] Tobacco abuse history should also be explored not only for the purposes of risk identification but also because physician counseling can significantly increase the likelihood of quitting.[50] Patients who are actively smoking have a nearly 5-fold increased risk of pulmonary complications following major surgery.[51] Cessation of 6 months to 1 year before major surgery essentially lowers pulmonary risks to consistent with the nonsmoking population.[52] A history of obstructive sleep apnea (OSA) further increases the risk of postoperative hypoxic events.[53] Though many patients with OSA are undiagnosed, utilization of risk evaluators such as the STOP-Bang score (snoring, tiredness, observed apnea, hypertension, neck circumference, and male sex) can help identify these patients.[54,55]

Chest radiography

Preoperative chest radiography (with plain film x-ray) is often conducted in patients in preparation for vascular surgery. Abnormal preoperative chest radiograph has been associated with increased pulmonary complication risk following major surgery.[51,56] Interestingly, a thorough history and physical exam are often independently able to predict an abnormal chest radiograph.[57] Additionally, abnormal chest radiography only variably drives a change in operative plan or preoperative risk management beyond what was already determined from history, physical and functional assessment.[58] Currently, guidelines only support obtaining chest radiography in patients older than 50 years of age undergoing abdominal, thoracic or surgery for aneurysmal disease or those with known cardiopulmonary disease.

Spirometry
In patients with known lung disease, spirometry (pulmonary function testing) is often obtained to investigate the extent of the disease. There is limited evidence to provide specific thresholds for vascular surgery. In a study of patients undergoing abdominal surgery (not specifically vascular surgery), FEV1 values less than 61% predicted were independently associated with pulmonary complications.[59] Hyper-inflation and low DLCO also appear predictive of increased risk of pulmonary complications following abdominal surgery.[60] However, spirometry alone is not an accurate tool to predict the risk of postoperative pulmonary complication due to high rates of misdiagnosis.[61] As such, spirometry is likely best used for patients with either a confirmed diagnosis of COPD and functional limitations or those at high risk for COPD based on history and physical.[62]

Coronavirus testing
The coronavirus-19 (COVID-19) pandemic has affected the preoperative pulmonary evaluation of vascular patients in evolving ways. Patients with a history of COVID-19 infection have increased fatigue, breathlessness and reduced pulmonary function even 4 to 6 months following their infection, regardless of whether the primary infection required hospitalization.[63] Timing of nonemergent operations after COVID-19 infection and vaccination status appear to affect surgical outcomes. Patients who are not fully vaccinated and present shortly after COVID-19 infection (within 4 weeks) are at particularly high risk for surgery that involves general anesthesia.[64] In a Veterans Affairs study blinded to vaccination status, the increased risk of perioperative mortality was higher among patients with a positive test within the past 8 weeks.[65] Though acute respiratory distress syndrome is one common postoperative complication, non-pulmonary complications, such as increased risk of shock and stroke, should be considered as well.[66] Vascular surgery patients should be considered a particularly at-risk population. In the COVER study, increased mortality rates among following all vascular surgery were observed, regardless of infection status.[67] Among vascular surgery patients who test positive for COVID-19 within 7 days of their operation, mortality is exceedingly high (27.2%) and pulmonary complications occur in nearly half of these patients.[68] Vascular patients with active respiratory tract infections and COPD are at increased risk beyond what was seen in prepandemic cohorts.[67] Taken together, these data suggest that patients with vascular disease who are anticipating undergoing a procedure should be tested for COVID-19 and treatment in the early infectious phase should be avoided, if possible. The timeline at which point it will be safer to operate on these patients is uncertain and actively being researched.

Diabetic Evaluation

Diabetes mellitus has both systemic and vascular-specific effects that place these patients at increased risk for the complication following vascular surgery. Preoperative evaluation to determine the severity and degree of glycemic control are important predictors of postoperative complication and can help guide the method of management (diet control, oral hypoglycemic, and/or insulin therapy) after the operation. The combination of perioperative surges in catecholamines and cortisol as well as the baseline impaired insulin production or response of diabetic patients places them at particular risk for postoperative hyperglycemia and ketosis.[69] Hyperglycemia in the preoperative setting has numerous impacts on vascular disease, including endothelial dysfunction, plaque instability, intimal changes from advanced glycation end products, and increased reactive oxygen species.[70] In carotid surgery, perioperative hyperglycemia has been associated with higher rates of stroke and POMI.[71] As such, hyperglycemic control of the diabetic vascular patient is a markedly important goal that falls under the purview of multiple specialists, including vascular surgeons.

Hemoglobin A1C

All diabetic patients should have hemoglobin A1c (HBA1c) testing completed every 3 to 6 months. All patients with cardiovascular disease should have diabetic screening testing (with either HbA1c or fasting glucose measurement).[72] However, many preoperative patients do not have recent testing and, of those that do, many proceed to surgery without optimization.[73] This has specific implications for vascular surgery patients.[74] Elevated HbA1c levels have been identified as a risk factor in studies of both cardiac and noncardiac operations. Supranormal HbA1c is predictive of increased perioperative mortality among patients undergoing cardiac surgery.[75] Likewise, elevated HbA1c levels have been strongly correlated with major complications following major abdominal surgery.[76] In vascular surgery patients specifically, elevated preoperative HbA1c levels are predictive of 30-day cardiac complications.[77] Preoperative HbA1c levels are associated with increased adverse limb events in patients undergoing lower extremity revascularization.[78] The association of elevated HbA1c with worse outcomes also appears to hold true when long-term mortality is examined among vascular surgery patients and those with peripheral artery disease.[77,79] Ultimately, HbA1c testing may be a reliable mechanism to both evaluate for preoperative diabetic control and drive the consideration for aggressive hyperglycemic control in the perioperative period. However, data are lacking regarding specific targets for vascular patients and overly aggressive management has not been associated with a reduction in wound complications, as initially thought.[74] This represents an important area of ongoing research.

Renal Evaluation

Renal impairment is common among vascular surgery patients. Chronic kidney disease (CKD) is a well-recognized cardiovascular risk factor. Patients undergoing vascular surgery with CKD have an elevated long-term cardiovascular mortality risk of nearly 30% at 10 years, regardless of perioperative acute kidney injury (AKI).[80] Multivariate regression of risk factors for AKI after aortic reconstruction has identified baseline severe CKD (OR 15) and moderate CKD (OR 2.8) as predictors of AKI with a subsequent increased risk of late mortality.[81] Moderate or severe preoperative CKD increases the risk of mortality in patients undergoing carotid artery surgery.[82] Similarly, coronary bypass patients with CKD have a significantly increased risk for multiple perioperative complications, including POMI, stroke and death within 30 days.[83] Despite these concerning outcomes, the need to operate on patients with CKD is common and, therefore, an appreciation of the severity of disease and impact on perioperative plan is essential.

The increased use of endovascular therapy has helped to drive near ubiquitous assessment of preoperative baseline creatinine levels and estimated glomerular filtration rate (eGFR). Preoperatively, vascular surgery patients with CKD should be additionally evaluated for anemia, a common comorbidity in this population. Discussion of bleeding risk during surgery is another major component of the preoperative evaluation of patients with CKD. Patients on antiplatelet therapy with end-stage renal disease (ESRD) have a well-recognized increased risk of bleeding.[84] Holding antiplatelet therapy in the anticipation of vascular surgery should be carefully considered in this population and weighed against the risk of cardiovascular or cerebrovascular complication. Interestingly, patients with CKD and albuminuria appear to be at a higher risk for bleeding than those without albuminuria.[85] Bleeding risk can be complicated by polypharmacy in CKD as well. For instance, pentoxifylline, intermittently used for symptomatic management in patients with PAD, in CKD is associated with a high rate of spontaneous major bleeding.[86]

Contrast-induced nephropathy (CIN) is an important consideration as an increasing number of patients are undergoing either computed tomographic angiography (CTA) for either diagnosis of disease or surveillance of endografts.[87] In many patients, vascular surgeons can be instrumental in reducing this risk by using limited contrast during conventional angiography or the use of carbon dioxide-based angiography. To date, strategies to reduce or eliminate iodinated contrast altogether are more effective than adjunctive measures such as sodium bicarbonate.[87] Gadolinium use in this population has also been associated with nephrogenic systemic fibrosis. Unenhanced magnetic resonance imaging (MRI), including ECG-gated fast spin and black blood models, can successfully be used to image both central and peripheral vasculature with high fidelity.[88]

Frailty Assessment

Decreasing physiologic reserve, or "frailty," is increasingly common among an aging population with vascular disease. Emerging evidence has shown it can be predictive of poor response to vascular surgery.[89] Measures of frailty variably include multiple phenotypic and comorbid factors such as slow gait, decreased hand grip strength and sarcopenia.[90,91] Patients with vascular disease who meet frailty criteria are at risk both pre and perioperatively. Frail patients with intermittent claudication have a much higher rate of major adverse cardiac events.[92] Likewise, frail patients also have increased 30-day mortality and morbidity risk after abdominal aortic operations.[93] One area of concern for these patients is the discharge disposition, with many requiring increased nursing care following vascular surgery. Frail patients especially are at increased risk of nonhome discharge or loss of independence after vascular surgery.[94] Interventions geared toward reducing frailty are being investigated to potentially reduce the risk of complication following vascular surgery.[89] Many of these, such as improved nutrition, prehabilitation, and increased social aspects of care, represent laudable goals regardless of vascular status but will very likely have an important impact on future outcomes after vascular surgery.

The role of preparing the "at-risk" patient for the OR has garnered increased interest under the moniger "prehabilitation." The aim of these efforts is to increase a patient's functional capacity and address modifiable risk factors in advance of surgery to reduce postoperative complications. In many vascular disease processes (ie, PAD), the specific methods (increased walking, dietary changes, tobacco cessation, and so forth) to achieve these goals are indistinguishable from aggressive medical management in everything but intent. Indeed, the goal of prehabilitation is to *survive an operation rather than avoid it.* Despite the connection between poor preoperative functional status and poor postoperative outcomes, data are limited to support that operative complication rate can be meaningfully modified through exercise or nutritional changes in the preoperative setting.[95] In particular, patients with PAD present a unique challenge due to many patients' inability to change exercise tolerance *until* surgery is completed. Even in the face of equivocal reports, there is very likely to be value in instilling lifestyle changes focused on increased mobility, improved diet, and even psychological intervention specifically in the vascular surgery population.

SUMMARY

Patients undergoing vascular surgery are the highest risk surgical patients. The comorbid conditions found in vascular patients, such as CAD, CHF, ESRD, and DM,

17. Heart Outcomes Prevention Evaluation Study Investigators, Yusuf S, Sleight P, Pogue J, et al. Effects of an angiotensin-converting-enzyme inhibitor, ramipril, on cardiovascular events in high-risk patients. N Engl J Med 2000;342(3): 145–53. Available at: https://pubmed.ncbi.nlm.nih.gov/10639539/. Accessed December 2, 2022.

18. Kertai MD, Westerhout CM, Varga KS, et al. Dihydropiridine calcium-channel blockers and perioperative mortality in aortic aneurysm surgery. Br J Anaesth 2008;101(4):458–65. Available at: https://pubmed.ncbi.nlm.nih.gov/18556693/. Accessed December 2, 2022.

19. Beaulieu RJ, Sutzko DC, Albright J, et al. Association of High Mortality with Post-operative Myocardial Infarction after Major Vascular Surgery Despite Use of Evidence-Based Therapies. JAMA Surgery 2020;131–7.

20. Sorber R, Lehman A, Alshaikh HN, et al. Metabolic syndrome is associated with increased cardiac morbidity after infrainguinal bypass surgery irrespective of the use of cardiovascular risk-modifying agents. J Vasc Surg 2019;69(1):190–8. Available at: https://pubmed.ncbi.nlm.nih.gov/30292611/. Accessed December 2, 2022.

21. Steely AM, Callas PW, Hohl PK, et al. Underutilization of antiplatelet and statin therapy after postoperative myocardial infarction following vascular surgery. J Vasc Surg 2018;67(1):279–86.e2. Available at: http://www.ncbi.nlm.nih.gov/pubmed/28830706. Accessed March 22, 2019.

22. Bauer SM, Cayne NS, Veith FJ. New developments in the preoperative evaluation and perioperative management of coronary artery disease in patients undergoing vascular surgery. J Vasc Surg 2010;51(1):242–51. Available at: https://pubmed.ncbi.nlm.nih.gov/19954922/. Accessed December 2, 2022.

23. Columbo JA, Barnes JA, Jones DW, et al. Adverse cardiac events after vascular surgery are prevalent despite negative results of preoperative stress testing. J Vasc Surg 2020;72(5):1584–92. Available at: https://pubmed.ncbi.nlm.nih.gov/32247699/. Accessed December 2, 2022.

24. McFalls EO, Ward HB, Moritz TE, et al. Coronary-Artery Revascularization before Elective Major Vascular Surgery. N Engl J Med 2004;351(27):2795–804. Available at: http://www.ncbi.nlm.nih.gov/pubmed/15625331. Accessed DecembeMarch 22, 2019.

25. Thomas D, Sharmila S, Saravana Babu MS, et al. Perioperative cardiovascular outcome in patients with coronary artery disease undergoing major vascular surgery: A retrospective cohort study. Ann Card Anaesth 2022;25(3):297–303. Available at: https://pubmed.ncbi.nlm.nih.gov/35799557/. Accessed December 2, 2022.

26. Bertges DJ, Goodney PP, Zhao Y, et al. The Vascular Study Group of New England Cardiac Risk Index (VSG-CRI) predicts cardiac complications more accurately than the Revised Cardiac Risk Index in vascular surgery patients. J Vasc Surg 2010;52(3):674–83, e3. Available at: http://www.ncbi.nlm.nih.gov/pubmed/20570467. Accessed March 15, 2019.

27. Moses DA, Johnston LE, Tracci MC, et al. Estimating risk of adverse cardiac event after vascular surgery using currently available online calculators. J Vasc Surg 2018;67(1):272–8. Available at: https://pubmed.ncbi.nlm.nih.gov/29066242/. Accessed December 2, 2022.

28. Lurati Buse GAL, Puelacher C, Menosi Gualandro D, et al. Association between self-reported functional capacity and major adverse cardiac events in patients at elevated risk undergoing noncardiac surgery: a prospective diagnostic cohort

study. Br J Anaesth 2021;126(1):102–10. Available at: https://pubmed.ncbi.nlm. nih.gov/33081973/. Accessed December 2, 2022.

29. Wiklund RA, Stein HD, Rosenbaum SH. Activities of daily living and cardiovascular complications following elective, noncardiac surgery. Yale J Biol Med 2001; 74(2):75. Available at: /pmc/articles/PMC2588693/?report=abstract. Accessed December 2, 2022.

30. LA F, JA B, KA B, et al. ACC/AHA 2007 guidelines on perioperative cardiovascular evaluation and care for noncardiac surgery: a report of the American College of Cardiology/American Heart Association Task Force on Practice Guidelines (Writing Committee to Revise the 2002 Guidelines on Perioperative Cardiovascular Evaluation for Noncardiac Surgery): developed in collaboration with the American Society of Echocardiography, American Society of Nuclear Cardiology, Heart Rhythm Society, Society of Cardiovascular Anesthesiolog. Circulation 2007; 116(17). Available at: https://pubmed.ncbi.nlm.nih.gov/17901357/. Accessed December 2, 2022.

31. Ganapathi AM, Englum BR, Schechter MA, et al. Role of cardiac evaluation before thoracic endovascular aortic repair. J Vasc Surg 2014;60(5):1196–203. Available at: https://pubmed.ncbi.nlm.nih.gov/24973286/. Accessed December 2, 2022.

32. Lee TH, Marcantonio ER, Mangione CM, et al. Derivation and prospective validation of a simple index for prediction of cardiac risk of major noncardiac surgery. Circulation 1999;100(10):1043–9. Available at: https://pubmed.ncbi.nlm.nih.gov/ 10477528/. Accessed December 2, 2022.

33. Rohde LE, Polanczyk CA, Goldman L, et al. Usefulness of transthoracic echocardiography as a tool for risk stratification of patients undergoing major noncardiac surgery. Am J Cardiol 2001;87(5):505–9. Available at: https://pubmed.ncbi.nlm. nih.gov/11230829/. Accessed December 2, 2022.

34. Fleisher LA, Fleischmann KE, Auerbach AD, et al. 2014 ACC/AHA guideline on perioperative cardiovascular evaluation and management of patients undergoing noncardiac surgery: a report of the American College of Cardiology/American Heart Association Task Force on practice guidelines. J Am Coll Cardiol 2014; 64(22):e77–137. Available at: https://pubmed.ncbi.nlm.nih.gov/25091544/. Accessed December 2, 2022.

35. Fleisher LA, Fleischmann KE, Auerbach AD, et al. 2014 ACC/AHA guideline on perioperative cardiovascular evaluation and management of patients undergoing noncardiac surgery: executive summary: a report of the American College of Cardiology/American Heart Association Task Force on Practice Guidelines. Circulation 2014;130(24):2215–45. Available at: https://pubmed.ncbi.nlm.nih.gov/ 25085962/. Accessed December 2, 2022.

36. Etchells E, Meade M, Tomlinson G, et al. Semiquantitative dipyridamole myocardial stress perfusion imaging for cardiac risk assessment before noncardiac vascular surgery: A metaanalysis. J Vasc Surg 2002;36(3):534–40. Available at: https://pubmed.ncbi.nlm.nih.gov/12218978/. Accessed December 2, 2022.

37. McFalls EO, Doliszny KM, Grund F, et al. Angina and persistent exercise thallium defects: independent risk factors in elective vascular surgery. J Am Coll Cardiol 1993;21(6):1347–52. Available at: https://pubmed.ncbi.nlm.nih.gov/8473640/. Accessed December 2, 2022.

38. Priebe HJ. Perioperative myocardial infarction–aetiology and prevention. Br J Anaesth 2005;95(1):3–19. Available at: https://pubmed.ncbi.nlm.nih.gov/ 15665072/. Accessed December 2, 2022.

39. Walsh M, Berwanger O, Villar JC, et al. Association between postoperative troponin levels and 30-day mortality among patients undergoing noncardiac surgery. JAMA 2012;307(21):2295–304. Available at: https://pubmed.ncbi.nlm.nih.gov/22706835/. Accessed December 2, 2022.

40. Humble CAS, Huang S, Jammer I, et al. Prognostic performance of preoperative cardiac troponin and perioperative changes in cardiac troponin for the prediction of major adverse cardiac events and mortality in noncardiac surgery: A systematic review and meta-analysis. PLoS One 2019;(4):14. Available at: https://pubmed.ncbi.nlm.nih.gov/31009468/. Accessed December 2, 2022.

41. Park J, Hyeon CW, Lee SH, et al. Preoperative cardiac troponin below the 99th-percentile upper reference limit and 30-day mortality after noncardiac surgery. Sci Rep 2020;(1):10. Available at: https://pubmed.ncbi.nlm.nih.gov/33046756/. Accessed December 2, 2022.

42. Karthikeyan G, Moncur RA, Levine O, et al. Is a pre-operative brain natriuretic peptide or N-terminal pro-B-type natriuretic peptide measurement an independent predictor of adverse cardiovascular outcomes within 30 days of noncardiac surgery? A systematic review and meta-analysis of observational studies. J Am Coll Cardiol 2009;54(17):1599–606. Available at: https://pubmed.ncbi.nlm.nih.gov/19833258/. Accessed December 2, 2022.

43. Levine GN, Bates ER, Blankenship JC, et al. 2011 ACCF/AHA/SCAI Guideline for Percutaneous Coronary Intervention: a report of the American College of Cardiology Foundation/American Heart Association Task Force on Practice Guidelines and the Society for Cardiovascular Angiography and Interventions. Circulation 2011;(23):124. Available at: https://pubmed.ncbi.nlm.nih.gov/22064601/. Accessed December 2, 2022.

44. McAlister FA, Bertsch K, Man J, et al. Incidence of and risk factors for pulmonary complications after nonthoracic surgery. Am J Respir Crit Care Med 2005;171(5):514–7. Available at: https://pubmed.ncbi.nlm.nih.gov/15563632/. Accessed December 2, 2022.

45. Canver CC, Chanda J. Intraoperative and postoperative risk factors for respiratory failure after coronary bypass. Ann Thorac Surg 2003;75(3):853–7. Available at: https://pubmed.ncbi.nlm.nih.gov/12645706/. Accessed December 2, 2022.

46. Arozullah AM, Khuri SF, Henderson WG, et al. Development and validation of a multifactorial risk index for predicting postoperative pneumonia after major noncardiac surgery. Ann Intern Med 2001;135(10):847–57. Available at: https://pubmed.ncbi.nlm.nih.gov/11712875/. Accessed December 2, 2022.

47. Pasin L, Nardelli P, Belletti A, et al. Pulmonary Complications After Open Abdominal Aortic Surgery: A Systematic Review and Meta-Analysis. J Cardiothorac Vasc Anesth 2017;31(2):562–8. Available at: https://pubmed.ncbi.nlm.nih.gov/27988091/. Accessed December 2, 2022.

48. Elkouri S, Gloviczki P, McKusick MA, et al. Perioperative complications and early outcome after endovascular and open surgical repair of abdominal aortic aneurysms. J Vasc Surg 2004;39(3):497–505. Available at: https://pubmed.ncbi.nlm.nih.gov/14981437/. Accessed December 2, 2022.

49. Vaz Fragoso CA, Beavers DP, Hankinson JL, et al. Respiratory impairment and dyspnea and their associations with physical inactivity and mobility in sedentary community-dwelling older persons. J Am Geriatr Soc 2014;62(4):622–8. Available at: https://pubmed.ncbi.nlm.nih.gov/24635756/. Accessed December 2, 2022.

50. Stead LF, Buitrago D, Preciado N, et al. Physician advice for smoking cessation. Cochrane Database Syst Rev 2013;(5):2013. Available at: https://pubmed.ncbi.nlm.nih.gov/23728631/. Accessed December 2, 2022.

51. Bluman LG, Mosca L, Newman N, et al. Preoperative smoking habits and postoperative pulmonary complications. Chest 1998;113(4):883–9. Available at: https://pubmed.ncbi.nlm.nih.gov/9554620/. Accessed December 2, 2022.

52. Musallam KM, Rosendaal FR, Zaatari G, et al. Smoking and the risk of mortality and vascular and respiratory events in patients undergoing major surgery. JAMA Surg 2013;148(8):755–62. Available at: https://pubmed.ncbi.nlm.nih.gov/23784299/. Accessed December 2, 2022.

53. Liao P, Yegneswaran B, Vairavanathan S, et al. Postoperative complications in patients with obstructive sleep apnea: a retrospective matched cohort study. Can J Anaesth 2009;56(11):819–28. Available at: https://pubmed.ncbi.nlm.nih.gov/19774431/. Accessed December 2, 2022.

54. Vasu TS, Grewal R, Doghramji K. Obstructive sleep apnea syndrome and perioperative complications: a systematic review of the literature. J Clin Sleep Med 2012;8(2):199–207. Available at: https://pubmed.ncbi.nlm.nih.gov/22505868/. Accessed December 2, 2022.

55. Nagappa M, Liao P, Wong J, et al. Validation of the STOP-Bang Questionnaire as a Screening Tool for Obstructive Sleep Apnea among Different Populations: A Systematic Review and Meta-Analysis. PLoS One 2015;(12):10. Available at: https://pubmed.ncbi.nlm.nih.gov/26658438/. Accessed December 2, 2022.

56. Lawrence VA, Dhanda R, Hilsenbeck SG, et al. Risk of pulmonary complications after elective abdominal surgery. Chest 1996;110(3):744–50. Available at: https://pubmed.ncbi.nlm.nih.gov/8797421/. Accessed December 2, 2022.

57. Smetana GW, Lawrence VA, Cornell JE. Preoperative pulmonary risk stratification for noncardiothoracic surgery: systematic review for the American College of Physicians. Ann Intern Med 2006;144(8):581–95. Available at: https://pubmed.ncbi.nlm.nih.gov/16618956/. Accessed December 2, 2022.

58. Archer C, Levy AR, McGregor M. Value of routine preoperative chest x-rays: a meta-analysis. Can J Anaesth 1993;40(11):1022–7. Available at: https://pubmed.ncbi.nlm.nih.gov/8269561/. Accessed December 2, 2022.

59. Fuso L, Cisternino L, Di Napoli A, et al. Role of spirometric and arterial gas data in predicting pulmonary complications after abdominal surgery. Respir Med 2000;94(12):1171–6. Available at: https://pubmed.ncbi.nlm.nih.gov/11192952/. Accessed December 2, 2022.

60. Barisione G, Rovida S, Gazzaniga GM, et al. Upper abdominal surgery: does a lung function test exist to predict early severe postoperative respiratory complications? Eur Respir J 1997;10(6):1301–8. Available at: https://pubmed.ncbi.nlm.nih.gov/9192933/. Accessed December 2, 2022.

61. Miller MR, Levy ML. Chronic obstructive pulmonary disease: missed diagnosis versus misdiagnosis. BMJ 2015;351. Available at: https://pubmed.ncbi.nlm.nih.gov/26136356/. Accessed December 2, 2022.

62. Bevacqua BK. Pre-operative pulmonary evaluation in the patient with suspected respiratory disease. Indian J Anaesth 2015;59(9):542–9. Available at: https://pubmed.ncbi.nlm.nih.gov/26556912/. Accessed December 2, 2022.

63. Abdallah SJ, Voduc N, Corrales-Medina VF, et al. Symptoms, Pulmonary Function, and Functional Capacity Four Months after COVID-19. Ann Am Thorac Soc 2021;18(11):1912–7. Available at: https://pubmed.ncbi.nlm.nih.gov/33872135/. Accessed December 2, 2022.

64. Le ST, Kipnis P, Cohn B, et al. COVID-19 Vaccination and the Timing of Surgery Following COVID-19 Infection. Ann Surg 2022;276(5):E265–72. Available at: https://pubmed.ncbi.nlm.nih.gov/35837898/. Accessed December 2, 2022.

65. Kougias P, Sharath SE, Zamani N, et al. Timing of a Major Operative Intervention After a Positive COVID-19 Test Affects Postoperative Mortality: Results From a Nationwide, Procedure-matched Analysis. Ann Surg 2022;276(3):554–61. Available at: https://pubmed.ncbi.nlm.nih.gov/35837893/. Accessed December 2, 2022.

66. Lal BK, Prasad NK, Englum BR, et al. Periprocedural complications in patients with SARS-CoV-2 infection compared to those without infection: A nationwide propensity-matched analysis. Am J Surg 2021;222(2):431–7. Available at: https://pubmed.ncbi.nlm.nih.gov/33384154/. Accessed December 2, 2022.

67. Benson RA, Nandhra S. Outcomes of Vascular and Endovascular Interventions Performed During the Coronavirus Disease 2019 (COVID-19) Pandemic. Ann Surg 2021;273(4):630–5. Available at: https://pubmed.ncbi.nlm.nih.gov/33378307. Accessed December 2, 2022.

68. Hitchman L, Machin M. Impact of COVID-19 on vascular patients worldwide: analysis of the COVIDSurg data. J Cardiovasc Surg 2021;62(6):558–70. Available at: https://pubmed.ncbi.nlm.nih.gov/35037445/. Accessed December 2, 2022.

69. Sudhakaran S, Surani SR. Guidelines for Perioperative Management of the Diabetic Patient. Surg Res Pract 2015;2015. Available at: https://pubmed.ncbi.nlm.nih.gov/26078998/. Accessed December 2, 2022.

70. Duwayri Y, Jordan WD. Diabetes, dysglycemia, and vascular surgery. J Vasc Surg 2020;71(2):701–11. Available at: https://pubmed.ncbi.nlm.nih.gov/31327619/. Accessed December 2, 2022.

71. McGirt MJ, Woodworth GF, Brooke BS, et al. Hyperglycemia independently increases the risk of perioperative stroke, myocardial infarction, and death after carotid endarterectomy. Neurosurgery 2006;58(6):1066–72. Available at: https://pubmed.ncbi.nlm.nih.gov/16723885/. Accessed December 2, 2022.

72. Handelsman Y, Bloomgarden ZT, Grunberger G, et al. American association of clinical endocrinologists and American college of endocrinology - Clinical practice guidelines for developing a diabetes mellitus comprehensive care plan - 2015 -. Endocr Pract 2015;21(4):413–37. Available at: https://pubmed.ncbi.nlm.nih.gov/25869408/. Accessed December 2, 2022.

73. Fletcher E, Askari A, Yang Y, et al. Diabetes in day case general and vascular surgery: A multicentre regional audit. Int J Clin Pract 2020;(4):74. Available at: https://pubmed.ncbi.nlm.nih.gov/31884722/. Accessed December 2, 2022.

74. Bock M, Johansson T, Fritsch G, et al. The impact of preoperative testing for blood glucose concentration and haemoglobin A1c on mortality, changes in management and complications in noncardiac elective surgery: a systematic review. Eur J Anaesthesiol 2015;32(3):152–9. Available at: https://pubmed.ncbi.nlm.nih.gov/25046561/. Accessed December 2, 2022.

75. Halkos ME, Puskas JD, Lattouf OM, et al. Elevated preoperative hemoglobin A1c level is predictive of adverse events after coronary artery bypass surgery. J Thorac Cardiovasc Surg 2008;136(3):631–40. Available at: https://pubmed.ncbi.nlm.nih.gov/18805264/. Accessed December 2, 2022.

76. Goodenough CJ, Liang MK, Nguyen MT, et al. Preoperative Glycosylated Hemoglobin and Postoperative Glucose Together Predict Major Complications after Abdominal Surgery. J Am Coll Surg 2015;221(4):854–61.e1. Available at: https://pubmed.ncbi.nlm.nih.gov/26272016/. Accessed December 2, 2022.

77. Feringa HHH, Vidakovic R, Karagiannis SE, et al. Impaired glucose regulation, elevated glycated haemoglobin and cardiac ischaemic events in vascular surgery patients. Diabet Med 2008;25(3):314–9. Available at: https://pubmed.ncbi.nlm.nih.gov/18201208/. Accessed December 2, 2022.

78. Arya S, Binney ZO, Khakharia A, et al. High hemoglobin A1c associated with increased adverse limb events in peripheral arterial disease patients undergoing revascularization. J Vasc Surg 2018;67(1):217–28, e1. Available at: https://pubmed.ncbi.nlm.nih.gov/28844470/. Accessed December 2, 2022.
79. Hjellestad ID, Søfteland E, Husebye ES, et al. HbA1c predicts long-term postoperative mortality in patients with unknown glycemic status at admission for vascular surgery: An exploratory study. J Diabetes 2019;11(6):466–76. Available at: https://pubmed.ncbi.nlm.nih.gov/30367557/. Accessed December 2, 2022.
80. Huber M, Ozrazgat-Baslanti T, Thottakkara P, et al. Cardiovascular-Specific Mortality and Kidney Disease in Patients Undergoing Vascular Surgery. JAMA Surg 2016;151(5):441–50. Available at: https://pubmed.ncbi.nlm.nih.gov/26720406/. Accessed December 2, 2022.
81. Patel VI, Lancaster RT, Ergul E, et al. Postoperative renal dysfunction independently predicts late mortality in patients undergoing aortic reconstruction. J Vasc Surg 2015;62(6):1405–12. Available at: https://pubmed.ncbi.nlm.nih.gov/26598117/. Accessed December 2, 2022.
82. Klarin D, Lancaster RT, Ergul E, et al. Perioperative and long-term impact of chronic kidney disease on carotid artery interventions. J Vasc Surg 2016;64(5):1295–302. Available at: https://pubmed.ncbi.nlm.nih.gov/27776697/. Accessed December 2, 2022.
83. Li X, Zhang S, Xiao F. Influence of chronic kidney disease on early clinical outcomes after off-pump coronary artery bypass grafting. J Cardiothorac Surg 2020;(1):15. Available at: https://pubmed.ncbi.nlm.nih.gov/32727495/. Accessed December 2, 2022.
84. Holden RM, Harman GJ, Wang M, et al. Major bleeding in hemodialysis patients. Clin J Am Soc Nephrol 2008;3(1):105–10. Available at: https://pubmed.ncbi.nlm.nih.gov/18003768/. Accessed December 2, 2022.
85. Ocak G, Rookmaaker MB, Algra A, et al. Chronic kidney disease and bleeding risk in patients at high cardiovascular risk: a cohort study. J Thromb Haemost 2018;16(1):65–73. Available at: https://pubmed.ncbi.nlm.nih.gov/29125709/. Accessed December 2, 2022.
86. Fang JH, Chen YC, Ho CH, et al. The risk of major bleeding event in patients with chronic kidney disease on pentoxifylline treatment. Sci Rep 2021;11(1):1–8. Available at: https://www.nature.com/articles/s41598-021-92753-4. Accessed December 2, 2022.
87. Weisbord SD, Gallagher M, Jneid H, et al. Outcomes after Angiography with Sodium Bicarbonate and Acetylcysteine. N Engl J Med 2018;378(7):603–14. Available at: https://pubmed.ncbi.nlm.nih.gov/29130810/. Accessed December 2, 2022.
88. Morita S, Masukawa A, Suzuki K, et al. Unenhanced MR angiography: Techniques and clinical applications in patients with chronic kidney disease. Radiographics 2011;31(2):13–33. Available at: https://pubmed.ncbi.nlm.nih.gov/21415179/. Accessed December 2, 2022.
89. Czobor NR, Lehot JJ, Holndonner-Kirst E, et al. Frailty In Patients Undergoing Vascular Surgery: A Narrative Review Of Current Evidence. Ther Clin Risk Manag 2019;15:1217–32. Available at: https://pubmed.ncbi.nlm.nih.gov/31802876/. Accessed December 2, 2022.
90. Leng S, Chen X, Mao G. Frailty syndrome: an overview. Clin Interv Aging 2014;9:433. Available at: https://pubmed.ncbi.nlm.nih.gov/24672230/. Accessed December 2, 2022.

91. Vetrano DL, Landi F, Volpato S, et al. Association of sarcopenia with short- and long-term mortality in older adults admitted to acute care wards: results from the CRIME study. J Gerontol A Biol Sci Med Sci 2014;69(9):1154–61. Available at: https://pubmed.ncbi.nlm.nih.gov/24744390/. Accessed December 2, 2022.

92. Schaller MS, Ramirez JL, Gasper WJ, et al. Frailty Is Associated with an Increased Risk of Major Adverse Cardiac Events in Patients with Stable Claudication. Ann Vasc Surg 2018;50:38–45. Available at: https://pubmed.ncbi.nlm.nih.gov/29477684/. Accessed December 2, 2022.

93. Arya S, Kim SI, Duwayri Y, et al. Frailty increases the risk of 30-day mortality, morbidity, and failure to rescue after elective abdominal aortic aneurysm repair independent of age and comorbidities. J Vasc Surg 2015;61(2):324–31. Available at: https://pubmed.ncbi.nlm.nih.gov/25312534/. Accessed December 2, 2022.

94. Donald GW, Ghaffarian AA, Isaac F, et al. Preoperative frailty assessment predicts loss of independence after vascular surgery. J Vasc Surg 2018;68(5):1382–9. Available at: https://pubmed.ncbi.nlm.nih.gov/29773431/. Accessed December 2, 2022.

95. Shovel L, Morkane C. Prehabilitation for Vascular Surgery Patients: Challenges and Opportunities. Can J Cardiol 2022;38(5):645–53.

Infrarenal Abdominal Aortic Aneurysm

Simon De Freitas, MD, Nicole D'Ambrosio, MD,
Javairiah Fatima, MD*

KEYWORDS

- Abdominal aortic aneurysm • Endovascular • Open repair

KEY POINTS

- Endovascular abdominal aortic aneurysm repair has replaced open surgery as the primary modality for aneurysm repair.
- Screening programs are effective in reducing aneurysm-associated mortality in selected populations.
- Rutuptured aneurysms are are almost uniformaly fatal, irrespecive of the type of repair used and mortality reduction is acheived by repair in the asymptomatic stage.

INTRODUCTION

Abdominal aortic aneurysms are found in up to 6% of men and 1.7% of women over the age of 65 years and are usually asymptomatic.[1,2] The natural history of aortic aneurysms is continued dilation leading to rupture, which is associated with an overall 80% mortality. Of the patients with ruptured aneurysms that undergo intervention, half will not survive their hospitalization.[3] Reduction in aneurysm mortality is therefore achieved by prophylactic repair during the asymptomatic period. On a population-based level, this is supported by abdominal aortic aneurysm screening programs. Approximately 60% of abdominal aortic aneurysms are confined to the infrarenal portion of the aorta and are amenable to repair with off-the-shelf endovascular devices. Endovascular techniques have now replaced open surgery as the primary modality for aneurysm repair.[4] Several devices are available, and each has unique features that the operator must be familiar with when selecting the most suitable device. One major limitation of endovascular repair is the development of endoleaks, which may require reintervention over time. Currently in the United States, over 80% of infrarenal aneurysms are treated with endovascular techniques.[5] Open

Department of Vascular Surgery, Georgetown University Hospital, MedStar Health, Washington, DC, USA
* Corresponding author. 106th Irving Street Northwest, Suite 3150, POB N, Washington, DC 20010.
E-mail address: Javairiah.Fatima@MedStar.net

Surg Clin N Am 103 (2023) 595–614
https://doi.org/10.1016/j.suc.2023.05.001
0039-6109/23/© 2023 Elsevier Inc. All rights reserved.

surgical.theclinics.com

surgical repair is preferably limited to high-volume centers and is reserved for aneurysms with complex anatomy that have a high risk of failure with endovascular intervention.

EPIDEMIOLOGY AND NATURAL HISTORY OF ABDOMINAL AORTIC ANEURYSM

The true incidence of abdominal aortic aneurysms is uncertain, but detection continues to increase in developed countries as the population ages and more screening programs become established.[1] Increased age, tobacco smoking, biological male gender, and family history remain the most important risk factors for the development of abdominal aortic aneurysm. Additional risk factors include hypertension, dyslipidemia, coronary artery disease, and connective tissue disease. Diabetes mellitus is somewhat protective for uncertain reasons.[6] The overall incidence of abdominal aortic aneurysm in patients below 55 years of age is very low. From 55 to 64 years, there is a roughly 1% prevalence and this increases by 3% per decade thereafter.[7-9] Each year, approximately 10,000 deaths occur in the United States due to ruptured abdominal aortic aneurysm.[10] Tobacco use serves as the primary modifiable risk factor linked to the development and rupture of abdominal aortic aneurysms. One in four patients enrolled in screening programs are active smokers and these patients are seven times more likely to develop an aneurysm when compared to non-smokers. The association between smoking and aneurysm development is particularly strong for women.[11] The duration of smoking rather than the total number of cigarettes smoked appears to determine risk.[12] Smoking cessation is associated with a significant risk reduction and after 25 years of cessation the risk is similar to that observed in non-smokers.[13] Caucasian race is the most frequently associated with the development of AAA, whereas there is decreased risk among Hispanics (OR 0.69), African Americans (OR 0.72), and Asians (OR 0.72).[14] First-degree family history of an abdominal aortic aneurysm increases risk by two-fold and is not gender-specific.[15] Lastly, the finding of peripheral arterial aneurysms confers increased risk and necessitates prompt evaluation of the abdominal aorta for aneurysmal disease.[16] Once an aneurysm develops, dilation continues slowly, albeit progressively. In accordance with the law of Laplace, smaller aneurysms increase at a slower rate, whereas larger aneurysms in the 4–5 cm range expand faster, at an approximate rate of 0.3–0.5 cm/year[17] The rate of expansion is, however, nonlinear in that most will progress but some do not, making individual predictions difficult.

SCREENING AND SURVEILLANCE OF ABDOMINAL AORTIC ANEURYSM

Population-based screening reduces abdominal aortic aneurysm-related mortality and rates of rupture. Screening is supported by data from four population-based randomized controlled trials (**Table 1**). Targeted screening programs have proven to be both cost-effective and logistically simple to implement.[22] The modality of choice for aneurysm screening is ultrasound, which is inexpensive and non-invasive and has sensitivity and specificity of 94% and 98% for the detection of aortic aneurysm.[23] The benefit of a single ultrasound screen extends out to 15 years follow-up.[24] United States Preventive Services Task Force (USPSTF) recommends screening be offered to men who have ever smoked, between the ages of 65 and 75 years.[25] Medicare beneficiaries who meet these inclusion criteria qualify for screening under the SAAVE act passed in 2007. Societal recommendations have somewhat broader inclusion recommendations and are summarized in **Table 2**. There is growing support for the expansion of screening programs beyond those outlined above.[14,30] One rationale is that screening trials proved effective during the era of open surgery when perioperative

Table 1
Landmark trials of population-based screening for AAA

Randomized Trial	Journal/ Year	Population Screened (n = no. Screened)	Positive Screens (n = Aneurysms)	Reduction from Aneurysm Mortality
MASS[18]	Lancet 2002	Men 65–74 yrs (n = 27,147)	4.9% (n = 1333)	Risk reduction 42% (95% CI 22–58)
Chichester[19]	Br J Surg 1995	Men and women 65–80 yrs (n = 5,394)	4.0% (n = 218)	Risk reduction 42% (95% CI NR)
Viborg[20]	BMJ 2005	Men 64–73 yrs (n = 6,333)	4.0% (n = 191)	Risk reduction 67% (95% CI 29–84)
Western Australia[21]	BMJ 2004	Men 65–79 yrs (n = 12,203)	7.2% (n = 875)	Risk ratio 0.61 (95% CI 0.33–1.11)

mortality rates were significantly higher than those seen in contemporary endovascular practice. Another driving force for expansion is the lower rates of repair in females and non-smokers.[31] The lower prevalence of comorbidities such as smoking and more advanced age at presentation are possible explanations why screening women under similar inclusion parameters to men has not proven beneficial.[11,32] Future directions aim at understanding which groups beyond the traditional scope need to be targeted for expansion of screening. Over 90% of aneurysms detected through screening will be below the size threshold for repair. These aneurysms instead undergo periodic ultrasound surveillance. Recommended surveillance intervals vary slightly among societal guidelines. In general, aneurysms under 4 cm should undergo imaging at 3-year intervals and those between 4.0 cm and 4.9 cm should be imaged annually. Once at the 5 cm mark, screening should be performed every 3 to 6 months until the threshold for repair is met. In women, 6-monthly screening may begin at 4.5 cm. Adherence to surveillance guidelines is fundamental for screening programs to be effective and has been reported to be as low as 65%.[19]

THRESHOLDS FOR ELECTIVE REPAIR OF ABDOMINAL AORTIC ANEURYSM

The decision to intervene should consider the likelihood of rupture, the individualized risks associated with repair and life expectancy of the patient. The diameter of an aneurysm is a surrogate for radial wall stress and remains the most accurate predictor of rupture. The cumulative five-year rate of rupture beyond 5 cm is approximately 30 to 40%, while smaller aneurysms in the sub-5 cm range have a much lower rupture rate at 1 to 5% per year.[33–35] Repair should be considered for small aneurysms that demonstrate expansion >0.5 cm in a 6 mth period. Such rapid growth is often representative of an unstable aortic wall. Heavy smokers and patients with poorly controlled hypertension are more likely to demonstrate rapid growth whereas this phenomenon is seen less often in diabetic patients.[36] The most widely accepted size threshold for intervention is $\geq$ 5.5 cm in men and between 5.0 cm and 5.4 cm for women.[4,26,27,37] Symptomatic aneurysms, typically in the form of abdominal or back pain, may be a sign of impending rupture and warrant urgent repair even if below the recommended size threshold.

REPAIR OF SMALL ABDOMINAL AORTIC ANEURYSMS

Repair of small aneurysms has been evaluated in several randomized trials. The UKSAT study randomized patients to either early open repair in the 4.0 cm to 5.5 cm range, or continued surveillance and open repair at the >5.5 cm threshold.

Table 2
Summary of AAA screening recommendations from major cardiovascular societies

Society	Year	Summary of AAA Screening Guidance
Society for Vascular Surgery (SVS)[4]	2018	Men or women aged 65–75 yrs with history of tobacco use First-degree relatives of patient with AAA aged 65–75 yrs or >75rs and in good health Men or women >75 yrs in good health if not screened prior
European Society for Vascular Surgery (ESVS)[26]	2019	Men aged 65 yrs Men and women aged ≥50 yrs who have first deg relative with AAA Population based screening for women not recommended
American College of Cardiology (ACC)/American Heart Association (AHA)[27]	2005	Men aged 65–75 yrs with history of smoking Men 60 years of age who are either siblings or offspring of patients with AAAs
American College of Preventive Medicine (ACPM)[28]	2011	Men aged 65–75 yrs with history of smoking
Canadian Society for Vascular Surgery (CSVS)[29]	2007	Men aged 65–75 yrs of age who are candidates for surgery, including those without significant smoking history

There was no difference in long-term mortality and the early surgery group experienced a perioperative mortality of 5.8%.[38] These findings were subsequently confirmed by the ADAM study, even at a lower operative mortality rate of 2%.[39] The CESAR trial compared surveillance to repair at 4.1 cm to 5.4 cm, but used EVAR instead of open repair.[40] There was no difference in all-cause mortality at 54 months; 14.5% in the EVAR group and 10.1% in the surveillance group, p = 0.6. Rates of aneurysm-related mortality, aneurysm rupture, and major morbidity were similar in both groups. The PIVOTAL trial enrolled patients with 4 cm to 5 cm abdominal aortic aneurysms and similarly found no mortality benefit of early endovascular intervention. Furthermore, across each of the trials, the endovascular repair of small aneurysms now mandated lifelong surveillance and was associated with reintervention. Beyond the outcomes of survival, repair of aneurysms in the small range does not offer improve quality of life or reduce costs.[41]

HISTORICAL PERSPECTIVES ON ENDOVASCULAR ANEURYSM REPAIR

The high perioperative morbidity and mortality associated with open aneurysm repair anticipated an early alternative. Suggestions of an intraluminal repair, thereby negating the need to open the abdomen, surfaced by the mid-1980s.[42] These initiatives in the aorta were based on an existing knowledge of stents in animals, used either alone or in combination with a polyester lining.[43,44] In 1987, Nocolai Volodos and his team in Soviet Ukraine performed the first EVAR in a human patient, successfully repairing a traumatic thoracic aortic pseudoaneurysm.[45] Four years later in Buenos Aires, Juan Parodi together with Julio Palmaz documented five successful infrarenal aneurysm repairs by retrograde deployment of a stent-anchored straight tubular endograft.[46] Thereafter, numerous similar successes were documented in the United States, Europe and Australia. Operator-designed endografts with monoiliac and bi-iliac configurations were introduced by the mid-1990s and commercial input followed as the industry recognized the potential of the new technology. Concurrent with the refinement of infrarenal EVAR, the treatment of more complex aortic anatomy began, inspired by fenestrated concepts in Australia.[47] By 1999, the Food and Drug Administration (FDA) approved the first two stent-grafts for commercial use; the Medtronic AneuRx and the Guidant Ancure. With the turn of the century, multiple manufacturers received approvals and there were significant improvements in delivery systems, fixation apparatus, and conformability, while simultaneously allowing for smaller sheath sizes. In the year 2000, more than half of all aneurysm repairs in the United States were performed with an endograft.[48] A fenestrated endograft received FDA approval in 2012 and an iliac-branched device in 2016. Today, EVAR accounts for almost 85% of aneurysm repairs in the United States and approximately 25,000 procedures are performed annually.[49] Seven devices are available for off-the-shelf repair of infrarenal aneurysmal disease, each of which has undergone several iterations since its initial approval, with ongoing research sustaining continued evolution.

EVIDENCE FOR ENDOVASCULAR REPAIR OF ABDOMINAL AORTIC ANEURYSMS

EVAR-1 was the first randomized prospective trial to demonstrate a reduction in perioperative mortality in patients undergoing EVAR comparted to traditional open surgical repair.[50] This UK-based multicenter trial enrolled 1082 patients who were deemed fit for open repair and demonstrated a reduction in aneurysm-related deaths in patients who underwent EVAR (4% vs 7%, HR 0.55), but no difference in all-cause mortality. The DREAM trial in the Netherlands was a smaller trial with 345 patients and used a threshold of 5.0 cm for intervention.[51] The trial reported a reduction in operative mortality in patients with EVAR (1.2% vs 4.6%) and reduced major perioperative complications (4.7% vs 9.8%). The OPEN trial similarly compared open repair and EVAR in 881 patients in the Veterans Affairs healthcare system in the United States.[52] Perioperative mortality was significantly lower for endovascular repair (0.5% vs 3%) and EVAR was associated with improvement in other hospital metrics including procedural time, ICU stay and total length of hospitalization. The ACE trial in France compared EVAR to open surgery in a much lower risk group of patients and found that in these patients there was no mortality benefit, and those who received endovascular treatment required more reinterventions.[53] The EVAR-2 trial enrolled patients who were unfit for open repair, and randomized to either EVAR or no intervention.[54] Survival was not improved with EVAR and was associated with a considerable 30-day mortality. Mortality benefits of endovascular repair were most profound in the early postoperative period and in all three of the EVAR-1, DREAM, and OVER trials, this survival advantage was lost in the mid-term. In EVAR-1, after 2 years there was no difference in all-cause mortality, at least in part because of fatal endograft ruptures, but also from more cardiovascular deaths in those undergoing endovascular repair.[55] In the DREAM trial, the perioperative survival benefit of EVAR did not extend beyond one year after randomization, but there was sustained benefit in aorta-related mortality. Similarly to EVAR-1, rates of reintervention were higher. Noninferiority of endovascular repair in the DREAM trial was maintained to six years and twelve years from randomization.[56,57] In the OVER trial, the benefit of endovascular repair was sustained at two three years, and after a mean follow-up of 5.2 years the survival was similar.[58]

EVAR DEVICE CHARACTERISTICS AND SELECTION

There are no prospective data comparing outcomes among EVAR devices and all are cost-comparable. Operator device selection is based upon knowledge of device characteristics and the unique anatomy of the aneurysm being repaired. While each EVAR device has features that may either limit or support its use, there are several overarching principles for device selection. First, all devices will perform adequately in patients with straightforward anatomy i.e., disease-free access vessels of adequate caliber, minimal iliac tortuosity and healthy, minimally-angulated aortic neck without prohibitive calcification or mural thrombus. Second, the user should stay within the confines of the instructions for use (IFU).[59,60] Nonadherence, in particular with respect to the proximal neck IFU, bears relationship to the development of 1a endoleak, reinterventions, EVAR failure, and possibly aortic-related mortality.[61] Third, operative familiarity with all available FDA devices will facilitate selection decisions based on technical nuances of the individual devices that cannot be otherwise obtained from the literature. Evolutionary timelines, anatomic requirements, and material characteristics for each of the seven FDA-approved EVAR devices are presented in **Tables 3–5**.

PREPROCEDURAL PLANNING AND EVAR DEVICE SIZING

Endovascular repair begins with patient selection, risk stratification, and additional pre-operative planning through device sizing. Computed tomography angiography is the cornerstone of imaging, ideally with 1 mm cuts in the axial plane. Postprocessing three-dimensional reconstructions with centerline technology facilitate more precise measurements for sizing and planning. The overarching principle of sizing is to stay within the anatomic constraints of the IFU for the selected device. Review of the CT angiogram begins with a close examination of the seal zone. The presence of an angulated or conical neck, mural thrombus, or a high calcium burden is considered hostile neck features that may compromise proximal seal and result in EVAR failure. Healthy-appearing, parallel aortic neck is necessary to avoid failure of proximal seal. Ten to 20% oversizing to the aortic neck diameter is recommended. The neck diameter is measured from adventitia to adventitia for all endografts, except the Excluder C3 and Excluder Conformable (W.L. Gore) which is measured from intima to intima. Neck angulation in the craniocaudal axis is calculated to assist with the orthogonal orientation of the C-arm. Length measurements are then obtained from the lowest renal to the hypogastric arteries, ideally on using the centerline of flow to minimize inaccuracies in measurements. These measurements may also be obtained with a marker catheter during angiography. Next, the common iliac diameters are measured, and limbs are sized 10 to 20% beyond the diameters of the distal fixation sites. The common femoral arteries are evaluated for percutaneous access suitability, along with external iliac artery diameters to ensure sheath sizes of the selected device will be easily accommodated.

TECHNICAL APPROACH TO ENDOVASCULAR AORTIC ANEURYSM REPAIR

Endovascular aneurysm repair is most effectively performed in an operating room with fixed-mount imaging supported by staff trained in both open and endovascular techniques. The procedure can be performed under local anesthesia with conscious sedation or general anesthesia. The choice of anesthesia is tailored to the individual case at hand. Pedal Doppler signals are marked and recorded. The patient is then positioned supine and draped from nipples to knees for optimal exposure. Endovascular operators must be mindful of approaches to reduce radiation exposure throughout the

Table 3
FDA-approved EVAR devices available for use in the United States

Device	Excluder C3	Zenith Flex	AFX2	Endurant II	Alto	Excluder Conformable	Treo
Manufacturer	W. L. Gore & Associates	Cook Inc	Endologix LLC	Medtronic	Endologix LLC	W. L. Gore & Associates	Terumo Aortic
Device Name as Marketed	Excluder C3 conformable endoprosthesis	Zenith Flex AAA Endovascular Graft	AFX2 Endovascular AAA System	Endurant II Stent Graft System	Alto Abdominal Stent Graft System	Excluder Conformable AAA Endoprosthesis	TREO Abdominal Stent Graft System
Initial FDA Premarket Approval	2002	2003	2004	2010	2012	2020	2020
Current Iteration and year of Approval	3rd gen 2010	2nd gen 2008	3rd gen 2016	3rd gen 2017	4th gen 2020	1st gen 2020	1st gen 2020
Notable Revisions to prior Generations	Reduction in graft porosity to reduce type IV endoleak	Increase in conformability of iliac limbs	Change in fabric to reduce tears causing type III endoleak	Anchoring pins added to suprarenal fixation	Revision of filling channel to mitigate polymer leaks	Evolution of Excluder C3; reconstrainable with improved angulation control	NA

Table 4
Sizing requirements per the instructions for use (IFU) for FDA-approved EVAR devices

Device	Excluder C3	Zenith Flex	AFX2	Endurant II	Alto	Excluder Conformable	Treo
Proximal Neck Length	≥15 mm	≥15 mm	≥15 mm	≥10 mm	≥7 mm	≥10 mm, ≥15 mm	15 mm
Range of Neck Diameters	19–32 mm	18–32 mm	18–32 mm	19–32 mm	16–30 mm	16–32 mm	17–32 mm
Infrarenal Neck Angulation	≤60°	≤60°	≤60°	≤60°	≤60°	≤60° ≤90°	≤60°
Suprarenal Neck Angulation	N/A	≤45°	N/A	N/A	N/A	N/A	≤45°
Distal Fixation Length	≥10 mm	≥10 mm	≥15 mm	≥15 mm	≥10 mm	≥10 mm	≥10 mm
Range of Iliac Diameters	8–13.5 mm	7.5–20 mm	10–23 mm	8–25 mm	8–25 mm	8–25 mm	8–20 mm

Table 5
Material components and characteristics of FDA-approved EVAR devices

Device	Excluder C3	Zenith Flex	AFX2	Endurant II	Alto	Excluder Conformable	Treo
Graft Material	ePTFE and FEP	Woven polyester	Multilayered ePTFE	High-density woven polyester	ePTFE	ePTFE	Woven polyester
Stent Material	Nitinol	Stainless steel main body, nitinol limbs	Cobalt chromium alloy	Nitinol	Nitinol	Nitinol	Nitinol
Fixation Features	Infrarenal fixation with barbs	Suprarenal fixation with barbs	Anatomical fixation on bifurcation and suprarenal fixation with barbs	Suprarenal fixation with barbs	Suprarenal fixation with barbs and polymer rings	Infrarenal fixation with barbs	Suprarenal and infrarenal
Main Body Access Profile	18–20Fr	18–22 Fr	17 Fr	18–20 Fr	15 Fr	15–18 Fr	18–19 Fr
Delivery System	Sheath required	Ensheathed	Sheath required	Sheathless	Ensheathed	Sheath required	Sheathless

procedure.[62] Bilateral percutaneous femoral access is achieved using a combination of ultrasound and fluoroscopic guidance. Using the preclose technique, suture-mediated closure devices are deployed. In the setting of diseased access vessels, open femoral exposure remains preferable to percutaneous access. The patient is heparinized and introducer sheaths are exchanged for large-bore sheaths. The device is introduced in the aorta over a super-stiff wire. Gantry angles are adjusted to remove parallax errors. Aortography is performed under apnea, and the inferior margin of the renal arteries is marked with roadmap guidance. Intravascular ultrasound and image-fusion software are useful adjuncts in device positioning and reduce radiation exposure and contrast use. The device is repositioned and consideration is given to gate orientation in an effort to facilitate favorable cannulation, including the need for limb crossing. The device is then deployed with the top of the fabric at or marginally below (eg, 1 to 2 mm) the lowest renal artery, based on the IFU for each device. Next, the gate is cannulated. Confirmatory maneuvers are mandatory to ensure wire position is truly within the graft and avoid potential deployment of the limb outside the gate and within the aneurysm sac. An oblique pelvic arteriogram is performed to mark the hypogastric artery before the deployment of the contralateral iliac limb. The remainder of the main body and ipsilateral limb are then deployed in a similar fashion. Seal zones and modular junctions are apposed with a compliant molding balloon. Stiff wires are withdrawn to allow the device to sit naturally in the aorta and completion arteriography is performed to evaluate for endoleak. Sheaths are removed and percutaneous sutures are fastened to close the arteriotomy. Soft tissues and skin incisions are closed. Technical approaches for complex endovascular repairs are beyond the scope of this review and have been expertly addressed elsewhere.[63]

POST-EVAR IMAGING SURVEILLANCE

Postoperative surveillance facilltates the detection of endoleaks, sac expansion, limb kinks, stent fractures, and graft migration, each of which must be addressed to maintain long-term success of the endovascular repair. Surveillance protocols have generally followed early randomized trials and used computed tomography angiography at 1-month, 6-month, and 12-month intervals, followed by yearly thereafter. The preferred protocol is a triphasic scan in the unenhanced, arterial, and delayed venous phases. The major downsides of computed tomography are contrast nephrotoxicity and the increased cost and radiation exposure when compared to ultrasound. Currently, data demonstrates that adherence to surveillance protocols is highly variable and less than half of patients will follow published guidance.[64] Furthermore, when guidelines are followed it results in more interventions but does not improve mortality.[65] As a result, there has been a movement toward less-intense post-EVAR surveillance, or perhaps even no surveillance in select patients.[66] One of the first modifications to traditional surveillance included the omission of the first 6-month scan if the 1-month CT angiogram was satisfactory, and this has now been widely incorporated into guidelines.[4,67] If the 12-month computed tomography angiogram demonstrates no endoleak, with either a stable sac size or sac regression, the patient may be enrolled in yearly duplex ultrasound instead of computed tomography. Limitations of ultrasound include operator dependence and poor visualization of the aorta in patients with large body habitus or overlying bowel gas. Duplex can accurately determine sac size and detect endoleaks, at a sensitivity similar or better than CT when enhanced with microbubbles.[68,69] Indeed, rigorous contrast-enhanced ultrasonography protocols will suffice in selected patients as the sole imaging modality post-EVAR.

CLASSIFICATION AND MANAGEMENT OF ENDOLEAKS

An endoleak is defined by persistent flow into an aneurysm sac after repair with a stent-graft device, leading to pressurization and potential expansion of the aneurysm sac, **Fig. 1**.[70] Late complications of EVAR are largely attributable to endoleaks, and the rates of reintervention are relatively high at 10–15%.[71]

Type I endoleaks refer to persistent blood flow around the graft at the proximal aortic neck seal (Type IA) or distally at the iliac seal zones (Type IB). Loss of proximal seal confers markedly elevated sac pressures and increased risk of rupture, and every attempt should be made to address type 1 endoleaks identified intraoperatively.[72] If there is sufficient length of uncovered aortic neck between the graft fabric and the lowest renal, proximal cuff extension is the most straightforward maneuver. Beyond this, proximal extension will involve the management of renal and visceral vessels, including fenestrated or branch endografts or open repair with explant.[73] With proximal leaks from inadequate radial apposition, for example in the setting of thrombus or calcium, buttressing with a Palmaz bare metal stent, can be effective.[74] Type 1 A endoleaks detected later are often due to caudal device migration in the setting of progressive natural or degenerative dilation of the aortic neck. Distal type 1b endoleaks are treated with the extension of the iliac limb and commonly this involves coil embolization and coverage of the hypogastric artery, or ideally extension with an iliac branched device in order to preserve hypogastric flow. If endovascular approaches do not offer resolve, consideration must be given to open conversion.

Type II endoleaks are caused by back-bleeding from vessels that originate from the wall of the sealed aorta, such as the inferior mesenteric artery, lumbar arteries, or middle sacral artery. Type II endoleaks are present in 10–20% of EVARs on post-operative computed tomography scans and follow an overall benign course when compared to type I and type III endoleaks.[75] The main factors consistently associated with type II endoleaks include a patent inferior mesenteric artery, increased number of lumbar arteries and maximum aneurysm diameter. With these factors accounted for, the use of anticoagulation or antiplatelets does not confer added risk of a type II endoleak.[76] The rates of rupture are very low at approximately 1%, but as many as one-third occur without documented sac expansion. Resolution of the endoleak without intervention

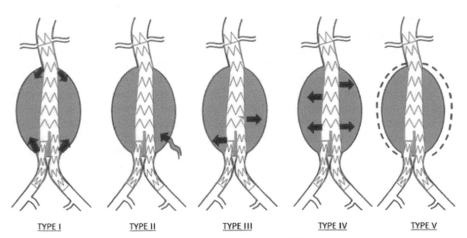

TYPE I   TYPE II   TYPE III   TYPE IV   TYPE V

Fig. 1. Endoleak classification system. (A. England, R. McWilliams Endovascular Aortic Aneurysm Repair (EVAR) Ulster Med J, 82 (1) (2013), pp. 3-10.)

occurs in 35% of cases.[77] The current approach is to intervene when there is documented sac enlargement. The Society of Vascular Surgery recommends intervention for aneurysm sac expansion of $\geq$5 mm, whereas the European Society of Vascular Surgery guidelines recommend treatment for sac expansion of $\geq$10 mm, both based on level C evidence.[4,26] One must be mindful that sac enlargement thought to be secondary to type II endoleaks may be the harbinger of an obscure type 1a endoleak and careful review is warranted. Embolization of the inflow and outflow vessels has a high success rate and may be performed with liquid embolic agents or coils. Routes to access the aneurysm sac include translumbar, transcaval or via the SMA-IMA arcade.

Type III endoleaks result from component separation in modular grafts (Type IIIa) or from tears in the graft fabric (Type IIIb). Component separation is caused by insufficient overlap between endograft modules, often precipitated by geometric changes in the aneurysm over time or from device migration. Fabric tears may be caused by stent fractures, calcific lesions, or erosion points. Most type III leaks therefore develop months to years beyond the index procedure.[78] The overall incidence is low across all devices, ranging from 3 to 5% in registry data.[79] Since type III endoleaks result in direct flow into the aortic sac, rates of secondary rupture are high and urgent repair is indicated.

Type IV endoleaks are caused by leakage into the sac across blood-porous fabric, classically seen as a blush across the fabric. It is no longer seen with newer-generation endografts. Type IV endoleaks self-resolve as the graft interstices thrombose and normal coagulation pathways resume.

Type V endoleak is somewhat of a misnomer and refers to continued sac expansion with increased pressures, but without demonstrable endoleak. The phenomenon may also be termed "endotension."The mainstay of treatment remains explant and open repair, although relining may be considered for higher-risk patients.

ENDOVASCULAR REPAIR OF RUPTURED ABDOMINAL AORTIC ANEURYSMS

Ruptured abdominal aortic aneurysm is a catastrophic event with an overall mortality of 80–90%.[80] Of those that survive until the point of hospital contact, the 30-day mortality is approximately 50%.[3] Mortality from ruptured AAA follows bimodal distribution. Death within the first 48 hrs is typically from hemorrhagic shock. Death beyond this immediate period, often in spite of successful repair, is related to sequelae of the initial critical illness compounded by comorbid conditions.[81] Several retrospective studies have noted a trend toward increased survival for ruptured abdominal aortic aneurysms in contemporary practice.[82–84] Arguably, the most major advancement is the use of EVAR for ruptured aneurysms. Endovascular therapy offers rapid balloon control of the proximal aorta, an overall shorter operative time and the ability for the procedure to be done under local anesthesia. This prompted several large single-center series, national registry, studies and randomized trials to evaluate the benefit of EVAR over open surgical repair for ruptured abdominal aortic aneurysm. US Medicare data derived from approximately 1100 propensity-matched pairs reported a significantly lower mortality with EVAR compared to open surgery (34% vs 48%, p < 0.001).[85] Similar findings were seen from an analysis of 21,206 ruptured abdominal aortic aneurysms across the United States as part of the Nationwide Inpatient Sample (NIS) database.[86] EVAR demonstrated a benefit over open repair for both mortality (OR 0.54) and major complications (OR 0.49). One of the major limitations of the aforementioned observational data is selection bias, whereby patients plausibly received an open operation because of highly unfavorable EVAR anatomy. The bias lies in the fact that patients with challenging landing zones will often require a more complex open operation, for example necessitating suprarenal exposure and clamping. That the mortality benefit of EVAR was not reproduced under the rigor randomized trial was un-surprising. However, close attention to each of these trials offers important insights into understanding the role of EVAR for rAAA. The AJAX trial, based across three cen-ters in Amsterdam, randomized 116 ruptured infrarenal AAAs that were fit for either type of repair. The primary endpoint was a composite of death and major complica-tions, which occurred in 42% of the EVAR group and 47% of the open surgical repair group (95% CI -13% – 23%).[87] There was a significant reduction in renal failure in the EVAR group (ARR 20%). One key limitation of the AJAX trial was the exclusion of pa-tients hemodynamically unfit for CTA. The IMPROVE trial included 316 patients which were randomized into open and endovascular groups after computed tomography im-aging was obtained.[88] The design allowed crossover to the open group if aortic morphology was unsuitable for endovascular repair, closely mirroring the reality of clinical practice. The 30-day mortality was not significantly different between groups (35.4% vs 37.4%, p = 0.62), although in the subset of women a significant mortality reduction was observed. Important secondary outcomes included a shorter ICU length of stay and higher rates of discharge to home in the endovascular group. Of note, the endovascular approach was not more cost-effective. The French ECAR trial randomized hemodynamically unstable ruptured AAAs that were suitable to both open and endovascular repair.[89] Mortality at 30 days and 1 year were not different between the groups (18% in the endovascular group vs. 24% in the open group at 30 days, and 30% vs. 35% respectively at 1 year). Pulmonary complications, need for transfusion and ICU length of stay were lower in the endovascular group.

CONTEMPORARY OUTCOMES OF OPEN ABDOMINAL AORTIC ANEURYSM REPAIR

Open surgical repair of abdominal aortic aneurysms became a routine part of vascular practice by the 1970s and has undergone continued technical refinement and evolution. It is the gold standard to which EVAR is compared and remains one of the most academically scrutinized surgical procedures. The leading cause of mortality after open aneurysm repair is related to comorbid coronary artery dis-ease and efforts to stratify and reduce this risk are paramount.[90] Management of pre-operative obstructive lung disease, including smoking cessation, and optimization of renal function also significantly reduces risk.[91–93] Historically, the post-operative mortality of open abdominal aortic aneurysm repair has been quoted at 5–8%.[94,95] These figures continue to improve and contemporary mortality, supported by figures from the UK National Vascular and US Nationwide Inpatient Sample databases are best estimated in the 3 to 5% range.[96,97] The open arms of DREAM, OVER and EVAR-1 also reports similar mortality.[50–52] Data from tertiary-level aortic centers, which largely include high-risk patients have consistently reported a ≤3% mortal-ity.[98,99] These data support the practice whereby younger patients with low anes-thetic risk and few comorbidities are offered open repair as first-line treatment for infrarenal aneurysms, provided the procedure is done in a center of expertise. Contemporary open outcomes occur in an era of unprecedented endovascular inno-vation whereby the open solution inherently involves a more challenging operation such as suprarenal clamping, explant of a failed endovascular device, or dealing with concomitant aortoiliac occlusive disease.

SUMMARY

Abdominal aortic aneurysms continue to pose considerable challenges in the daily practice of vascular surgery. Ruptured aortic aneurysms are almost uniformly fatal, irrespective of the type of repair used, and mortality reduction is achieved by repair in the asymptomatic stage. Advancements in endovascular technology have significantly reduced perioperative mortality and remain noninferior to open repair in the mid-term, but with higher rates of reintervention. Longer term trial data are not available for endovascular repair but the durability of an open repair is definite. An intricate understanding of the natural history of the disease and the patient at hand is imperative when deciding on the best modality of treatment. Each of the endovascular devices available is comparable in performance and selection is based on the anatomic features of the aneurysm. Device failure is frequent when the devices are used outside of the instructions for use and this has been a major failing of the endovascular revolution to date.

CLINICS CARE POINTS

- Abdominal aortic aneurysms are found in 5% of men over the age of 65 years.
- Screening programs reduce aneurysm-related mortality in selected populations.
- Endovascular repair is the primary modality of repair in contemporary practice.
- Endovascular repair is limited in anatomically more complex aneurysms.
- Open surgery may be offered as first-line treatment in younger patients with low anesthestic risk.
- Ruptured aneurysms continue to have very high mortality irrespecitve of approach used.

REFERENCES

1. Sampson UK, Norman PE, Fowkes FG, et al. Estimation of global and regional incidence and prevalence of abdominal aortic aneurysms 1990 to 2010. Glob Heart 2014;9(1):159–70.
2. Scott RA, Ashton HA, Kay DN. Abdominal aortic aneurysm in 4237 screened patients: prevalence, development and management over 6 years. Br J Surg 1991; 78(9):1122–5.
3. Bown MJ, Sutton AJ, Bell PR, et al. A meta-analysis of 50 years of ruptured abdominal aortic aneurysm repair. Br J Surg 2002;89(6):714–30.
4. Chaikof EL, Dalman RL, Eskandari MK, et al. The Society for Vascular Surgery practice guidelines on the care of patients with an abdominal aortic aneurysm. J Vasc Surg 2018;67(1):2–77 e2.
5. Dua A, Kuy S, Lee CJ, et al. Epidemiology of aortic aneurysm repair in the United States from 2000 to 2010. J Vasc Surg 2014;59(6):1512–7.
6. De Rango P, Farchioni L, Fiorucci B, et al. Diabetes and abdominal aortic aneurysms. Eur J Vasc Endovasc Surg 2014;47(3):243–61.
7. Pleumeekers HJ, Hoes AW, van der Does E, et al. Aneurysms of the abdominal aorta in older adults. The Rotterdam Study. Am J Epidemiol 1995;142(12): 1291–9.
8. Singh K, Bonaa KH, Jacobsen BK, et al. Prevalence of and risk factors for abdominal aortic aneurysms in a population-based study : the Tromso Study. Am J Epidemiol 2001;154(3):236–44.
9. Lederle FA, Johnson GR, Wilson SE, et al. Prevalence and associations of abdominal aortic aneurysm detected through screening. Aneurysm Detection

and Management (ADAM) Veterans Affairs Cooperative Study Group. Ann Intern Med 1997;126(6):441–9.

10. Go AS, Mozaffarian D, Roger VL, et al. Heart disease and stroke statistics–2013 update: a report from the American Heart Association. Circulation 2013;127(1): e6–245.

11. Carter JL, Morris DR, Sherliker P, et al. Sex-specific associations of vascular risk factors with abdominal aortic aneurysm: findings from 1.5 million women and 0.8 million men in the United States and United Kingdom. J Am Heart Assoc 2020; 9(4):e014748.

12. Wilmink TB, Quick CR, Day NE. The association between cigarette smoking and abdominal aortic aneurysms. J Vasc Surg 1999;30(6):1099–105.

13. Aune D, Schlesinger S, Norat T, et al. Tobacco smoking and the risk of abdominal aortic aneurysm: a systematic review and meta-analysis of prospective studies. Sci Rep 2018;8(1):14786.

14. Kent KC, Zwolak RM, Egorova NN, et al. Analysis of risk factors for abdominal aortic aneurysm in a cohort of more than 3 million individuals. J Vasc Surg 2010;52(3):539–48.

15. Larsson E, Granath F, Swedenborg J, et al. A population-based case-control study of the familial risk of abdominal aortic aneurysm. J Vasc Surg 2009;49(1): 47–50 [discussion: 1].

16. Diwan A, Sarkar R, Stanley JC, et al. Incidence of femoral and popliteal artery aneurysms in patients with abdominal aortic aneurysms. J Vasc Surg 2000;31(5): 863–9.

17. Powell JT, Sweeting MJ, Brown LC, et al. Systematic review and meta-analysis of growth rates of small abdominal aortic aneurysms. Br J Surg 2011;98(5):609–18.

18. Ashton HA, Buxton MJ, Day NE, et al. The Multicentre Aneurysm Screening Study (MASS) into the effect of abdominal aortic aneurysm screening on mortality in men: a randomised controlled trial. Lancet 2002;360(9345):1531–9.

19. Scott RA, Wilson NM, Ashton HA, et al. Influence of screening on the incidence of ruptured abdominal aortic aneurysm: 5-year results of a randomized controlled study. Br J Surg 1995;82(8):1066–70.

20. Lindholt JS, Juul S, Fasting H, et al. Screening for abdominal aortic aneurysms: single centre randomised controlled trial. BMJ 2005;330(7494):750.

21. Norman PE, Jamrozik K, Lawrence-Brown MM, et al. Population based randomised controlled trial on impact of screening on mortality from abdominal aortic aneurysm. BMJ 2004;329(7477):1259.

22. Glover MJ, KIm LG, Sweeting MJ, et al. Cost-effectiveness of the national health service abdominal aortic aneurysm screening programme in England. Br J Surg 2014;101(8):976–82.

23. Guirguis-Blake JM, Beil TL, Senger CA, et al. Ultrasonography screening for abdominal aortic aneurysms: a systematic evidence review for the U.S. Preventive Services Task Force. Ann Intern Med 2014;160(5):321–9.

24. Ali MU, Fitzpatrick-Lewis D, Miller J, et al. Screening for abdominal aortic aneurysm in asymptomatic adults. J Vasc Surg 2016;64(6):1855–68.

25. Force USPST, Owens DK, Davidson KW, Krist AH, et al. Screening for abdominal aortic aneurysm: US preventive services task force recommendation statement. JAMA 2019;322(22):2211–8.

26. Wanhainen A, Verzini F, Van Herzeele I, et al. Editor's Choice - European Society for Vascular Surgery (ESVS) 2019 clinical practice guidelines on the management of abdominal aorto-iliac artery aneurysms. Eur J Vasc Endovasc Surg 2019; 57(1):8–93.

27. Hirsch AT, Haskal ZJ, Hertzer NR, et al. ACC/AHA 2005 Practice Guidelines for the management of patients with peripheral arterial disease (lower extremity, renal, mesenteric, and abdominal aortic): a collaborative report from the American association for vascular surgery/society for vascular surgery, society for cardiovascular angiography and interventions, society for vascular medicine and biology, society of interventional radiology, and the ACC/AHA task force on practice guidelines (writing committee to develop guidelines for the management of patients with peripheral arterial disease): endorsed by the American association of cardiovascular and pulmonary rehabilitation; national heart, lung, and blood institute; society for vascular nursing; transatlantic inter-society consensus; and vascular disease foundation. Circulation 2006;113(11):e463–654.

28. Lim LS, Haq N, Mahmood S, et al, Committee APP, American College of Preventive M. Atherosclerotic cardiovascular disease screening in adults: American college of preventive medicine position statement on preventive practice. Am J Prev Med 2011;40(3):381 e1–e10.

29. Mastracci TM, Cina CS, Canadian Society for Vascular S. Screening for abdominal aortic aneurysm in Canada: review and position statement of the Canadian Society for Vascular Surgery. J Vasc Surg 2007;45(6):1268–76.

30. O'Donnell TFX, Landon BE, Schermerhorn ML. The case for expanding abdominal aortic aneurysm screening. J Vasc Surg 2020;71(5):1809–12.

31. Levin SR, Farber A, Goodney PP, et al. The U.S. preventive services task force abdominal aortic aneurysm screening guidelines negligibly impacted repair rates in male never-smokers and female smokers. Ann Vasc Surg 2022;82:87–95.

32. Duncan A, Maslen C, Gibson C, et al. Ultrasound screening for abdominal aortic aneurysm in high-risk women. Br J Surg 2021;108(10):1192–8.

33. Johansson G, Nydahl S, Olofsson P, et al. Survival in patients with abdominal aortic aneurysms. Comparison between operative and nonoperative management. Eur J Vasc Surg 1990;4(5):497–502.

34. Lederle FA, Johnson GR, Wilson SE, et al. Rupture rate of large abdominal aortic aneurysms in patients refusing or unfit for elective repair. JAMA 2002;287(22):2968–72.

35. Nevitt MP, Ballard DJ, Hallett JW Jr. Prognosis of abdominal aortic aneurysms. A population-based study. N Engl J Med 1989;321(15):1009–14.

36. Brady AR, Thompson SG, Fowkes FG, et al, Participants UKSAT. Abdominal aortic aneurysm expansion: risk factors and time intervals for surveillance. Circulation 2004;110(1):16–21.

37. Chaikof EL, Brewster DC, Dalman RL, et al. SVS practice guidelines for the care of patients with an abdominal aortic aneurysm: executive summary. J Vasc Surg 2009;50(4):880–96.

38. Mortality results for randomised controlled trial of early elective surgery or ultrasonographic surveillance for small abdominal aortic aneurysms. The UK Small Aneurysm Trial Participants. Lancet 1998;352(9141):1649–55.

39. Lederle FA, Johnson GR, Wilson SE, et al. The aneurysm detection and management study screening program: validation cohort and final results. Aneurysm detection and management veterans affairs cooperative study investigators. Arch Intern Med 2000;160(10):1425–30.

40. Cao P, De Rango P, Verzini F, et al. Comparison of surveillance versus aortic endografting for small aneurysm repair (CAESAR): results from a randomised trial. Eur J Vasc Endovasc Surg 2011;41(1):13–25.

41. Filardo G, Powell JT, Martinez MA, et al. Surgery for small asymptomatic abdominal aortic aneurysms. Cochrane Database Syst Rev 2015;(2):CD001835.

42. Balko A, Piasecki GJ, Shah DM, et al. Transfemoral placement of intraluminal polyurethane prosthesis for abdominal aortic aneurysm. J Surg Res 1986;40(4): 305–9.
43. Charnsangavej C, Wallace S, Wright KC, et al. Endovascular stent for use in aortic dissection: an in vitro experiment. Radiology 1985;157(2):323–4.
44. Wright KC, Wallace S, Charnsangavej C, et al. Percutaneous endovascular stents: an experimental evaluation. Radiology 1985;156(1):69–72.
45. Volodos NL, Karpovich IP, Shekhanin VE, et al. A case of distant transfemoral endoprosthesis of the thoracic artery using a self-fixing synthetic prosthesis in traumatic aneurysm. Grudn Khir 1988;(6):84–6.
46. Parodi JC, Palmaz JC, Barone HD. Transfemoral intraluminal graft implantation for abdominal aortic aneurysms. Ann Vasc Surg 1991;5(6):491–9.
47. Browne TF, Hartley D, Purchas S, et al. A fenestrated covered suprarenal aortic stent. Eur J Vasc Endovasc Surg 1999;18(5):445–9.
48. Anderson PL, Arons RR, Moskowitz AJ, et al. A statewide experience with endovascular abdominal aortic aneurysm repair: rapid diffusion with excellent early results. J Vasc Surg 2004;39(1):10–9.
49. Suckow BD, Goodney PP, Columbo JA, et al. National trends in open surgical, endovascular, and branched-fenestrated endovascular aortic aneurysm repair in Medicare patients. J Vasc Surg 2018;67(6):1690–1697 e1.
50. EVAR trial participants. Endovascular aneurysm repair versus open repair in patients with abdominal aortic aneurysm (EVAR trial 1): randomised controlled trial. Lancet 2005;365(9478):2179–86.
51. Prinssen M, Verhoeven EL, Buth J, et al. A randomized trial comparing conventional and endovascular repair of abdominal aortic aneurysms. N Engl J Med 2004;351(16):1607–18.
52. Lederle FA, Freischlag JA, Kyriakides TC, et al. Outcomes following endovascular vs open repair of abdominal aortic aneurysm: a randomized trial. JAMA 2009; 302(14):1535–42.
53. Becquemin JP, Pillet JC, Lescalie F, et al. A randomized controlled trial of endovascular aneurysm repair versus open surgery for abdominal aortic aneurysms in low- to moderate-risk patients. J Vasc Surg 2011;53(5):1167–11673 e1.
54. EVAR trial participants. Endovascular aneurysm repair and outcome in patients unfit for open repair of abdominal aortic aneurysm (EVAR trial 2): randomised controlled trial. Lancet 2005;365(9478):2187–92.
55. United Kingdom ETI, Greenhalgh RM, Brown LC, et al. Endovascular versus open repair of abdominal aortic aneurysm. N Engl J Med 2010;362(20):1863–71.
56. De Bruin JL, Baas AF, Buth J, et al. Long-term outcome of open or endovascular repair of abdominal aortic aneurysm. N Engl J Med 2010;362(20):1881–9.
57. van Schaik TG, Yeung KK, Verhagen HJ, et al. Long-term survival and secondary procedures after open or endovascular repair of abdominal aortic aneurysms. J Vasc Surg 2017;66(5):1379–89.
58. Lederle FA, Freischlag JA, Kyriakides TC, et al. Long-term comparison of endovascular and open repair of abdominal aortic aneurysm. N Engl J Med 2012; 367(21):1988–97.
59. Herman CR, Charbonneau P, Hongku K, et al. Any nonadherence to instructions for use predicts graft-related adverse events in patients undergoing elective endovascular aneurysm repair. J Vasc Surg 2018;67(1):126–33.
60. Abbruzzese TA, Kwolek CJ, Brewster DC, et al. Outcomes following endovascular abdominal aortic aneurysm repair (EVAR): an anatomic and device-specific analysis. J Vasc Surg 2008;48(1):19–28.

61. AbuRahma AF, Campbell J, Stone PA, et al. The correlation of aortic neck length to early and late outcomes in endovascular aneurysm repair patients. J Vasc Surg 2009;50(4):738–48.

62. Maurel B, Hertault A, Sobocinski J, et al. Techniques to reduce radiation and contrast volume during EVAR. J Cardiovasc Surg 2014;55(2 Suppl 1):123–31.

63. Oderich GS. Endovascular aortic repair: current techniques with fenestrated, Branched and parallel stent-grafts. 1e edition. Switzerland: Springer; 2017. p. 745.

64. Garg T, Baker LC, Mell MW. Adherence to postoperative surveillance guidelines after endovascular aortic aneurysm repair among Medicare beneficiaries. J Vasc Surg 2015;61(1):23–7.

65. Antoniou GA, Kontopodis N, Rogers SK, et al. Meta-analysis of compliance with endovascular aneurysm repair surveillance: The EVAR surveillance paradox. Eur J Vasc Endovasc Surg 2022;65(2):244–54.

66. Geraedts ACM, Mulay S, Vahl AC, et al. Editor's choice - post-operative surveillance and long term outcome after endovascular aortic aneurysm repair in patients with an initial post-operative computed tomography angiogram without abnormalities: the multicentre retrospective ODYSSEUS study. Eur J Vasc Endovasc Surg 2022;63(3):390–9.

67. Go MR, Barbato JE, Rhee RY, et al. What is the clinical utility of a 6-month computed tomography in the follow-up of endovascular aneurysm repair patients? J Vasc Surg 2008;47(6):1181–6 [discussion: 6-7].

68. Harky A, Zywicka E, Santoro G, et al. Is contrast-enhanced ultrasound (CEUS) superior to computed tomography angiography (CTA) in detection of endoleaks in post-EVAR patients? A systematic review and meta-analysis. J Ultrasound 2019;22(1):65–75.

69. Karaolanis GI, Antonopoulos CN, Georgakarakos E, et al. Colour duplex and/or contrast-enhanced ultrasound compared with computed tomography angiography for endoleak detection after endovascular abdominal aortic aneurysm repair: a systematic review and meta-analysis. J Clin Med 2022;11(13):3628.

70. Kassen T. Follow up CT angiography post EVAR: endoleaks detection, classification and manegement planning. Egypt J Radiol Nucl Med 2017;48(3):621–6.

71. Conrad MF, Adams AB, Guest JM, et al. Secondary intervention after endovascular abdominal aortic aneurysm repair. Ann Surg 2009;250(3):383–9.

72. Harris PL, Vallabhaneni SR, Desgranges P, et al. Incidence and risk factors of late rupture, conversion, and death after endovascular repair of infrarenal aortic aneurysms: the EUROSTAR experience. European Collaborators on Stent/graft techniques for aortic aneurysm repair. J Vasc Surg 2000;32(4):739–49.

73. Scali ST, Beck AW, Chang CK, et al. Defining risk and identifying predictors of mortality for open conversion after endovascular aortic aneurysm repair. J Vasc Surg 2016;63(4):873–881 e1.

74. Arthurs ZM, Lyden SP, Rajani RR, et al. Long-term outcomes of Palmaz stent placement for intraoperative type Ia endoleak during endovascular aneurysm repair. Ann Vasc Surg 2011;25(1):120–6.

75. Gelfand DV, White GH, Wilson SE. Clinical significance of type II endoleak after endovascular repair of abdominal aortic aneurysm. Ann Vasc Surg 2006;20(1):69–74.

76. Guo Q, Du X, Zhao J, et al. Prevalence and risk factors of type II endoleaks after endovascular aneurysm repair: a meta-analysis. PLoS One 2017;12(2):e0170600.

77. Sidloff DA, Stather PW, Choke E, et al. Type II endoleak after endovascular aneurysm repair. Br J Surg 2013;100(10):1262–70.

78. Maleux G, Poorteman L, Laenen A, et al. Incidence, etiology, and management of type III endoleak after endovascular aortic repair. J Vasc Surg 2017;66(4): 1056–64.

79. Hobo R, Buth J, collaborators E. Secondary interventions following endovascular abdominal aortic aneurysm repair using current endografts. A EUROSTAR report. J Vasc Surg 2006;43(5):896–902.

80. Reimerink JJ, van der Laan MJ, Koelemay MJ, et al. Systematic review and meta-analysis of population-based mortality from ruptured abdominal aortic aneurysm. Br J Surg 2013;100(11):1405–13.

81. Reitz KM, Phillips AR, Tzeng E, et al. Characterization of immediate and early mortality after repair of ruptured abdominal aortic aneurysm. J Vasc Surg 2022; 76(6):1578–87.e5.

82. Norman PE, Spilsbury K, Semmens JB. Falling rates of hospitalization and mortality from abdominal aortic aneurysms in Australia. J Vasc Surg 2011;53(2): 274–7.

83. Sandiford P, Mosquera D, Bramley D. Trends in incidence and mortality from abdominal aortic aneurysm in New Zealand. Br J Surg 2011;98(5):645–51.

84. Bartek MA, Kessler LG, Talbott JM, et al. Washington State abdominal aortic aneurysm-related mortality shows a steady decline between 1996 and 2016. J Vasc Surg 2019;70(4):1115–22.

85. Edwards ST, Schermerhorn ML, O'Malley AJ, et al. Comparative effectiveness of endovascular versus open repair of ruptured abdominal aortic aneurysm in the Medicare population. J Vasc Surg 2014;59(3):575–82.

86. Park BD, Azefor N, Huang CC, et al. Trends in treatment of ruptured abdominal aortic aneurysm: impact of endovascular repair and implications for future care. J Am Coll Surg 2013;216(4):745–54 [discussion: 54-5].

87. Reimerink JJ, Hoornweg LL, Vahl AC, et al. Endovascular repair versus open repair of ruptured abdominal aortic aneurysms: a multicenter randomized controlled trial. Ann Surg 2013;258(2):248–56.

88. Investigators IT, Powell JT, Sweeting MJ, et al. Endovascular or open repair strategy for ruptured abdominal aortic aneurysm: 30 day outcomes from IMPROVE randomised trial. BMJ 2014;348:f7661.

89. Desgranges P, Kobeiter H, Katsahian S, et al. Editor's Choice - ECAR (Endovasculaire ou Chirurgie dans les Anevrysmes aorto-iliaques Rompus): a French Randomized Controlled Trial of Endovascular Versus Open Surgical Repair of Ruptured Aorto-iliac Aneurysms. Eur J Vasc Endovasc Surg 2015;50(3):303–10.

90. Fleisher LA, Beckman JA, Brown KA, et al. 2009 ACCF/AHA focused update on perioperative beta blockade incorporated into the ACC/AHA 2007 guidelines on perioperative cardiovascular evaluation and care for noncardiac surgery: a report of the American college of cardiology foundation/American heart association task force on practice guidelines. Circulation 2009;120(21):e169–276.

91. Upchurch GR Jr, Proctor MC, Henke PK, et al. Predictors of severe morbidity and death after elective abdominal aortic aneurysmectomy in patients with chronic obstructive pulmonary disease. J Vasc Surg 2003;37(3):594–9.

92. Lee SM, Takemoto S, Wallace AW. Association between withholding angiotensin receptor blockers in the early postoperative period and 30-day mortality: a cohort study of the veterans affairs healthcare system. Anesthesiology 2015;123(2): 288–306.

93. Peterson L, Schweitzer G, Simone A, et al. The effect of smoking status on perioperative morbidity and mortality after open and endovascular abdominal aortic aneurysm repair. Ann Vasc Surg 2022;88:373–84.
94. Bradbury AW, Adam DJ, Makhdoomi KR, et al. A 21-year experience of abdominal aortic aneurysm operations in Edinburgh. Br J Surg 1998;85(5):645–7.
95. Heller JA, Weinberg A, Arons R, et al. Two decades of abdominal aortic aneurysm repair: have we made any progress? J Vasc Surg 2000;32(6):1091–100.
96. Hicks CW, Canner JK, Arhuidese I, et al. Comprehensive assessment of factors associated with in-hospital mortality after elective abdominal aortic aneurysm repair. JAMA Surg 2016;151(9):838–45.
97. Grant SW, Grayson AD, Mitchell DC, et al. Evaluation of five risk prediction models for elective abdominal aortic aneurysm repair using the UK National Vascular Database. Br J Surg 2012;99(5):673–9.
98. Hicks CW, Black JH 3rd, Arhuidese I, et al. Mortality variability after endovascular versus open abdominal aortic aneurysm repair in a large tertiary vascular center using a Medicare-derived risk prediction model. J Vasc Surg 2015;61(2):291–7.
99. Conrad MF, Crawford RS, Pedraza JD, et al. Long-term durability of open abdominal aortic aneurysm repair. J Vasc Surg 2007;46(4):669–75.

Thoracic Aortic Aneurysms and Arch Disease

Ryan Gedney, MD[a], Mathew Wooster, MD, MBA[b],*

KEYWORDS

- Aorta • TEVAR • Aortic arch • Aortic dissection • Aneurysm • Arch branch

KEY POINTS

- Thoracic aortic and aortic arch disease involves a spectrum of pathology, including primarily aneurysm and acute aortic syndrome, the pathogenesis of which is multifactorial.
- Other than medical based risk factor modification, medical based therapies for thoracic aneurysm have not proven to be successful at preventing growth.
- Medical management of acute aortic syndrome, on the other hand, involving goal directed antiimpulse therapy, is classically recommended.
- Surgical management of thoracic aortic pathology has historically been performed from an open approach, but given recent technological advancements in endovascular surgery and research in the space, endovascular approaches are increasingling showing success.

INTRODUCTION

The aorta is the largest artery in the body, with the thoracic component extending from the annulus to the diaphragmatic hiatus.[1] Various disease processes occur in the thoracic component of the aorta, most commonly thoracic aortic aneurysms, in addition to pseudoaneurysm, dissection, intramural hematoma, trauma, and infection. Thoracic aortic disease as a whole has been increasing in prevalence in reported literature since the 1980s, with an increase in incidence of 52% in men and 28% in women between 1987 and 2002. In general, thoracic aortic disease is more common in men.[2]

Thoracic aortic aneurysms are defined as dilation in the diameter of the blood vessel to 50% larger than the normal size (**Fig. 1**).[3] Most of the thoracic aortic aneurysms involve the aortic root and ascending thoracic aorta (60%), whereas roughly 40% involve the descending thoracic aorta.[4] Thoracic aortic aneurysms can involve the aortic arch as well, but the incidence is relatively low.[3] In a population-based study done in the 1980s, the incidence of thoracic aortic aneurysms was roughly 5.9 cases per 100,000 persons per year.[5] Since that time, the incidence of thoracic aneurysm

[a] Medical University of South Carolina, 30 Courtenay Drive, MSC 25, STE 654, Charleston, SC 29924, USA; [b] Division of Vascular Surgery, Medical University of South Carolina, 30 Courtenay Drive, MSC 25, Suite 654, Charleston, SC 29924, USA
* Corresponding author.
E-mail address: woosterm@musc.edu

Surg Clin N Am 103 (2023) 615–627
https://doi.org/10.1016/j.suc.2023.04.013
0039-6109/23/© 2023 Elsevier Inc. All rights reserved.

surgical.theclinics.com

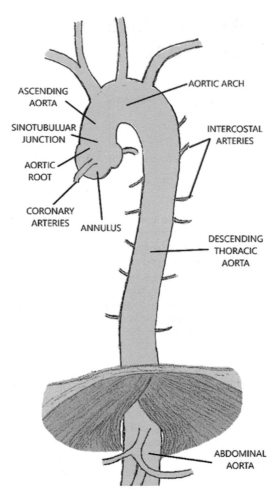

Fig. 1. Thoracic aortic anatomy.

has increased significantly with recent reported numbers as high as 10.4 cases per 100,000 persons per year in the United States.[6]

Acute aortic syndromes are a spectrum of disease involving intimal tears of the aorta and progressing to dissection, intramural hematoma, or penetrating aortic ulcer. Patients presenting on the spectrum of acute aortic syndrome occur with an incidence of 2.6 to 3.5 cases per 100,000 persons per year, with most patients (70%–80%) presenting with acute aortic dissection.[7] Type A acute aortic dissection involves the ascending thoracic aorta and is more common than other acute dissections, occurring in roughly 53% of cases, and has elevated associated mortality. Type B acute aortic dissection is less common, occurring in about 46% of cases, and involves the descending thoracic aorta.[8] Intramural hematoma accounts for 5% to 25% of these acute aortic syndrome cases, and penetrating aortic ulcer makes up 2% to 7% of cases.[9] Roughly half of patients presenting with acute aortic syndrome have a concurrent aortic aneurysm as well.[10]

Anatomically, thoracic aneurysms can be categorized as ascending, arch, descending, or thoracoabdominal aneurysms. Thoracoabdominal aneurysms are further

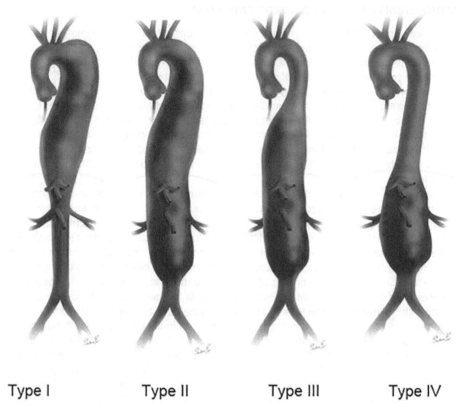

Type I   Type II   Type III   Type IV

Fig. 2. Crawford TAAA classification.

classified by the extent of the aneurysm based on the Crawford type, originally described by Crawford and colleagues in 1986 in the Journal of Vascular Surgery (**Fig. 2**).[11]

Further describing thoracic aneurysms by cause is important to understanding each patient's individual disease process, as well as clinical management. Aneurysms can be degenerative and related to chronic atherosclerosis and elastic breakdown or related to chronic dissection, infections, inflammation, or connective tissue disorder.[11]

Aortic dissection has historically been associated with separate classification systems than aneurysm, but the focus is similar in describing both the location and extent of the dissection. The Debakey classification groups aortic dissection based on location of intimal injury and how far the dissection flap extended longitudinally down the aorta. The Stanford classification simplified the Debakey system into 2 groups based on whether or not the ascending aorta is involved but did not describe how far the dissection extends; this was the predominant classification system until 2020, when the SVS/STS Aortic Dissection Classification system was published, focusing on aortic zones of involvement.[12] As endovascular treatment methods have increased, requiring landing zone and coverage considerations, there was a need for more specific description of the anatomic involvement of dissection. This system describes the location of the dissection entry tear as either type A or type B and then involves a subtext descriptor that further describes the distal extent and proximal extent.[12]

PATHOGENESIS OF THORACIC AORTIC ANEURYSM

The development of thoracic aortic aneurysm has been linked to multiple risk factors, including risk factors of vascular inflammation, chronic dissection, bicuspid aortic valve, family history, and connective tissue disorders. All of these risk factors contribute to the pathogenesis of aneurysm in different ways.[13]

Aneurysms of the descending aorta are more likely to have developed from chronic atherosclerotic degeneration, whereas more proximal aneurysms are due to breakdown of the elastic media. Ascending aortic vascular smooth muscle cells (VSMCs) arise from neural crest cells embryonically, and descending aortic VSMCs arise from mesoderm. The different origins of the cells that make up each part of the thoracic aorta contribute to variability in cell signaling and the cellular response to insult in each region.[14,15]

Biochemical and mechanical factors contribute to the pathogenesis of thoracic aortic aneurysm. The cause of each individual aneurysm accounts for different inciting events to the aortic wall, but once the stage has been set, the general pathway of aneurysm development is similar. Matrix metalloproteinase and other extracellular matrix inflammatory and degenerative signaling molecules are triggered in these settings, leading to a discrepancy between key components of the structural support of the aortic wall. These discrepancies cause weakness in the aortic wall and subsequent expansion of the diameter of the vessel.[3,16] This process is called cystic medial degeneration, leading to the loss of smooth muscle cells and elastic fibers.

In the case of mycotic aneurysm, there may be an initial vascular insult, but the ultimate pathophysiologic cause is bacterial seeding of the arterial wall. Blood cultures are positive in up to 85% of cases. Initial bacterial seeding is thought to involve the intima first at a location of injury and then progress to medial infection; this produces an inflammatory environment that attracts cells and matrix degenerative signalers that result in extracellular matrix breakdown and vessel wall weakness, leading to aneurysm.[17] The most common organisms involved in mycotic aneurysm are *Staphylococcus aureus* and *Salmonella*.[18]

PATIENT EVALUATION FOR THORACIC AORTIC ANEURYSM

Most thoracic aneurysms are discovered incidentally, often when a computed tomography (CT) scan is obtained for another medical or surgical reason. Patients can develop chest pain, difficulty breathing or swallowing, and hoarseness from compression of the recurrent laryngeal nerve.[3] A diastolic murmur noticed on physical examination, sometimes associated with a widened pulse pressure, can be a sign of aortic root aneurysm.[19]

Cross-sectional imaging is the most effective form of imaging in diagnosing thoracic aortic aneurysm, with electrocardiographically gated CT angiography (CTA) reaching nearly 100% sensitivity and specificity. Magnetic resonance angiography (MRA) can also be effective, but issues with blood flow artifact, the need for spin echo sequencing in order to perform the most specific evaluation, and the need for black and bright blood imaging protocols make CTA more desirable.[20] The Society for Vascular Surgery recommends using thin-cut CTA, with slices less than 0.25 mm, of the entire aorta, including bilateral iliofemoral vessels for diagnosis and interventional planning.[21]

Four-dimensional (4D) MRA may offer some unique insights into the evaluation of thoracic aortic aneurysm, although not standard of care currently. Wall shear stress assessment with 4D MRI has demonstrated a direct relationship with elastic fiber degeneration of the ascending aorta in bicuspid aortic valve patients, which suggests that patients who exhibit increased wall shear stress in 4D MRI may be at elevated risk of developing aortic pathology.[22]

In an elective setting, surgical repair is indicated for ascending aortic aneurysm sized greater than 5.5 cm or descending aortic aneurysm sized greater than 6 cm, although these size criteria are often modified for surgery at smaller diameters in patients with elevated risk syndromes including Marfan syndrome and Loeys Dietz syndrome.[16] Patients with a 6-cm thoracic aortic aneurysm have a roughly 3.7% risk of rupture per year, with a 5-year survival of 54%.[21] The Society for Vascular Surgery currently recommends TEVAR as first-line treatment of thoracic aortic aneurysms that meet surgical criteria.[21] It is recommended with class II evidence that patients with Marfan syndrome undergo prophylactic ascending aorta replacement when the ascending aortic to patient height ratio exceeds 10.[16]

PATIENT EVALUATION FOR ACUTE AORTIC SYNDROME

Acute aortic syndrome classically presents as an intense, sudden onset chest pain, although nearly 5% of patients present atypically with no pain.[9] Hypertension is the inciting event in 70% of cases.[23] Patients with type A dissection will more often associate their pain with an anterior distribution, where type B dissection patients complain of deeper back and abdominal pain.[24] Patients with type A dissection will present with syncope 12.7% of the time.[24]

Critical to the evaluation of patients with acute aortic syndromes is consideration of malperfusion syndromes, which are the result of obstruction of flow to aortic branch vessels due to intimal flap or false lumen propagation. In patients with a malperfusion syndrome secondary to aortic dissection, 70% of the time extremity malperfusion is involved and is often concomitant with other malperfusion syndromes; these present with acute limb ischemia of the affected extremity. In thoracic dissection, a difference in brachial blood pressure between arms is a clear indicator of subclavian artery involvement. Identifying limb ischemia is a strong predictor that other forms of malperfusion are present as well.[23] Limb ischemia as a malperfusion syndrome of aortic dissection is associated with higher rates of in-hospital mortality. Suzuki and colleagues demonstrated a 17.5% in-hospital mortality in patients from the International Registry of Acute Aortic Dissection (IRAD) registry that presented with limb ischemia.[25] Stroke secondary to malperfusion of the great vessels happens at a rate of 0.3% to 10% and occurs more frequently in type A dissection.[24]

The most devastating malperfusion syndrome in type B dissection is mesenteric ischemia, with a mortality of 30% associated with presentation. Laboratory evaluation of these patients will demonstrate a metabolic acidosis, increasing lactate, electrolyte derangement, elevated white blood cell count, or elevated creatinine.[23] The kidneys are the most common organ involved in dissection-related malperfusion syndromes; this presents as acute kidney injury, and elucidating that the acute kidney injury is directly related to renal malperfusion can be challenging. Imaging will suggest malperfusion, and often kidneys will demonstrate asymmetric enhancement on contrasted imaging, but the positive predictive value of renal malperfusion with CTA is only 70%.[23] Patients who have associated kidney malperfusion will end up on temporary hemodialysis 28.1% of the time and permanent hemodialysis roughly 2% of the time.[26]

Recognize that obstruction of flow to branch vessels can occur in a static or dynamic manner. Dynamic obstruction occurs far more often, nearly 80% of the time,[27] and is due to changes in where the intimal flap lies relative to branch arteries due to pulse propagation. Static obstruction occurs due to branches involving a thrombosed false lumen.[23]

When acute aortic syndrome is suspected, chest radiograph demonstrating widening of the mediastinum, prominent aortic notch, tracheal shift, or double density of the aortic shadow has a 64% sensitivity and 86% specificity in diagnosis.[28] However, CT is the most specific in identifying true and false lumen, reaching 95% sensitivity and 100% specificity.[29] It is important to keep in mind that CT imaging, although the gold standard in diagnosis of acute aortic syndrome, will not have the same sensitivity and specificity in identifying dynamic obstruction as it does in diagnosing dissection.

Urgent open surgery is indicated in patients with acute type A dissection, unless the patients is not medically appropriate for surgery. IRAD registry data demonstrated decreased rates of surgical success of repairing type A dissection when the patient is older than 70 years; has a history of end-stage renal disease (ESRD), myocardial infarction (MI), or prior aortic valve replacement; abnormal electrocardiography; associated hemorrhagic stroke; hyperacute presentation; associated acute cardiac failure or tamponade; or associated malperfusion syndromes.[24]

In patients with type B dissection, surgical repair, most often endovascular surgical repair, has classically not been indicated unless the patient presents with complicated type B dissection. Complicated dissection accounts for roughly 25% of acute type B thoracic aortic dissections and are defined as dissection associated with a malperfusion syndrome, evidence of dissection progression on follow-up imaging, pain that does not subside, or uncontrolled severe hypertension.[30]

MEDICAL MANAGEMENT OF THORACIC ANEURYSM

Chronic thoracic aortic disease is directly related to clinical risk factors that are often modifiable. Medical management, particularly in aneurysmal disease of the thoracic aorta, is focused on these modifiable risk factors, much like the treatment of chronic vascular disease elsewhere in the human body.

Smoking is the greatest associated with thoracic aortic aneurysm, and therefore, smoking cessation counseling should be the top priority.[31] Other risk factor modification that is pertinent not only for thoracic aortic disease, but all vascular disease, is "best medical therapy" for cardiovascular disease, including aspirin as an antiplatelet agent, a statin medication for oxidative stress reduction and plaque stabilization, and life-style modifications including smoking cessation, exercise, healthy diet, and control of blood pressure.[3]

The renin-angiotensin-aldosterone pathway is thought to relate to vascular inflammation, most directly with the proinflammatory cellular and extracellular matrix effects of angiotensin II. Although angiotensin-converting enzyme inhibitors and angiotensin receptor blockers (ARBs) have demonstrated some effects in animal models at reducing aneurysm progression, this has not been sustained in prospective treatment in humans. Interestingly, however, both β-blockers and ARBs have demonstrated slowing of aneurysm growth in humans.[13,32]

Because of the known inhibition of matrix metalloproteinase by tetracyclines, the drug class has been extensively studied in thoracic aortic aneurysm literature, including animal models, as well as a randomized control trial done between 2013 and 2017 that measured doxycycline effects on aneurysm size over 2 years. Results thus far have demonstrated no effect on aneurysm growth.[33]

Fluoroquinolones are contraindicated in patients with thoracic aortic aneurysm. They are thought to increase aortic wall degeneration. A meta-analysis done in 2019 showed fluoroquinolones more than doubles the risk of both dissection and rupture in patients with thoracic aortic aneurysm.[34]

In patients being medically managed for thoracic aortic aneurysm not yet indicated for surgery, it is recommended that reimaging be performed at 6 months after diagnosis of thoracic aortic aneurysm and then annually thereafter in order to monitor the progression of aneurysm appropriately.[3]

MEDICAL MANAGEMENT OF ACUTE AORTIC SYNDROME

In uncomplicated acute aortic type B dissection, it is classically recommended that patients not undergo surgical intervention initially, although recent studies have shown a positive effect of early TEVAR on long-term aortic remodeling and prevention of aortic degeneration.[35] In type B aortic dissection, in-hospital mortality is around 8.8% with goal-directed antiimpulse medical therapy.[36]

Goal-directed antiimpulse medical therapy seeks to decrease the high impulse, or high change in pressure over a very short time frame, that the aortic wall experiences with hypertension and tachycardia. Therapy involves the use of intravenous β-blockade, calcium channel blockade, and sometimes nitroglycerin and sodium nitroprusside in order to reduce the systolic blood pressure to less than 120 mm Hg and the heart rate to less than 80 beats per minute.[37]

SURGERY OF THE THORACIC AORTA

Surgical exposure of the thoracic aorta depends on its location, with median sternotomy being the typical preference for exposure of the ascending and transverse arch, and the descending thoracic aorta is most readily visualized from a posterolateral approach. Aortic arch reconstruction may be performed with complete replacement using multiple branches, island reimplantation, or debranching from more proximal aorta followed by endovascular exclusion.[38] Advanced endovascular repair of the arch has been more frequently described recently but will be excluded from this article, as it is presented elsewhere in this volume.[21,39–47] Decision for type of surgical repair is driven by a multitude of factors including extent of disease, health of ascending aorta, patient body habitus, cardiopulmonary reserve, and surgeon experience. Total arch replacement is the most complex repair, with requirement of total cardiopulmonary bypass and hypothermic arrest with targeted cerebral perfusion. Ascending debranching, although more straightforward, requires a healthy ascending aortic segment from which to debranch but avoids the need for hypothermic arrest. Generally, these procedures carry significant risk with an overall operative mortality up to 15% and complication rate of roughly 3%, including bleeding, stroke, and MI.[38,48]

As disease extends more distally down the thoracic aorta, often multistage procedures must be used to treat the entirety of the aortic condition. Conventionally, the elephant trunk technique used during arch repair involves extending an intraluminal portion of prosthetic graft with a free-floating distal end terminating in the descending thoracic aorta, no more than 7 to 8 cm distally from the arch repair; this offers either a landing zone for descending thoracic TEVAR placement or an adequate proximal anastomosis site for future open descending aortic repair. The elephant trunk technique can also be used in conjunction with descending TEVAR in an antegrade fashion during the index operation, which is often termed the frozen elephant technique (**Fig. 3**).[39]

Isolated descending thoracic aortic pathology is most frequently treated via endovascular approach, as this has been shown to be associated with lower morbidity and mortality as well as significantly faster recovery.[30] Despite these improvements, TEVAR does carry significant risks of spinal cord ischemia, stroke, endoleaks,

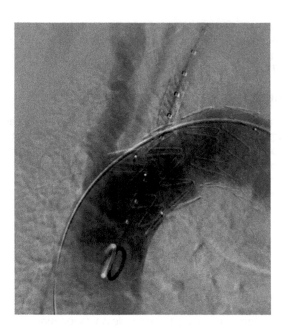

Fig. 3. TEVAR

vascular access complications, and graft failure. Reported rates of spinal cord ischemia range from 2% to 10%, and the risks factors that increase the incidence of spinal cord injury mainly includes the extent of aneurysm requiring endograft coverage, but other risk factors include perioperative hypotension, advanced age, ESRD, chronic obstructive pulmonary disease, and hypertension. Coverage of the left subclavian artery or hypogastric arteries due to the extent of the aneurysm carries significant risk of spinal cord ischemia due to obstructed flow to collateral networks of spinal cord blood supply.[40] Spinal cord ischemia protection modalities include maintaining mean arterial perfusion pressure greater than 80 mm Hg, hemoglobin levels greater than 10 mg/dL, and oxygen saturation levels of 100%.[49] Stroke rates range from 1.2% to 8.2% and are largely due to wire manipulation in the aortic arch. Patients with heavy atherosclerotic disease in the aortic arch should undergo careful consideration before introducing wires for TEVAR, as this elevates the risk of stroke significantly.[40] Endoleak rates range from 5% to 10% in reported TEVAR literature.[40] With access complication rates up to 4.7%, care must be taken to evaluate the iliofemoral segment.[40] Special care should be taken when iliac vessels are particularly tortuous or calcified or when femoral access vessels are small, aneurysmal, or calcified. In reported literature, 15% of the time a common iliac conduit is required for appropriate access.

It is recommended to plan for elective TEVAR with centerline imaging software analysis using CTA with less than 1 mm slice thickness (**Fig. 4**).[21] Imaging should demonstrate at least a 2 cm healthy aortic segment proximally and distally as landing zones for the endovascular device. The device diameter should use a roughly 10% to 20% oversizing for aneurysm pathology and 0% to 10% for dissections. Landing zone inner wall aortic diameter should be no larger than 42 mm and no smaller than 16 mm based on commercially available device sizes.[40] Other considerations in planning for TEVAR involve vascular access and proximal extent requiring coverage of great vessels, as up to 40% of thoracic pathology involves the aortic arch.[50]

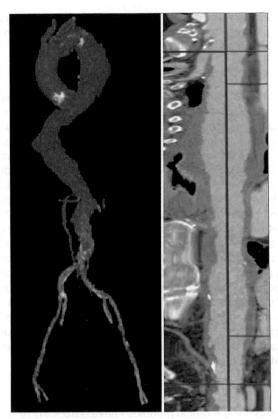

Fig. 4. Centerline imaging for TEVAR planning.

Although the literature remains controversial, Zone 2 aortic aneurysms or aortic dissection that involves the region around the left subclavian artery require revascularization of the left subclavian artery.[51] The rates of stroke have been reported to be elevated in patients undergoing elective TEVAR without left subclavian artery revascularization. Of note, coverage of the left subclavian artery is contraindicated in patients with coronary artery bypass using the left internal mammary artery, patients with a dominant left vertebral artery, or patients with working left arm dialysis access. In the emergent setting, and if no contraindication exists, coverage of the left subclavian artery in order to obtain appropriate seal is appropriate with interval revascularization.[52] Although open surgical carotid-subclavian artery bypass has been the standard of care in left subclavian artery revascularization, an investigational device study comparing branched endoprosthesis for left subclavian revascularization with open revascularization did not show any differences in upper extremity ischemic events, stroke, or reinterventions.[52] These branching endoprostheses have demonstrated technical success and safety with several different devices, including the Medtronic Mona Lisa device, Gore TAG thoracic branch device, Terumo arch branch device, the Nexus endograft, and Cook custom-made devices, although there remains the need for long-term data.[43–45]

In infected aneurysms, TEVAR should only be used as a temporizing measure. Some studies have reported good results with antibiotic pretreated endografts, but this is not standard practice. TEVAR for symptomatic or ruptured infected aneurysm should only be considered as a life-saving treatment in order to bridge to definitive repair.[21] In these patients, consideration must be taken to maintain perfusion of the great vessels branching off the aortic arch.

POSTOPERATIVE SURVEILLANCE

Long-term surveillance of patients after thoracic aortic intervention is critical to monitoring for long-term complications that would require further intervention. Following open surgical repair of the ascending aorta, with or without reconstruction of the aortic valve, the Society of Thoracic Surgery recommends regular contrasted imaging and echocardiographic surveillance every 6 months for the first year postoperatively and then annually for life thereafter.[53] In patients who have received endovascular repair, serial imaging for surveillance can identify endoleaks, stent migration, or failure. Therefore, postoperatively patients should be reimaged with cross-sectional imaging at 1 month, 12 months, and yearly thereafter based on Society for Vascular Surgery guidelines. Patients should undergo more frequent imaging if an abnormality is noted on follow-up imaging.[21] Late complications of thoracic aortic surgery occurring greater than 1 year postoperatively that can be identified with appropriate surveillance include endoleak (3.9%), device migration (2.8%), device failure, including fracture or barb separation (<1%), or loss of patency, including kinking or compression (1.6%).[54] Further aneurysmal degeneration at the proximal and distal ends of the graft can occur, as well as anastamotic pseudoaneurysm in the case of open repair, with reported rates ranging from 0.5% to 13%.[55] If used to treat dissection, stent-induced new entry tear can occur during follow-up roughly 3.4% of the time and is a life-threatening condition with an associated 26.1% mortality.[56]

SUMMARY

Aortic arch and descending thoracic pathology have historically remained in the realm of open surgical repair. Technology is quickly pushing to bring these under the endovascular umbrella, with lower morbidity repairs proving safe in their early experience. Much work remains particularly for acute aortic syndromes, however, to understand who is best treated medically, surgically, endovascularly, or with hybrid approaches.

CLINICS CARE POINTS

- Acute aortic syndrome occurs at a rate of 2.6-3.5 cases per 100,000 persons per year with >70% presenting as aortic dissection.

- IMH, PAH, and aortic dissection all represent one spectrum of disease with varied degree of separation of layers of the wall of the aorta.

- All acute aortic syndromes should initially be treated with impulse control. Surgical management follows electively, urgently, or emergently dependent upon location and complicating factors.

- TEVAR is broadly first line therapy for acute aortic pathology distal to the left carotid artery.

DISCLOSURE

R. Gedney: no disclosures. M. Wooster: receives research support from Shockwave Medical. Is on Speakers Bureau for Cook, Gore, Medtronic, Shockwave, and Penumbra.

REFERENCES

1. Bolen MA, Abbara S. Chapter 16 - Aortic disease. In: Taylor AJ, editor. Atlas of cardiovascular computed tomography. Imaging techniques to braunwald's heart disease. Philadelphia, PA: W.B. Saunders; 2010. p. 188–203. https://doi.org/10.1016/B978-1-4160-6136-6.00016-6.
2. Olsson C, Thelin S, Ståhle E, et al. Thoracic Aortic Aneurysm and Dissection. Circulation 2006;114(24):2611–8.
3. Faiza Z, Sharman T. Thoracic Aorta Aneurysm. In: StatPearls. StatPearls Publishing; 2022. Available at: http://www.ncbi.nlm.nih.gov/books/NBK554567/. Accessed September 8, 2022.
4. Isselbacher EM. Thoracic and Abdominal Aortic Aneurysms. Circulation 2005; 111(6):816–28.
5. Bickerstaff LK, Pairolero PC, Hollier LH, et al. Thoracic aortic aneurysms: a population-based study. Surgery 1982;92(6):1103–8.
6. Ellahi A, Shaikh FN, Kashif H, et al. Effectiveness of endovascular repair versus open surgery for the treatment of thoracoabdominal aneurysm: A systematic review and meta analysis. Ann Med Surg 2022;81:104477.
7. Tsai TT, Nienaber CA, Eagle KA. Acute Aortic Syndromes. Circulation 2005; 112(24):3802–13.
8. Appelbaum A, Karp RB, Kirklin JW. Ascending vs descending aortic dissections. Ann Surg 1976;183(3):296–300.
9. Vignaraja V, Thapar A, Dindyal S. Acute Aortic Syndrome. In: StatPearls. StatPearls Publishing; 2022. Available at: http://www.ncbi.nlm.nih.gov/books/NBK576402/. Accessed September 8, 2022.
10. Bossone E, Eagle KA. Epidemiology and management of aortic disease: aortic aneurysms and acute aortic syndromes. Nat Rev Cardiol 2021;18(5):331–48.
11. Fillinger MF, Greenberg RK, McKinsey JF, et al. Society for Vascular Surgery Ad Hoc Committee on TEVAR Reporting Standards. Reporting standards for thoracic endovascular aortic repair (TEVAR). J Vasc Surg 2010;52(4):1022–33, 1033.e15.
12. Lombardi JV, Hughes GC, Appoo JJ, et al. Society for Vascular Surgery (SVS) and Society of Thoracic Surgeons (STS) reporting standards for type B aortic dissections. J Vasc Surg 2020;71(3):723–47.
13. Danyi P, Elefteriades JA, Jovin IS. Medical therapy of thoracic aortic aneurysms. Trends Cardiovasc Med 2012;22(7):180–4.
14. Elefteriades JA, Farkas EA. Thoracic aortic aneurysm clinically pertinent controversies and uncertainties. J Am Coll Cardiol 2010;55(9):841–57.
15. Saeyeldin AA, Velasquez CA, Mahmood SUB, et al. Thoracic aortic aneurysm: unlocking the "silent killer" secrets. Gen Thorac Cardiovasc Surg 2019; 67(1):1–11.
16. Booher AM, Eagle KA. Diagnosis and management issues in thoracic aortic aneurysm. Am Heart J 2011;162(1):38–46.e1.
17. McCready RA, Bryant MA, Divelbiss JL, et al. Arterial infections in the new millennium: an old problem revisited. Ann Vasc Surg 2006;20(5):590–5.
18. Majeed H, Ahmad F. Mycotic Aneurysm. In: StatPearls. StatPearls Publishing; 2022. Available at: http://www.ncbi.nlm.nih.gov/books/NBK560736/. Accessed September 9, 2022.
19. Kuzmik GA, Sang AX, Elefteriades JA. Natural history of thoracic aortic aneurysms. J Vasc Surg 2012;56(2):565–71.
20. Bhave NM, Nienaber CA, Clough RE, et al. Multimodality Imaging of Thoracic Aortic Diseases in Adults. JACC Cardiovasc Imaging 2018;11(6):902–19.

21. Upchurch GR, Escobar GA, Azizzadeh A, et al. Society for Vascular Surgery clinical practice guidelines of thoracic endovascular aortic repair for descending thoracic aortic aneurysms. J Vasc Surg 2021;73(1):55S–83S.
22. Guzzardi DG, Barker AJ, van Ooij P, et al. Valve-Related Hemodynamics Mediate Human Bicuspid Aortopathy: Insights From Wall Shear Stress Mapping. J Am Coll Cardiol 2015;66(8):892–900.
23. Crawford TC, Beaulieu RJ, Ehlert BA, et al. Malperfusion Syndromes in Aortic Dissection. Vasc Med Lond Engl 2016;21(3):264–73.
24. Hagan PG, Nienaber CA, Isselbacher EM, et al. The International Registry of Acute Aortic Dissection (IRAD)New Insights Into an Old Disease. JAMA 2000; 283(7):897–903.
25. Suzuki T, Mehta RH, Ince H, et al. Clinical profiles and outcomes of acute type B aortic dissection in the current era: lessons from the International Registry of Aortic Dissection (IRAD). Circulation 2003;108(Suppl 1):II312–7.
26. Nishigawa K, Fukui T, Uemura K, et al. Preoperative renal malperfusion is an independent predictor for acute kidney injury and operative death but not associated with late mortality after surgery for acute type A aortic dissection. Eur J Cardio Thorac Surg 2020;58(2):302–8.
27. Williams DM, Lee DY, Hamilton BH, et al. The dissected aorta: percutaneous treatment of ischemic complications–principles and results. J Vasc Interv Radiol 1997;8(4):605–25.
28. Kodolitsch Y von, Nienaber CA, Dieckmann C, et al. Chest radiography for the diagnosis of acute aortic syndrome. Am J Med 2004;116(2):73–7.
29. Sommer T, Fehske W, Holzknecht N, et al. Aortic dissection: a comparative study of diagnosis with spiral CT, multiplanar transesophageal echocardiography, and MR imaging. Radiology 1996;199(2):347–52.
30. Moulakakis KG, Mylonas SN, Dalainas I, et al. Management of complicated and uncomplicated acute type B dissection. A systematic review and meta-analysis. Ann Cardiothorac Surg 2014;3(3):234–46.
31. Bonser RS, Pagano D, Lewis ME, et al. Clinical and patho-anatomical factors affecting expansion of thoracic aortic aneurysms. Heart 2000;84(3):277–83.
32. Brooke BS, Habashi JP, Judge DP, et al. Angiotensin II blockade and aortic-root dilation in Marfan's syndrome. N Engl J Med 2008;358(26):2787–95.
33. Baxter BT, Matsumura J, Curci JA, et al. Effect of Doxycycline on Aneurysm Growth Among Patients With Small Infrarenal Abdominal Aortic Aneurysms. JAMA 2020;323(20):2029–38.
34. Rawla P, El Helou ML, Vellipuram AR. Fluoroquinolones and the Risk of Aortic Aneurysm or Aortic Dissection: A Systematic Review and Meta-Analysis. Cardiovasc Hematol Agents Med Chem 2019;17(1):3–10.
35. Tadros RO, Tang GHL, Barnes HJ, et al. Optimal Treatment of Uncomplicated Type B Aortic Dissection: JACC Review Topic of the Week. J Am Coll Cardiol 2019;74(11):1494–504.
36. Harrington PB, Davies JE, Melby SJ. Diagnosis and clinical management of aortic dissection. Res Rep Clin Cardiol 2014;5:123–32.
37. Estrera AL, Miller CC, Safi HJ, et al. Outcomes of Medical Management of Acute Type B Aortic Dissection. Circulation 2006;114(1_supplement):I–384.
38. Alonso Pérez M, Llaneza Coto JM, del Castro Madrazo JA, et al. Debranching aortic surgery. J Thorac Dis 2017;9(Suppl 6):S465–77.
39. De Paulis R, Di Bartolomeo R, Murana G, et al. Frozen versus conventional elephant trunk technique: application in clinical practice. Eur J Cardio Thorac Surg 2017;51(suppl_1):i20–8.

40. Chen SW, Lee KB, Napolitano MA, et al. Complications and Management of the Thoracic Endovascular Aortic Repair. AORTA J 2020;8(3):49–58.
41. Marcos FÁ. Access Related Complications in TEVAR: The Roads to Success Are Rougher for Women. Eur J Vasc Endovasc Surg 2020;60(2):210.
42. Fairman AS, Beck AW, Malas MB, et al. Reinterventions in the modern era of thoracic endovascular aortic repair. J Vasc Surg 2020;71(2):408–22.
43. Ibrahim M, Lindsay TF, Chung JCY, et al. Endovascular arch repair using the NEXUS arch endograft. Ann Cardiothorac Surg 2022;11(1):62.
44. Ee R, Fr A, Mm T. Results of the Valiant Mona LSA early feasibility study for descending thoracic aneurysms. J Vasc Surg 2015;62(6).
45. Dake MD, Fischbein MP, Bavaria JE, et al. Evaluation of the Gore TAG thoracic branch endoprosthesis in the treatment of proximal descending thoracic aortic aneurysms. J Vasc Surg 2021;74(5). https://doi.org/10.1016/j.jvs.2021.04.025.
46. Tsilimparis N, Detter C, Law Y, et al. Single-center experience with an inner branched arch endograft. J Vasc Surg 2019;69(4):977–85.e1.
47. Voskresensky I, Scali S, Feezor RJ, et al. Outcomes of Thoracic Endovascular Aortic Repair Using Aortic Arch Chimney Stents in High Risk Patients. J Vasc Surg 2017;66(1):9.
48. Cohn LH, Rizzo RJ, Adams DH, et al. Reduced mortality and morbidity for ascending aortic aneurysm resection regardless of cause. Ann Thorac Surg 1996;62(2):463–8.
49. Aucoin VJ, Eagleton MJ, Farber MA, et al. Spinal cord protection practices used during endovascular repair of complex aortic aneurysms by the U.S. Aortic Research Consortium. J Vasc Surg 2021;73(1):323–30.
50. D D, Ts M. Left subclavian artery coverage during TEVAR: is revascularization necessary? J Cardiovasc Surg (Torino). 2012;53(2). Available at: https://pubmed.ncbi.nlm.nih.gov/22456634/. Accessed September 15, 2022.
51. Matsumura JS, Rizvi AZ. Left subclavian artery revascularization: Society for Vascular Surgery® Practice Guidelines. J Vasc Surg 2010;52(4):65S–70S.
52. Squiers JJ, DiMaio JM, Schaffer JM, et al. Surgical debranching versus branched endografting in zone 2 thoracic endovascular aortic repair. J Vasc Surg 2022;75(6). https://doi.org/10.1016/j.jvs.2021.12.068.
53. Svensson LG, Adams DH, Bonow RO, et al. Aortic valve and ascending aorta guidelines for management and quality measures. Ann Thorac Surg 2013;95(6 Suppl):S1–66.
54. Matsumura JS, Cambria RP, Dake MD, et al. International controlled clinical trial of thoracic endovascular aneurysm repair with the Zenith TX2 endovascular graft: 1-year results. J Vasc Surg 2008;47(2):247–57 [discussion: 257].
55. Quevedo HC, Santiago-Trinidad R, Castellanos J, et al. Systematic Review of Interventions to Repair Ascending Aortic Pseudoaneurysms. Ochsner J 2014;14(4):576–85.
56. Dong Z, Fu W, Wang Y, et al. Stent graft-induced new entry after endovascular repair for Stanford type B aortic dissection. J Vasc Surg 2010;52(6):1450–7.

Contemporary Treatment of the Asymptomatic Carotid Patient

Caron B. Rockman, MD[a],*, Karan Garg, MD[b]

KEYWORDS

- Carotid artery stenosis • Asymptomatic • Optimal medical therapy
- Carotid endarterectomy • Carotid artery stenting

KEY POINTS

- All patient with asymptomatic carotid artery stenosis should be treated with medical management and risk factor modification to reduce their future risk of stroke and cardiovascular complications.
- Select patients with asymptomatic carotid artery stenosis with an increased risk of future stroke based on the degree of stenosis and other imaging or patient-related characteristics are appropriate to consider for carotid artery intervention.
- When performing carotid intervention for asymptomatic disease, the preponderance of evidence and guidelines suggest that carotid endarterectomy is most appropriate; however, the choice of intervention should be based on individual patient factors that may place them at an increased risk with a particular carotid revascularization technique.

BACKGROUND

Stroke is among the major causes of mortality and disability worldwide.[1] Stroke causes 5.5 million deaths and more than 44 million disabilities every year.[2] In the United States alone, a stroke occurs approximately every 40 seconds; this translates into about 2160 strokes each day. Each year, approximately 800,000 Americans suffer a stroke.[3] The treatment of acute ischemic stroke is generally and historically supportive and medical.[1] Improved functional outcome in stroke patients who receive endovascular intervention in conjunction with thrombolysis within a defined period of symptom onset has been widely reported and studied.[4] A meta-analysis of 5 trials that investigated the efficacy of endovascular intervention for stroke have provided

[a] Florence and Joseph Ritorto Professor of Surgery, Division of Vascular Surgery, NYU Langone Medical Center, NYU Grossman School of Medicine, 530 1st Avenue, 11th Floor, New York, NY 10016, USA; [b] Division of Vascular Surgery, NYU Langone Medical Center, 530 1st Avenue, 11th Floor, New York, NY 10016, USA
* Corresponding author.
E-mail address: Caron.rockman@nyulangone.org

Surg Clin N Am 103 (2023) 629–644
https://doi.org/10.1016/j.suc.2023.04.016
0039-6109/23/© 2023 Elsevier Inc. All rights reserved.

strong evidence to support the use of thrombolysis/thrombectomy procedures when initiated within 6 hours of stroke onset.[5] Although urgent thrombolytic therapy in combination with adjunctive endovascular therapy within several hours after an ischemic stroke is an attractive and important option, its widespread application is limited from a practical and logistical point of view. Therefore, the principal strategy against cerebrovascular disease and its role in causing ischemic stroke remains primary stroke prevention.[1]

Atherosclerotic plaque in the carotid artery causes a substantial proportion of ischemic strokes; however, the mechanisms are less well understood than those of acute coronary thrombosis.[6] Carotid artery plaque can cause transient ischemic attack (TIA) or stroke by 2 mechanisms: embolization and hypoperfusion. Due to the abundant collateral circulation in the brain, global cerebral hypoperfusion is rare; it occurs only in patients with severe multivessel occlusive disease in both the carotid and vertebral artery territories. Atheroembolization of debris originating from carotid artery plaque and traveling to the brain is thought to be the predominant cause of both TIA and ischemic stroke related to carotid artery disease. Evidence for the role of embolization comes from the early reports of Hollenhorst, who found embolic debris in the retinal vessels of patients with transient monocular blindness.[7] The severity of carotid artery stenosis is strongly associated with stroke risk in symptomatic patients.[6,8,9] Currently, it is the most important predictor of benefit from carotid artery intervention.[10] However, other factors predictive of stroke clearly exist, including an ulcerated appearance present on carotid arteriography or duplex ultrasonography, which is also a strong independent risk factor for acute stroke.[6,11,12]

The degree of carotid artery stenosis is a critical factor involved in identifying patients at an increased risk of future ischemic stroke; in fact, most asymptomatic patients with moderate degrees of carotid artery stenosis are at relatively low risk for future stroke.[1] However, only 15% of ischemic strokes are preceded by a warning TIA. Therefore, waiting for carotid stenosis to become symptomatic will fail to prevent most strokes caused by carotid artery disease.[13] Hence, there is a critical need to improve the selection of asymptomatic patients for carotid intervention so as to improve the potential effectiveness of treatment in stroke prevention.[14] Nevertheless, whether or not they are being considered for carotid intervention, all patients with atherosclerotic plaque identified at the carotid bifurcation need to be treated with appropriate medical management to prevent both stroke as well as other cardiovascular complications.

PATIENT EVALUATION OVERVIEW: HOW IS THE PATIENT WITH ASYMPTOMATIC CAROTID DISEASE IDENTIFIED?

Patients with asymptomatic carotid stenosis are typically identified following the performance of an imaging study, typically a Carotid Duplex ultrasound. This may have been performed for "screening" purposes; although the United States Preventive Services Task Force (USPSTF) clearly recommends against screening for occult carotid disease in the general population,[15] the recently updated Society for Vascular Surgery (SVS) guidelines on the management of extracranial cerebrovascular disease do recommend screening patients at high risk for disease.[16] Alternatively, imaging may have been performed either after hearing a carotid bruit on physical examination or as part of a workup for nonspecific, nonfocal cerebrovascular symptoms such as dizziness. In these cases, the symptoms that prompted the performance of imaging are not typically directly related to any carotid disease that is subsequently discovered. Carotid atherosclerosis can also be identified on axial imaging studies including computerized tomography (CT) and MRI scans performed for related or unrelated reasons.

Once the diagnosis of asymptomatic carotid artery stenosis has been made, 3 questions need to be addressed: What risk factors need to be addressed? Is the patient receiving optimal medical therapy (OMT)? Is there a need for intervention for severe disease with either carotid endarterectomy (CEA) or stenting procedures including transfemoral carotid artery stenting (TF-CAS) or transcarotid artery revascularization (TCAR)?[17]

PHARMACOLOGIC/MEDICAL TREATMENT OPTIONS
Medical Management of the Patient with Asymptomatic Carotid Disease

The potential effect of modern medical therapy on the possibly decreased incidence of stroke has received great attention in the recent literature and has resulted in challenges to the role of CEA and carotid stenting procedures for asymptomatic patients.[1] Previous randomized trials have demonstrated a clear benefit of surgical therapy with CEA over contemporaneous medical therapy regarding stroke prevention in both asymptomatic and previously symptomatic patients with severe extracranial carotid stenosis.[18–20] Some more recent analyses have additionally reported that the annual risk of stroke even in patients with known asymptomatic carotid stenosis is lower than that reported in the seminal CEA trials, presumably due to improved medical therapy.[21,22] Nevertheless, it remains clear that asymptomatic carotid stenosis continues to cause a significant number of strokes.[23] Data from the Greater Cincinnati Northern Kentucky Stroke Study has reported in conservative estimates that about 41,000 strokes may be attributed to previously asymptomatic carotid stenosis annually in the United States.[1,23]

Although many attribute the possibly decreased incidence of stroke to antilipid therapy, the epidemiologic association between elevated cholesterol levels and stroke is inconsistent and somewhat controversial.[24] Treatment with statins has generally shown stroke reduction, as reflected in the report of a meta-analysis of more than 90,000 patients.[25] It should be noted that many of the studies included in this meta-analysis involved secondary as opposed to primary stroke prevention. Nevertheless, the relative reduction in stroke risk was found to be 21%. Statins have also been demonstrated to be associated with a reduction in stroke incidence in a variety of specific patient populations, including those with known coronary artery disease,[26] hypercholesterolemia,[26] normocholesterolemia,[26] elderly patients,[26] and diabetics.[27] Statins have also been demonstrated to consistently reduce carotid intima-media thickness. Although data regarding the utility of statin medications for the primary prevention of stroke is less conclusive than for secondary prevention, current guidelines do in fact recommend statins for the prevention of first stroke in high-risk patients, including those with low-density lipoprotein (LDL) levels greater than 4.1 and for men aged older than 45 years and women aged older than 55 years with the following risk factors: a positive family history, smoking, hypertension, or left ventricular hypertrophy.[24] However, it is unclear what exact role and effect statins have in patients with known severe carotid occlusive disease with regard to stroke prevention.

In a report authored by Writing Group Members on behalf of the American Heart Association's Stroke Council, a clear decline in stroke mortality is in fact noted.[28] The authors think that this reduction is mainly due to the treatment of hypertension as opposed antilipid treatment. The authors note that epidemiologic studies have shown that elevated blood pressure is the most important determinant of the risk of stroke.[28] They also think that improved treatment of hypertension is likely the most important factor that has contributed to the decline in stroke mortality. This report echoes the Tromso Study, which noted that while changes in cardiovascular risk factors were found to account for 57% of the decrease in ischemic stroke incidence, the most important factor was thought to be improved control of hypertension.[29]

The INTERSTROKE Study, in 2010, reported a case-control study of 2337 ischemic stroke cases in 22 countries worldwide. Patients with an acute first stroke were compared with controls with no history of stroke and were matched for both age and sex.[30] The authors found that 5 factors accounted for more than 80% of the global risk of all ischemic strokes: hypertension, current smoking, abdominal obesity, poor diet, and physical inactivity.[30] Hypertension was the most important risk factor for all stroke subtypes.[30,31]

All patients with carotid artery atherosclerosis must be treated with OMT and risk factor modification.[32] Modifiable risk factors include smoking, alcohol, obesity, physical inactivity, hypertension, diabetes, and hyperlipidemia.[17]

Hypertension[1,17]: Hypertension is a significant risk factor for both ischemic stroke and intracranial hemorrhage.[33] Appropriate treatment of blood pressure in hypertensive patients is associated with a significant reduction in the risk of ischemic stroke; patients with a blood pressure less than 120/80 mmHg have half the lifetime risk of stroke than subjects with hypertension.[34,35] So-called intensive blood pressure control as opposed to standard treatment has also resulted in a significantly lower risk of stroke.[36] Strict blood pressure control can also reduce the risk of recurrent stroke.[37] There is no level 1 evidence assessing the influence of BP reduction on stroke prevention in patients with known asymptomatic carotid disease.[16] Target level for BP in patients with asymptomatic carotid disease in the 2017 guidelines from the American Heart Association (AHA) and the American College of Cardiology is 130/80 mmHg.[17]

Cigarette smoking[1,17]: Current cigarette smokers have a 2 to 4 times increased risk of stroke as compared with nonsmokers or those who have quit for more than 10 years.[35,38,39] Discontinuation of smoking reduces future stroke risk in multiple demographic patient categories.[40] In a large cohort of black patients, current cigarette smoking was associated with a dose-dependent higher risk of all stroke. Past smokers did not have a significantly increased risk of stroke compared with never smokers, suggesting that smoking cessation helped to reduce the incident of stroke.[41] Smoking cessation reduces stroke risk in both men and women.[16,42] Pharmacological therapy is superior to placebo in achieving successful quitting of cigarette smoking.[16]

Hypercholesterolemia[1,17,32]: The data regarding elevated cholesterol levels and their relationship with primary stroke risk in particular is once again somewhat conflicting.[16] However, there is compelling evidence that decreasing LDL levels with lipid-lowering therapy is effective in decreasing stroke risk in patients with known atherosclerotic disease.[16] A meta-analysis of randomized clinical trials including more than 100,000 patients demonstrated that in patients without an earlier history of stroke who had hyperlipidemia, statins were associated with up to a 30% decrease in stroke incidence.[16,43] More recent metanalysis of 26 trials in patients with coronary artery or other atherosclerotic disease demonstrated a greater than 15% decrease in the rate of stroke for every 10% reduction in serum LDL.[16,44] Although statins have been shown to demonstrate improvement in intima-media thickness in the carotid artery, there is no compelling evidence that statins are associated with significant plaque regression.[16,45] Recent evidence supports high-intensity statin therapy in patients aged 75 years or less with atherosclerosis, including carotid artery disease, or moderate-intensity statin therapy if high–intensity therapy is not tolerated.[16]

Trials specific to ischemic stroke have demonstrated that there may be a 25% increased risk of ischemic stroke with each 38.7 mg/dL increase in total cholesterol levels.[46] However, not all trials have consistently demonstrated a correlation between hypercholesterolemia and ischemic stroke.[3] An association between total cholesterol levels and ischemic stroke has been found in some studies but has not been confirmed in others.[33] There are no large randomized trials of statins in asymptomatic carotid stenosis patients.[17]

Physical activity[1]: Increased leisure-time physical activity is protective against stroke across race, sex, and age, and related to the level of intensity and the duration of activity.[47] In the Reasons for Geographic and Racial Differences in Stroke (REGARDS) study, participants who reported physical activity less than 4 times a week had a 20% increase in stroke risk as compared with those who exercised more than 4 times a week. However, it is possible that this is related to the fact that physical activity also improves traditional risk factors such as diabetes and obesity.[33,48]

Diabetes[1,17,32]: Diabetes is a risk factor for ischemic stroke at all ages but the most significant risk increase seems to occur among patients aged younger than 65 years.[33] Diabetes mellitus nearly doubles the risk of stroke among persons with diabetes as compared with others who have normal glucose levels.[49] The effect of diabetes on stroke risk seems to be more significant in women than in men.[50] Among patients with documented carotid artery disease in the Cardiovascular Health Study, elevated fasting blood glucose levels were associated with an increased stroke risk.[16,51] In the Northern Manhattan Study, diabetes was associated with a doubling of stroke risk.[52] However, other large studies have not confirmed that strict glucose control definitively decreases stroke risk among diabetics.[16,53] Nevertheless, in patients with carotid artery disease hemoglobin A1c of less than 7% is recommended.[16]

Diet[1]: A protective relationship between fruit and vegetable consumption and decreased ischemic stroke risk has been reported.[54] A Mediterranean-style diet higher in the consumption of nuts and olive oil has been shown to be associated with a reduced risk of stroke.[55]

Obesity[1]: Obesity is a specific risk factor for ischemic stroke in both men and women.[56,57] There is an additional association between abdominal obesity and ischemic stroke in men.[58]

Antiplatelet/antithrombotic therapy[1,17,32]

There is a paucity of quality randomized controlled trial (RCT) data regarding the need for antiplatelet therapy in asymptomatic carotid stenosis patients. Aspirin studies in patients with asymptomatic carotid stenoses show conflicting results, particularly with regard to primary prevention. Nevertheless, The USPSTF recommends initiating low-dose aspirin for primary prevention of cardiovascular disease in adults aged 50 to 59 years who have a 10-year risk of greater than 10% for cardiovascular disease, have a life expectancy of 10 years or more, and are not at increased risk of bleeding.[16,59] In the Asymptomatic Cervical Bruit study, there was no significant difference in the incidence of stroke between patients taking aspirin or placebo at 2 years.[60] However, in the Asymptomatic Carotid Embolism Study that followed asymptomatic patients with a 70% to 99% stenosis, antiplatelet therapy was in fact associated with lower risks of ipsilateral stroke, TIA, and any stroke.[16,61]

SURGICAL/INTERVENTIONAL TREATMENT OPTIONS
Which Asymptomatic Patient with Carotid Disease Warrant Carotid Intervention?

Whether carotid artery disease remains a significant cause of ischemic stroke, and whether OMT can decrease this risk to the same degree as proven carotid revascularization procedures, is currently a matter of significant controversy. Although mortality rates from stroke have declined globally in the past 2 decades, the absolute numbers of people affected has increased and the costs of caring for stroke survivors are increasing.[62,63]

Level I data support the superiority of CEA over medical management in the prevention of stroke in patients with severe asymptomatic carotid artery disease (**Table 1**). Nevertheless, the debate is ongoing in the case of asymptomatic carotid atherosclerosis in patients who have never experienced cerebrovascular symptoms. Challenges to the role of CEA in the treatment of asymptomatic carotid stenosis supported by level I data generally fall into 2 categories: (1) the view that modern OMT may allow better stroke protection, obviating CEA (or CAS) and (2) the argument that the degree of stenosis alone is a poor surrogate for vulnerable plaque and does not allow the accurate prediction of patients at high risk for stroke.[64] As carotid intervention in asymptomatic patients is a purely prophylactic procedure, it is clear that to achieve benefit in stroke prevention, intervention should only be performed in patients who are at the highest risk of future stroke. In addition to age, sex, the degree of stenosis, medical comorbidities, and life expectancy, relevant factors include the severity of the stenosis,[62,65] progression of stenosis,[62,66] evidence of infarction on brain imaging,[67] and plaque imaging characteristics.[68] From a practical perspective, the degree of stenosis is the most important factor influencing the choice of intervention, and most clinicians thought that 70% stenosis or greater defines severe stenosis warranting consideration of intervention. A consistent rate of stroke risk of approximately 2% per year in patients with high-grade asymptomatic stenosis was reported in Asymptomatic Carotid Atherosclerosis Study (ACAS), North American Symptomatic Carotid Endarterectomy Trial (NASCET), and European Carotid Surgery Trial (ECST). Although the ACAS study results have been criticized as obsolete in the current era of improved medical management of atherosclerosis, in the later years of ACST, 80% of patients in fact were on statins.[18–20,69] Additionally, the Reduction of Atherothrombosis for Continued Health Registry states that carotid stenosis of 70% or more was associated with a significantly increased stroke risk despite the fact that more than two-thirds of subjects were on statin medications.[70]

Progression of carotid stenosis has been shown to be a significant predictor of stroke risk in multiple natural history studies.[71–73] In a follow-up study from the Asymptomatic Carotid Stenosis and Risk of Stroke (ACSRS) group, 1121 patients with asymptomatic carotid stenosis of 50% to 99% were analyzed with a mean follow-up period of 4 years.[74] Progression occurred in 19.8% of patients. Independent

Table 1
Five-year and 10-year data for ipsilateral stroke and any stroke (including perioperative risks) in ACAS an ACST for CEA + OMT versus OMT alone

	30-Day Death or Stroke Rate After CEA	Ipsilateral Stroke (+ Perioperative Death/Stroke)			Any Stroke (+ Perioperative Death/Stroke)		
		CEA + OMT	OMT	ARR (%)	CEA + OMT	OMT	ARR%
ACAS[19]	2.3%	5.1% at 5 y	11% at 5 y	5.9%	12.4% at 5 y	17.8% at 5 y	5.4%
ACST[80]	2.8%				6.4% at 5 y	11.8% at 5 y	5.4%
ACST[20]	2.8%				13.4% at 10 y	17.9% at 10 y	4.5%

Abbreviations: ARR, absolute risk reduction; OMT, optimal medical therapy; Y, years.
Modified from Naylor AR, McCabe DJH. Decision Making Including Optimal Medical Therapy. In: Sidawy AN PB, ed. Rutherford's Vascular Surgery and Endovascular Therapy, 10th Edition. 10th Edition. Elsevier; 2023:1203-1220:chap 92; with permission.

predictors of progression included male sex, high creatinine, not taking lipid-lowering medications, low grade of stenosis, and increased plaque area. A total of 130 first ipsilateral cerebral of retinal events occurred, including 59 strokes. Forty strokes (67.8%) occurred in patients whose stenosis was not changed and 19 strokes (32.2%) occurred in those with progression. For patients with baseline 70% to 99% stenosis and in the absence of progression (n = 349), the 8-year cumulative ipsilateral ischemic stroke rate was 12%. In the presence of progression, it was 21% (n = 77).

Another report comprised 126 arteries with severe stenosis in patients who were treated medically.[64] Of this cohort, including 86% taking a statin medication with a mean follow-up period of 63 months, ipsilateral neurologic symptoms developed related to 25% of the arteries. Of these events, 14 (45%) were strokes and 17 (55%) were TIAs or retinal events. Of this cohort of patients who initially were not considered for carotid artery intervention or were refused, 33% ultimately underwent carotid revascularization during the follow-up period.

Conrad and colleagues[75] reported a study including 900 arteries in 794 patients with moderate stenosis. OMT included aspirin and a statin with documented LDL levels less than 100 mg/dL. Mean follow-up was 3.6 years. The 5-year freedom from progression to severe stenosis was 61.2% ± 2.6% with no benefit seen from OMT. Plaque progression occurred in 262 arteries, and 36 (13.7%) of these developed symptoms. Average time to plaque progression was 32 months. Of this cohort, 90 patients (11.3%) developed ipsilateral neurologic symptoms during follow-up; 58% of these were strokes. Average time to symptom onset was 36 months. A total of 36 (40%) symptomatic patients also showed plaque progression but the remaining 60% developed symptoms with a stable moderate stenosis. Five-year freedom from symptoms was 88.4%, with no benefit seen with OMT. Overall, the authors concluded that current medial therapy was unable to halt the progression from moderate to severe stenosis or the development of symptoms in 45% of the cohort. These results were echoed in an additional study performed in Korea.[76] Of patient with initial moderate (50%–79%) stenosis, progression of stenosis occurred in 31.8% and development of associated neurological symptoms occurred in 3.2% during a mean follow-up of 49 months. The authors concluded that the progression of disease was high despite the prevalent use of antiplatelet medications and statins.[76]

In a population-based cohort in Sweden, all 65-year-old men in a single county underwent a carotid Duplex scan and were reassessed 5 years later at the age of 70 years.[77] Among men with initially moderate (50%–79%) stenosis, 12.9% progressed to a severe stenosis, of whom 2 developed symptoms. Of 12 patients with initial 80% to 99% stenosis, 5 (42%) developed symptoms. In multivariable analysis, smoking, coronary artery disease, and hypercholesterolemia were associated with disease progression.[77] Progression of carotid stenosis along with the development of neurologic symptoms has been noted in patients with carotid stenosis despite OMT.[75]

Currently, the most important factor used to choose appropriate patients for carotid artery intervention is the degree of carotid stenosis. However, the degree of stenosis alone is likely an incomplete predictor of future stroke risk. With these issues in mind, there has been a great deal of focus on identifying other characteristics of both the patient and the carotid plaque itself in addition to the degree of stenosis alone that would be distinguishable on imaging studies and allow the clinician to identify patients at an increased risk who would most benefit from vascular intervention. The term "vulnerable" plaque is often used to denote unstable plaques, or plaques prone to complications, including embolization and subsequent stroke.[1]

THE VULNERABLE PLAQUE AND PATIENTS AT INCREASED RISK FOR ISCHEMIC STROKE

A strong attempt has been made to identify patients with carotid disease at an increased risk for stroke by combining both morphologic plaque features and clinical patient characteristics.[1] The ACSRS Study Group attempted to determine the cerebrovascular risk stratification potential of baseline degree of stenosis, clinical features, and ultrasonic plaque characteristics in patients with asymptomatic carotid artery stenosis.[68] This was a prospective cohort study involving 1121 patients with 50% to 99% asymptomatic internal carotid artery (ICA) stenosis who were followed for 6 to 96 months. The authors found that the following characteristics were associated with an increased risk for ipsilateral cerebral or retinal ischemic events: severity of stenosis, age, systolic blood pressure, increased creatinine, smoking history of more than 10 pack-years, history of contralateral TIA or stroke, low gray-scale median, increased plaque area, and the absence of discrete white areas without acoustic shadowing. Combinations of these characteristics could stratify patients into different levels of risk for stroke (**Table 2**). Of 923 patients with 70% or greater stenosis, the predicted cumulative 5-year stroke risk was less than 5% in 495, 5% to 9.9% in 202, 10% to 19.9% in 142, and 20% or more in 84. The authors concluded that cerebrovascular risk stratification related to carotid artery disease is possible using a combination of clinical and ultrasonic plaque features. In a more recent update from the ACSRS group,[78] the authors expounded on their earlier work and noted that the size of a juxtaluminal black hypoechoic area in ultrasound images of asymptomatic carotid artery plaques is linearly related to the risk of future stroke and is an additional factor that can be used to predict the risk of future ipsilateral ischemic stroke.

In addition to the above sonographic features, additional ultrasound features that imply an increased risk for stroke include plaque echolucency, neovascularity, a lipid rich necrotic core, a thin or ruptured fibrous cap, and intraplaque hemorrhage. Other patient-related factors that predict future stroke risk include the progression of stenosis during surveillance, impaired cerebrovascular reserve, spontaneous embolization noted on Transcranial Doppler examination, and the presence of silent brain infarction on brain imaging.[17,79]

SUMMARY/GUIDELINES

The SVS recently updated its guidelines for the management of extracranial cerebrovascular disease with both a clinical practice guideline and implementation document.[16,32] There are several recommendations relevant to the discussion of the current management of patients with asymptomatic carotid disease.

One of the key questions addressed in the clinical practice guideline document is the following: Is CEA recommended over maximal medical therapy for asymptomatic carotid stenosis in low-risk surgical patients?[16] An extensive literature review and systematic review was performed. In summarizing the evidence and rationale for the eventual recommendation, the authors note that several trials have compared CEA with best medical therapy. Both the ACAS[19] and ACST[80] trials favored CEA over medical management in treatment of low-risk surgical patients with severe asymptomatic carotid stenosis. In ACAS, the risk of stroke at 2 years was 5.1% for surgery as opposed to 11% for medical management, with an aggregate risk reduction of 53% (95% confidence interval, 22%–77%).[19] In the initial report of the ACST trial, CEA provided an advantage in limiting stroke and death at 5 years (4.1% vs 10%).[80] Long-term results of the ACST trial additionally noted that the CEA arm patients had significantly lower perioperative and 10-year stroke rates (13.3% vs 17.9%).[20] The guideline

Table 2
Stable and unstable plaque features

	Stable Plaque	Unstable Plaque
Core	Fibrous smooth muscle cells	Necrotic, lipid rich core
Cap	Stable fibrous cap	Thin/unstable fibrous cap
Intraplaque characteristics	Calcified, hard	Intraplaque hemorrhage/necrosis; soft; ulcerations
Cells	Smooth muscle cells	Macrophage infiltration
Biomarkers	High-density lipoprotein	Various inflammatory and cytokine mediators
Composition	Homogenous	Heterogeneous
Ultrasound characteristics	Echogenic	Echolucent

From Howell C, Zhou W. Cerebrovascular Disease: The Unstable Carotid Plaque. In: Sidawy AN, Perler BA, ed. Rutherford's Vascular Surgery and Endovascular Therapy. 10th Edition ed. Elsevier; 2023. Chapter 89, 1179-1185.e3; with permission.

discussion does note that the strength of conclusions from these 2 trials has been challenged due to several factors: the relatively modest absolute benefits of CEA, the fact that the medical arms of these trials did not use contemporaneous optimal medical management, and the fact that the overall incidence of stroke may in fact be decreasing, presumably due to more widespread medical management of atherosclerosis.[16] Clearly, the question of whether modern medical therapy including statins is equivalent or superior to CEA or CAS has not yet been adequately addressed by any prospective randomized trials.[16] However, in ACST, the outcomes among patients who were in fact receiving statins was separately analyzed; those who underwent CEA still had a lower stroke incidence annually as compared with patients who were treated with medical management alone. The benefit of CEA was not as great for those receiving lipid-lowering therapy (0.7% vs 1.3% annually for those on lipid lowering therapy compared with 1.8% vs 3.3% for patients not on lipid lower therapy).[16,20]

Additional relevant data comes from the Howard Oxford Vascular study,[81] which analyzed the correlation between ipsilateral stroke and the degree of asymptomatic carotid stenosis in patients treated with best medical therapy.[16] The authors reported that the ipsilateral stroke rate at 5 years for patients with 70% to 99% stenosis was 14.6% as opposed to 0% for those patients with 50% to 69% stenosis. For patients with 80% to 99% stenosis, the ipsilateral stroke rate was significantly greater than that for those with 50% to 80% stenosis (18.3% vs 1%). In fact, ipsilateral stroke was linearly associated with the degree of ipsilateral carotid stenosis.[16,81] Conversely, the 5-year stroke risk was low for those patients with less than 70% stenosis on contemporary best medical therapy.[81] The authors conclude that the benefit of CEA in the prospective trials might have in fact been underestimated for the patients with the most severe stenosis.[16,81] Finally, the guidelines note that the role of TF-CAS and TCAR is even less clear because at this time no completed studies have compared these treatments for patients with asymptomatic stenosis compared with best medical therapy.[16]

The final recommendation from the SVS guidelines[16] is as follows.

- In low surgical risk patients with asymptomatic carotid bifurcation atherosclerosis and stenosis of greater than 70% documented by validated Duplex or computed tomography angiography (CTA), we recommend CEA with best

Table 3
Revascularization techniques with associated high-risk criteria

Revascularization Technique	High-Risk Criteria (Based on Clinical Judgment
CEA	Neck irradiation Previous CEA Previous neck surgery Tracheal stoma Lesion above C2 Contralateral vocal cord injury Hostile neck owing to obesity, immobility, or kyphosis Medical high risk
TCAR	Heavily calcified carotid lesion Lesion within 5 cm of clavicle CCA diameter <6 cm Neck irradiation Tracheal stoma Hostile neck owing to obesity, immobility, or kyphosis Medical high risk
TF-CAS	Age >75 years Heavily calcified carotid stenosis Complex bifurcation stenosis >15 mm length Tortuous ICA Tortuous CCA Type 3 or tortuous aortic arch Heavy atherosclerotic burden of arch

Abbreviations: CCA, common carotid artery; ICA, internal carotid artery.

From AbuRahma AF, Avgerinos ED, Chang RW, et al. The Society for Vascular Surgery implementation document for management of extracranial cerebrovascular disease. J Vasc Surg. 2022;75(1S):26S-98S; with permission.

medical therapy over maximal medical therapy alone for the long-term prevention of stroke and death.[16]

- The level of the grade of the recommendation is 1 (strong), and the quality of evidence is noted as B (moderate).[16]

Additional recommendations relevant to the treatment of patients with asymptomatic carotid artery disease are found in the corresponding SVS Guideline implementation document.[32] There are listed below.

- Neurologically asymptomatic patients with greater than 70% diameter stenosis should be considered for CEA, TCAR, or TF-CAS for the reduction of long-term risk of stroke, provided the patient has a 3 to 5-year life expectancy and perioperative stroke/death rates are less than 3%. The determination for which technique to use should be based on the presence or absence of high-risk criteria for CEA, TCAR, or TF-CAS (**Table 3**).
- Neurologically asymptomatic patients deemed high risk for CEA, TCAR, and TF-CAS should be considered for primary medical management.
- There are insufficient data to recommend TF-CAS as primary therapy for neurologically asymptomatic patients with 70% to 99% diameter stenosis.[32]

SUMMARY

Patients with asymptomatic carotid stenosis should be treated with aggressive risk factor modification and optimal medical management as appropriate for all patients with demonstrable significant atherosclerotic disease. Select patients with severe degrees of stenosis and/or other characteristics placing them at increased risk for future stroke are suitable to additionally consider for carotid artery intervention, which at this time is probably most appropriately performed with CEA, unless the patient has other medical or anatomical features that place them at an increased risk for CEA. At present, most guidelines advise that where carotid interventions are being considered in asymptomatic patients that CEA is currently the preferred option over TF-CAS.[16,17,32] No published comparative trials at this time have included the TCAR technique. It is likely that ACST-2[82] and CREST-2[83] will provide much more information on patient selection and the role of appropriate indications for and selection of carotid interventions for asymptomatic patients.[17,84,85]

DISCLOSURE

The authors have nothing to disclose.

REFERENCES

1. Rockman C, Maldonado T. Cerebrovascular disease: epidemiology and natural history. In: Sidawy AN, PB, editors. Rutherford's vascular surgery and endovascular therapy. 9th edition. Phildadelphia, PA: Elsevier; 2019. p. 1121–39, chap Section 13, Chapter 86.
2. Mukherjee D, Patil CG. Epidemiology and the global burden of stroke. World Neurosurg 2011;76(6 Suppl):S85–90.
3. Grysiewicz RA, Thomas K, Pandey DK. Epidemiology of ischemic and hemorrhagic stroke: incidence, prevalence, mortality, and risk factors. Neurol Clin 2008;26(4):871–95, vii.
4. Hui W, Wu C, Zhao W, et al. Efficacy and safety of recanalization therapy for acute ischemic stroke with large vessel occlusion: a systematic review. Stroke 2020;3. STROKEAHA119028624.
5. Mokin M, Rojas H, Levy EI. Randomized trials of endovascular therapy for stroke–impact on stroke care. Nat Rev Neurol 2016;12(2):86–94.
6. Redgrave JN, Lovett JK, Gallagher PJ, et al. Histological assessment of 526 symptomatic carotid plaques in relation to the nature and timing of ischemic symptoms: the Oxford plaque study. Circulation 2006;113(19):2320–8.
7. Hollenhorst RW. Significance of bright plaques in the retinal arterioles. JAMA 1961;178:23–9.
8. Barnett HJ, Taylor DW, Eliasziw M, et al. Benefit of carotid endarterectomy in patients with symptomatic moderate or severe stenosis. North American Symptomatic Carotid Endarterectomy Trial Collaborators. N Engl J Med 1998;339(20): 1415–25.
9. Rothwell PM, Gutnikov SA, Warlow CP. Reanalysis of the final results of the European Carotid Surgery Trial. Stroke 2003;34(2):514–23.
10. Rothwell PM, Eliasziw M, Gutnikov SA, et al. Endarterectomy for symptomatic carotid stenosis in relation to clinical subgroups and timing of surgery. Lancet 2004; 363(9413):915–24.
11. Eliasziw M, Streifler JY, Fox AJ, et al. Significance of plaque ulceration in symptomatic patients with high-grade carotid stenosis. North American Symptomatic Carotid Endarterectomy Trial. Stroke 1994;25(2):304–8.
12. Rothwell PM, Gibson R, Warlow CP. Interrelation between plaque surface morphology and degree of stenosis on carotid angiograms and the risk of ischemic stroke in patients with symptomatic carotid stenosis. On behalf of the

European Carotid Surgery Trialists' Collaborative Group. Stroke 2000;31(3): 615–21.

13. Markus HS, King A, Shipley M, et al. Asymptomatic embolisation for prediction of stroke in the Asymptomatic Carotid Emboli Study (ACES): a prospective observational study. Lancet Neurol 2010;9(7):663–71.

14. Jayasooriya G, Thapar A, Shalhoub J, et al. Silent cerebral events in asymptomatic carotid stenosis. J Vasc Surg 2011;54(1):227–36.

15. Tanner M. USPSTF recommends against screening adults in the general population for asymptomatic carotid artery stenosis. Ann Intern Med 2021;174(6):JC62.

16. AbuRahma AF, Avgerinos EM, Chang RW, et al. Society for vascular surgery clinical practice guidelines for management of extracranial cerebrovascular disease. J Vasc Surg 2021. https://doi.org/10.1016/j.jvs.2021.04.073.

17. Naylor AR, McCabe DJH. Decision making including optimal medical therapy. In: Sidawy AN, PB, editors. Rutherford's vascular surgery and endovascular therapy. 10th edition. Phildadelphia, PA: Elsevier; 2023. p. 1203–20, chap 92.

18. Beneficial effect of carotid endarterectomy in symptomatic patients with high-grade carotid stenosis. North American Symptomatic Carotid Endarterectomy Trial Collaborators. Clinical Trial Multicenter Study Randomized Controlled Trial Research Support, U.S. Gov't, P.H.S. N Engl J Med 1991;325(7):445–53.

19. Endarterectomy for asymptomatic carotid artery stenosis. Executive committee for the asymptomatic carotid atherosclerosis study. JAMA 1995;273(18):1421–8.

20. Halliday A, Harrison M, Hayter E, et al. 10-year stroke prevention after successful carotid endarterectomy for asymptomatic stenosis (ACST-1): a multicentre randomised trial. Lancet 2010;376(9746):1074–84.

21. Abbott AL. Medical (nonsurgical) intervention alone is now best for prevention of stroke associated with asymptomatic severe carotid stenosis: results of a systematic review and analysis. Stroke 2009;40(10):e573–83.

22. Marquardt L, Geraghty OC, Mehta Z, et al. Low risk of ipsilateral stroke in patients with asymptomatic carotid stenosis on best medical treatment: a prospective, population-based study. Stroke 2010;41(1):e11–7.

23. Flaherty ML, Kissela B, Khoury JC, et al. Carotid artery stenosis as a cause of stroke. Neuroepidemiology 2013;40(1):36–41.

24. Di Legge S, Koch G, Diomedi M, et al. Stroke prevention: managing modifiable risk factors. Stroke Res Treat 2012;2012:391538.

25. Amarenco P, Labreuche J, Lavallee P, et al. Statins in stroke prevention and carotid atherosclerosis: systematic review and up-to-date meta-analysis. Stroke 2004;35(12):2902–9.

26. MRC/BHF Heart Protection Study of cholesterol lowering with simvastatin in 20,536 high-risk individuals: a randomised placebo-controlled trial. Lancet 2002;360(9326):7–22.

27. Collins R, Armitage J, Parish S, et al. MRC/BHF Heart Protection Study of cholesterol-lowering with simvastatin in 5963 people with diabetes: a randomised placebo-controlled trial. Lancet 2003;361(9374):2005–16.

28. Lackland DT, Roccella EJ, Deutsch AF, et al. Factors influencing the decline in stroke mortality: a statement from the American Heart Association/American Stroke Association. Stroke 2014;45(1):315–53.

29. Vangen-Lonne AM, Wilsgaard T, Johnsen SH, et al. Declining incidence of ischemic stroke: what is the impact of changing risk factors? The Tromso Study 1995 to 2012. Stroke 2017;48(3):544–50.

30. O'Donnell MJ, Xavier D, Liu L, et al. Risk factors for ischaemic and intracerebral haemorrhagic stroke in 22 countries (the INTERSTROKE study): a case-control study. Lancet 2010;376(9735):112–23.
31. Lawes CM, Bennett DA, Feigin VL, et al. Blood pressure and stroke: an overview of published reviews. Stroke 2004;35(4):1024.
32. AbuRahma AF, Avgerinos EM, Chang RW, et al. The society for vascular surgery implementation document for management of extracranial cerebrovascular disease. J Vasc Surg 2021. https://doi.org/10.1016/j.jvs.2021.04.074.
33. Benjamin EJ, Blaha MJ, Chiuve SE, et al. Heart disease and stroke statistics-2017 update: a report from the American heart association. Circulation 2017;135(10): e146–603.
34. Cushman WC, Evans GW, Byington RP, et al. Effects of intensive blood-pressure control in type 2 diabetes mellitus. N Engl J Med 2010;362(17):1575–85.
35. Roger VL, Go AS, Lloyd-Jones DM, et al. Heart disease and stroke statistics–2012 update: a report from the American Heart Association. Circulation 3 2012; 125(1):e2–220.
36. Perkovic V, Rodgers A. Redefining blood-pressure targets–SPRINT starts the marathon. N Engl J Med 2015;373(22):2175–8.
37. Group SPSS, Benavente OR, Coffey CS, et al. Blood-pressure targets in patients with recent lacunar stroke: the SPS3 randomised trial. Lancet 2013;382(9891): 507–15.
38. Goldstein LB, Bushnell CD, Adams RJ, et al. Guidelines for the primary prevention of stroke: a guideline for healthcare professionals from the American Heart Association/American Stroke Association. Stroke 2011;42(2):517–84.
39. Shah RS, Cole JW. Smoking and stroke: the more you smoke the more you stroke. Expert Rev Cardiovasc Ther 2010;8(7):917–32.
40. Bhat VM, Cole JW, Sorkin JD, et al. Dose-response relationship between cigarette smoking and risk of ischemic stroke in young women. Stroke 2008;39(9): 2439–43.
41. Oshunbade AA, Yimer WK, Valle KA, et al. Cigarette smoking and incident stroke in blacks of the jackson heart study. j am Heart Assoc 2020;9(12):e014990.
42. Wannamethee SG, Shaper AG, Whincup PH, et al. Smoking cessation and the risk of stroke in middle-aged men. JAMA 1995;274(2):155–60.
43. Bucher HC, Griffith LE, Guyatt GH. Effect of HMGcoA reductase inhibitors on stroke. A meta-analysis of randomized, controlled trials. Ann Intern Med 1998; 128(2):89–95.
44. Baigent C, Keech A, Kearney PM, et al. Efficacy and safety of cholesterol-lowering treatment: prospective meta-analysis of data from 90,056 participants in 14 randomised trials of statins. Lancet 2005;366(9493):1267–78.
45. Crouse JR, Goldbourt U, Evans G, et al. Risk factors and segment-specific carotid arterial enlargement in the Atherosclerosis Risk in Communities (ARIC) cohort. Stroke 1996;27(1):69–75.
46. Zhang X, Patel A, Horibe H, et al. Cholesterol, coronary heart disease, and stroke in the Asia Pacific region. Int J Epidemiol 2003;32(4):563–72.
47. Sacco RL, Gan R, Boden-Albala B, et al. Leisure-time physical activity and ischemic stroke risk: the Northern Manhattan Stroke Study. Stroke 1998;29(2): 380–7.
48. McDonnell MN, Hillier SL, Hooker SP, et al. Physical activity frequency and risk of incident stroke in a national US study of blacks and whites. Stroke 2013;44(9): 2519–24.

49. Vermeer SE, Sandee W, Algra A, et al. Impaired glucose tolerance increases stroke risk in nondiabetic patients with transient ischemic attack or minor ischemic stroke. Stroke 2006;37(6):1413–7.
50. Peters SA, Huxley RR, Woodward M. Diabetes as a risk factor for stroke in women compared with men: a systematic review and meta-analysis of 64 cohorts, including 775,385 individuals and 12,539 strokes. Lancet 2014;383(9933): 1973–80.
51. Smith NL, Barzilay JI, Shaffer D, et al. Fasting and 2-hour postchallenge serum glucose measures and risk of incident cardiovascular events in the elderly: the Cardiovascular Health Study. Arch Intern Med 2002;162(2):209–16.
52. Banerjee C, Moon YP, Paik MC, et al. Duration of diabetes and risk of ischemic stroke: the Northern Manhattan Study. Stroke 2012;43(5):1212–7.
53. Zhang C, Zhou YH, Xu CL, et al. Efficacy of intensive control of glucose in stroke prevention: a meta-analysis of data from 59,197 participants in 9 randomized controlled trials. PLoS One 2013;8(1):e54465.
54. Joshipura KJ, Ascherio A, Manson JE, et al. Fruit and vegetable intake in relation to risk of ischemic stroke. JAMA 1999;282(13):1233–9.
55. Estruch R, Ros E, Salas-Salvado J, et al. Primary prevention of cardiovascular disease with a Mediterranean diet. N Engl J Med 2013;368(14):1279–90.
56. Kurth T, Gaziano JM, Berger K, et al. Body mass index and the risk of stroke in men. Arch Intern Med 2002;162(22):2557–62.
57. Rexrode KM, Hennekens CH, Willett WC, et al. A prospective study of body mass index, weight change, and risk of stroke in women. JAMA 1997;277(19):1539–45.
58. Hu G, Tuomilehto J, Silventoinen K, et al. Body mass index, waist circumference, and waist-hip ratio on the risk of total and type-specific stroke. Arch Intern Med 2007;167(13):1420–7.
59. Bibbins-Domingo K, Force USPST. Aspirin use for the primary prevention of cardiovascular disease and colorectal cancer: U.S. preventive services task force recommendation statement. Ann Intern Med 2016;164(12):836–45.
60. Cote R, Battista RN, Abrahamowicz M, et al. Lack of effect of aspirin in asymptomatic patients with carotid bruits and substantial carotid narrowing. The Asymptomatic Cervical Bruit Study Group. Ann Intern Med 1995;123(9):649–55.
61. King A, Shipley M, Markus H, et al. The effect of medical treatments on stroke risk in asymptomatic carotid stenosis. Stroke 2013;44(2):542–6.
62. DD DEW, Morris D, GJ DEB, et al. Asymptomatic carotid artery stenosis: who should be screened, who should be treated and how should we treat them? J Cardiovasc Surg 2017;58(1):3–12.
63. Feigin VL, Krishnamurthi RV, Parmar P, et al. Update on the global burden of ischemic and hemorrhagic stroke in 1990-2013: the GBD 2013 study. Neuroepidemiology 2015;45(3):161–76.
64. Conrad MF, Michalczyk MJ, Opalacz A, et al. The natural history of asymptomatic severe carotid artery stenosis. J Vasc Surg 2014;60(5):1218–25.
65. Nicolaides AN, Kakkos SK, Griffin M, et al. Severity of asymptomatic carotid stenosis and risk of ipsilateral hemispheric ischaemic events: results from the ACSRS study. Eur J Vasc Endovasc Surg 2005;30(3):275–84.
66. Hirt LS. Progression rate and ipsilateral neurological events in asymptomatic carotid stenosis. Stroke 2014;45(3):702–6.
67. Streifler JY, den Hartog AG, Pan S, et al. Ten-year risk of stroke in patients with previous cerebral infarction and the impact of carotid surgery in the Asymptomatic Carotid Surgery Trial. Int J Stroke 2016;11(9):1020–7.

68. Nicolaides AN, Kakkos SK, Kyriacou E, et al. Asymptomatic internal carotid artery stenosis and cerebrovascular risk stratification. J Vasc Surg 2010;52(6): 1486–96.e1-5.
69. Inzitari D, Eliasziw M, Gates P, et al. The causes and risk of stroke in patients with asymptomatic internal-carotid-artery stenosis. North American Symptomatic Carotid Endarterectomy Trial Collaborators. N Engl J Med 2000;342(23):1693–700.
70. Aichner FT, Topakian R, Alberts MJ, et al. High cardiovascular event rates in patients with asymptomatic carotid stenosis: the REACH Registry. Eur J Neurol 2009;16(8):902–8.
71. Muluk SC, Muluk VS, Sugimoto H, et al. Progression of asymptomatic carotid stenosis: a natural history study in 1004 patients. J Vasc Surg 1999;29(2):208–14 [discussion: 214-6].
72. Rockman CB, Riles TS, Lamparello PJ, et al. Natural history and management of the asymptomatic, moderately stenotic internal carotid artery. J Vasc Surg 1997; 25(3):423–31.
73. Sabeti S, Schlager O, Exner M, et al. Progression of carotid stenosis detected by duplex ultrasonography predicts adverse outcomes in cardiovascular high-risk patients. Stroke 2007;38(11):2887–94.
74. Kakkos SK, Nicolaides AN, Charalambous I, et al. Predictors and clinical significance of progression or regression of asymptomatic carotid stenosis. J Vasc Surg 2014;59(4):956–967 e1.
75. Conrad MF, Boulom V, Mukhopadhyay S, et al. Progression of asymptomatic carotid stenosis despite optimal medical therapy. J Vasc Surg 2013;58(1): 128–135 e1.
76. Park YJ, Kim DI, Kim GM, et al. Natural history of asymptomatic moderate carotid artery stenosis in the era of medical therapy. World Neurosurg 2016;91: 247–53.
77. Hogberg D, Bjorck M, Mani K, et al. Five year outcomes in men screened for carotid artery stenosis at 65 years of age: a population based cohort study. Eur J Vasc Endovasc Surg 2019;57(6):759–66.
78. Kakkos SK, Griffin MB, Nicolaides AN, et al. Size of juxtaluminal hypoechoic area in ultrasound images of asymptomatic carotid plaques predicts the occurrence of stroke. J Vasc Surg 2013.
79. Kamtchum-Tatuene J, Noubiap JJ, Wilman AH, et al. Prevalence of high-risk plaques and risk of stroke in patients with asymptomatic carotid stenosis: a meta-analysis. JAMA Neurol 2020;77(12):1524–35.
80. Halliday A, Mansfield A, Marro J, et al. Prevention of disabling and fatal strokes by successful carotid endarterectomy in patients without recent neurological symptoms: randomised controlled trial. Lancet 2004;363(9420):1491–502, published correction appears in Lancet. 2004 Jul 31;364(9432):416.
81. Howard DPJ, Gaziano L, Rothwell PM, et al. Risk of stroke in relation to degree of asymptomatic carotid stenosis: a population-based cohort study, systematic review, and meta-analysis. Lancet Neurol 2021;20(3):193–202.
82. Bulbulia R, Halliday A. The Asymptomatic Carotid Surgery Trial-2 (ACST-2): an ongoing randomised controlled trial comparing carotid endarterectomy with carotid artery stenting to prevent stroke. Health Technol Assess 2017;21(57):1–40.
83. Howard VJ, Meschia JF, Lal BK, et al. Carotid revascularization and medical management for asymptomatic carotid stenosis: Protocol of the CREST-2 clinical trials. Int J Stroke 2017;12(7):770–8.
84. Batchelder AJ, Saratzis A, Naylor AR. Corrigendum to 'overview of primary and secondary analyses from 20 randomised controlled trials comparing carotid

artery stenting with carotid endarterectomy'. Eur J Vasc Endovasc Surg 2020; 59(3):496. European Journal of Vascular & Endovascular Surgery 58/4 (2019) 479-493.

85. Kashyap VS, Schneider PA, Foteh M, et al. Early outcomes in the ROADSTER 2 Study of transcarotid artery revascularization in patients with significant carotid artery disease. Stroke 2020;51(9):2620–9.

Interventions in Carotid Artery Surgery

An Overview of Current Management and Future Implications

Charles Adam Banks, MD, Benjamin J. Pearce, MD*

KEYWORDS

- Carotid artery endarterectomy • Transfemoral carotid artery stent
- Transcarotid artery revascularization • Carotid artery disease
- Carotid artery shunting

KEY POINTS

- Interventions in carotid artery surgery have evolved over time to include carotid endarterectomy (CEA) as the gold standard, transfemoral carotid artery stenting (TFCAS), and hybrid transcarotid artery revascularization (TCAR).
- Surgical outcomes regarding neuromonitoring techniques and intraoperative shunting during CEA have remained relatively controversial.
- The primary outcome of perioperative stroke has remained superior in CEA and TCAR compared with TFCAS.

BRIEF HISTORY OF CAROTID ARTERY SURGERY

Carotid artery anatomy and the consequences of extracranial vascular compromise were described as early as 400 BC by Hippocrates in ancient Grecian literature.[1,2] Throughout early history extending from the Middle Ages to the late 1800s, neurovascular surgical experience was largely limited to military-related cervical trauma requiring arterial or venous ligation.[1,2] In the early 1900s, carotid artery surgery was expanded to more complex arterial reconstructions in trauma, oncological operations, and carotid occlusive disease.[1]

In the modern era, the technique of carotid endarterectomy (CEA) was first described by DeBakey and colleagues [3] and Cooley and colleagues[4] for symptomatic carotid artery stenosis. In their report, Cooley and colleagues described the utilization of an internal carotid artery (ICA) shunt to maintain cerebral perfusion during the procedure. These

Division of Vascular Surgery and Endovascular Therapy, University of Alabama at Birmingham, 1808 7th Avenue South, Boshell Diabetes Building 652, Birmingham, AL 35294, USA
* Corresponding author.
E-mail address: bjpearce@uabmc.edu

Surg Clin N Am 103 (2023) 645–671
https://doi.org/10.1016/j.suc.2023.05.003
surgical.theclinics.com
0039-6109/23/© 2023 Elsevier Inc. All rights reserved.

methods were refined over the next several decades with introduction of carotid artery patch angioplasty (1967), prosthetic interposition bypasses, transluminal angioplasty (1977), and carotid artery stenting (1993).[1] These treatment modalities have continued to evolve over the last several decades. In this article, the authors discuss the natural history of extracranial carotid artery occlusive disease, currently available operative therapy, and the future implications of evolving technologies.

NATURAL HISTORY OF CAROTID ATHEROSCLEROSIS

Stroke is one of the leading causes of disability and death with an estimated 25 million neurologic events annually worldwide.[5] The prevalence of cerebrovascular accident (CVA) in the United States is approximately 800,000 cases each year of which 23% are recurrent strokes.[6,7] The vast majority (87%) of all strokes are ischemic in nature with approximately 20% attributable to extracranial carotid artery atherosclerotic disease.[8,9] The prevalence of asymptomatic and symptomatic carotid artery atherosclerosis varies significantly with age, sex, and race (**Fig. 1**).[10–12] In patients less than 50 years old, the prevalence of moderate degree carotid artery atherosclerosis is 0.2% compared with 7.5% in patients greater than 79 years of age.[10] African American and Hispanic patients are at higher risk to experience ischemic strokes associated with intracranial vascular disease and hypertension.[11] However, Caucasian and Native American men are at a higher risk of experiencing moderate to severe extracranial carotid artery disease especially after age 65 years (see **Fig. 1**). Last, female patients demonstrate a lower prevalence of carotid artery disease but experience significantly greater 1-year mortality after index stroke at 36%.[6]

Risk factors associated with carotid artery occlusive disease are consistent with other sites of cardiovascular atherosclerosis. Primary modifiable risk factors include hypertension, diabetes mellltus (DM), tobacco smoking, and hyperlipidemia.[9] Hypertension is an independent risk factor for stroke with associated 35% to 45% increased risk of neurologic infarction with every 10 mm Hg elevation in systolic blood pressure (SBP).[13] The

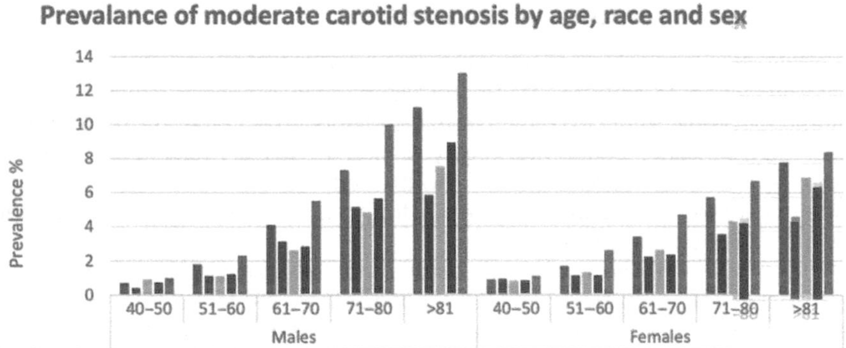

Prevalance of moderate carotid stenosis by age, race and sex

	40–50	51–60	61–70	71–80	>81	40–50	51–60	61–70	71–80	>81
			Males					Females		
■ Caucasian	0.7	1.8	4.1	7.3	11	0.9	1.7	3.4	5.7	7.8
■ Asian	0.4	1.1	3.1	5.1	5.8	0.9	1.1	2.2	3.5	4.6
■ African American	0.9	1.1	2.6	4.8	7.5	0.8	1.3	2.6	4.3	6.9
■ Hispanic	0.7	1.2	2.8	5.6	8.9	0.8	1.1	2.3	4.5	6.6
■ Native American	1	2.3	5.5	10	13	1.1	2.6	4.7	6.7	8.4

■ Caucasian   ■ Asian   ■ African American   ■ Hispanic   ■ Native American

Fig. 1. Prevalence of carotid artery stenosis (>50%). (*From* Rockman CB, Hoang H, Guo Y, et al. The prevalence of carotid artery stenosis varies significantly by race. J Vasc Surg 2013;57:327–37; with permission.)

relationship between DM and vascular disease has been well established.[9,14] DM is an independent risk factor for ischemic stroke with increased annual risk compared with the general population.[14] Studies have demonstrated that diabetic patients experience alterations in epithelial cell function with increased intima-medial hyperplasia accounting for accelerated progression of carotid artery disease.[9,14] Patients with fasting hyperglycemia are at a near twofold increased risk of stroke at all ages.[15]

Cigarette smoking is associated with accelerated plaque progression and increases the risk of stroke by fourfold when compared with nonsmokers.[16,17] Other significant risk factors include age, race, family history, obesity, diet, and renal insufficiency. As vascular patients are typically a highly comorbid population, these risk factors are often compounded with exponential increase in risk of disease progression and stroke (**Fig. 2**).

MEDICAL MANAGEMENT OF CAROTID ARTERY OCCLUSIVE DISEASE

Initial treatment for carotid artery disease is systemic and requires modulation of patient risk factors to limit disease progression and reduce risk of stroke. Aggressive antihypertensive regimens have been associated with significant stroke risk reduction. Maintaining SBP less than 120 provides a 50% decrease in overall risk of stroke.[6,18] The increase in stroke risk associated with tobacco smoking is dose-dependent, and patients who successfully stop smoking have similar risk of stroke compared with the general population.[19] Therefore, it is imperative that vascular surgeons counsel patients regarding increased stroke risk and plaque progression associated with cigarette smoking. Nicotine replacement therapy and medical management

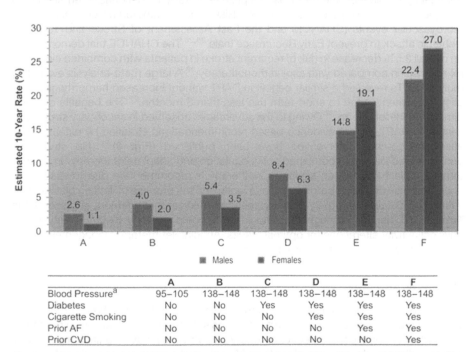

	A	B	C	D	E	F
Blood Pressure[a]	95–105	138–148	138–148	138–148	138–148	138–148
Diabetes	No	No	Yes	Yes	Yes	Yes
Cigarette Smoking	No	No	No	Yes	Yes	Yes
Prior AF	No	No	No	No	Yes	Yes
Prior CVD	No	No	No	No	No	Yes

Fig. 2. A 10 year estimated risk of stroke in males and females stratified by risk factors. [a]Closest range for women are: 95–104 and 115–124. (*From* Benjamin EJ, et al. Heart disease and stroke statistics; 2017 update: a report from the American Heart Association. Circulation. 2017;135:e146–e603; with permission.)

with bupropion, varenicline, and nortriptyline have demonstrated efficacy as adjunctive therapy in smoking cessation.[9] In our experience, however, no tobacco cessation adjunct is independently successful and ultimately works best when the patient is committed to quitting smoking.

Hyperlipidemia is a well-defined risk factor in coronary artery disease, but some uncertainty exists as to the direct role of lipid dysregulation in formation of carotid plaque.[9] However, decreasing low-density lipoprotein (LDL) levels and increasing high-density lipoprotein levels (HDL) have been associated with significant decrease in stroke and cardiovascular risk in several large studies.[20] More importantly, the beneficial effects of statin therapy have been demonstrated in the perioperative setting as well with significant decrease in perioperative stroke and mortality after CEA in symptomatic and asymptomatic cases.[21] In addition, statin therapy is associated with regression of intima-medial hyperplasia, slowing of plaque progression, and plaque stabilization.[22] In the Stroke Prevention by Aggressive Reduction of Cholesterol Levels randomized controlled trial (RCT), patients with carotid artery stenosis treated with atorvastatin had a decreased overall risk of stroke of 33%.[23] If patients are unable to tolerate statin therapy or if older (>75 years), moderate intensity statins are recommended (pravastatin or simvastatin).[9]

Antiplatelet therapy in patients with carotid artery stenosis has been well described for secondary prevention in symptomatic patients.[9] Multiple RCTs have demonstrated the efficacy of timely initiation of aspirin at the time of ischemic stroke with a 60% decrease in recurrent stroke at 6-weeks.[24] Owing to the increased plaque instability during acute ischemic stroke, maximum medical management has been considered with combining antiplatelet agents.[9] Dual antiplatelet therapy (DAPT) has been studied in multiple RCTs including Clopidogrel in High-Risk Patients with Acute Non-disabling Cerebrovascular events (CHANCE) and the Fast Assessment of Stroke and Transient ischemic attack to prevent Early Recurrence trials.[25,26] The CHANCE trial demonstrated an overall 3.5% decrease in risk of recurrent stroke in patients with combined clopidogrel and aspirin compared with aspirin monotherapy.[26] A large meta-analysis evaluating multiple RCTs revealed a similar benefit in DAPT without increased hemorrhagic complications when limited to short-term use less than 3 months.[27] The benefits of DAPT diminish in the long term.[27] Owing to the advantages observed in secondary stroke prevention in DAPT, recent evidence-based recommendations stratified by extent of disease and planned intervention have been published (**Fig. 3**).[28] No study has demonstrated benefit in combined anticoagulation and antiplatelet therapy. In asymptomatic patients, low-dose aspirin monotherapy is recommended due to associated decreased risk of stroke, cardiovascular events, and the premise of limiting platelet activation.[29] A detailed summary of recommended medical management is presented in **Table 1**. All medical management should be accompanied by dietary, lifestyle, and physical activity alterations for optimal results. Antiplatelet therapy management varies with modality of operative repair and will be discussed in later sections.

SCREENING AND IMAGING

There are no current guidelines recommending general population screening of asymptomatic patients for carotid artery stenosis. Screening should be limited to patients who are being considered for coronary artery bypass, have significant peripheral vascular disease, or who are older than 65 with multiple atherosclerotic risk factors including a history of current or prior smoking. Initially, digital subtraction angiography (DSA) was the only means for the detection of carotid artery stenosis. In the North American Symptomatic Carotid Endarterectomy Trial (NASCET), DSA was used as

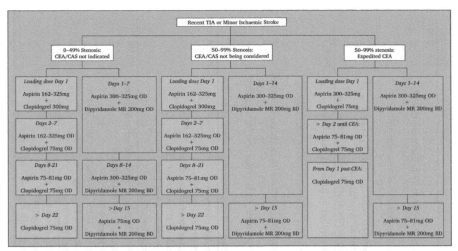

Fig. 3. Graphic representation of recommendations regarding DAPT after acute ischemic stroke or Transient Ischemic Attack (TIA). (*From* Naylor AR, McCabe DJH. New Data and the Covid-19 Pandemic Mandate a Rethink of Antiplatelet Strategies in Patients With TIA or Minor Stroke Associated With Atherosclerotic Carotid Stenosis. Eur J Vasc Endovasc Surg. 2020;59(6):861-865; with permission.)

the primary imaging modality by measuring the ratio between the luminal depression within the stenosis and the distal ICA.[30–32] The imaging guidelines derived from NAS-CET are the most widely accepted consensus criteria for determining extent of carotid artery disease. This trial also introduced the use of duplex ultrasonography (DUS) for carotid disease evaluation and provided a valuable repository to define correlation between DSA and DUS imaging of carotid stenosis. Owing to the invasive nature of DSA, risk of perioperative stroke, and intravenous contrast load, DUS has emerged as the primary imaging modality for screening and surveillance imaging of carotid artery disease.[9,32,33]

The utilization of DUS presents a noninvasive and cost-effective imaging alternative for carotid artery stenosis.[9] Prior studies have compared angiographic measurements of percent ICA stenosis to DUS peak systolic velocities (PSVs) to develop consensus criteria for diagnosing different degrees of carotid artery stenosis.[32] DUS produces a greyscale visual representation of the vessel and plaque morphology as well as Doppler color-flow allowing for visual depiction of non-laminar flow. In addition, DUS generates spectral analysis for graphical representation of flow pattern, systolic, and diastolic velocities (**Fig. 4**). Primary parameters for determining degree of carotid artery stenosis are ICA PSV and plaque morphology with percent of plaque occlusion estimated by B-mode imaging. Discriminating features of DUS can increase specificity for significant disease; these secondary parameters include end-diastolic velocity and ICA-to-common carotid artery (CCA).[32] Overall, DUS demonstrates high sensitivity and specificity at 89% and 84%, respectively.[34] However, DUS is not without limitations. Variability in operator, lower sensitivity/specificity in moderate degree stenosis, vessel tortuosity, and high lesions present significant challenge in obtaining reliable results.[32] In these cases, computed tomography angiogram (CTA) or magnetic resonance angiography may be necessary for complete evaluation arterial anatomy. CTA has excellent sensitivity/specificity similar to DSA and allow for evaluation of the aortic arch and detailed operative planning. Patient surveillance imaging frequency

Table 1
Current recommendations and evidence for optimal medical management of carotid artery disease

Modification	Regimen	Key Evidence	Sources
Antihypertensives	• ACE inhibitor, calcium-channel blockers, Beta-blockers, others • Permissive hypertension intraoperatively • Postoperatively is beneficial (SBP 140–160)	• Maintain BP 130/70 • 10 mm Hg SBP decrease affords 33% decrease risk of stroke • Permissive hypertension beneficial in symptomatic patients • ACE inhibitors associated with decrease in plaque progression and intimal hyperplasia • Beta-blockers afford perioperative stroke protection	13,19,37,96,97
Antiplatelet therapy	• Aspirin monotherapy • Some advocate for DAPT	• Daily aspirin recommended in patients >50 with cardiovascular risk • Approximately 15%–60% recurrent stroke reduction with aspirin alone • Anticoagulation combined with antiplatelet provides no benefit • CHANCE trial: DAPT affords 3.5% reduction in recurrent stroke • Postoperative dextran reduces embolic events after CEA	24,98–100
Lipid-lowering therapy	• High-intensity statin (atorvastatin 40–80 mg daily, rosuvastatin 20–40 mg daily) • LDL < 70 mg/dL; total cholesterol <170 mg/dL; HDL > 60 mg/dL	• 15%–30% decrease risk of stroke • Decreases recurrent stroke by 42% • Increased HDL reduces stroke risk 14% • 300% decrease in risk of stroke after CEA • Fourfold decrease in stroke after CAS • Superior survival after CAS/CEA	101–104
Smoking cessation	• Smoking cessation or reduction • Combination of counseling and medical adjuncts	• Smokers 5x more likely to develop carotid atherosclerosis • High risk of developing severe stenosis • Increases plaque progression • Varenicline, bupropion, Nicotine Replacement Therapy, nortriptyline show similar efficacy • Diabetes is risk factor for stroke	105,106
Diabetes control	• Maintain A1C < 7.0 to minimize micro- and macro-vascular disease	• No evidence showing decreased risk with improved A1C or aggressive glycemic control • Diabetes is associated with intimal hyperplasia	14,15,107

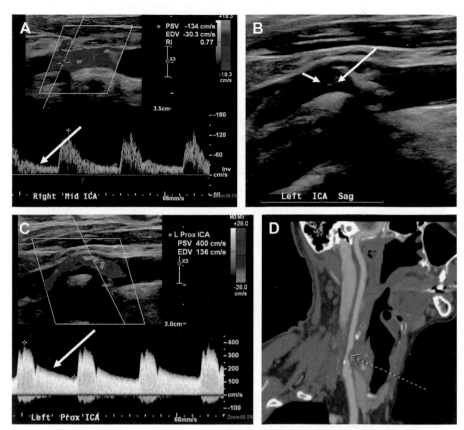

Fig. 4. Duplex Ultrasonography (DUS) diagnostic imaging. (*A*) Normal carotid DUS with preservation of spectral window (*arrow*) and laminar flow. (*B*) ICA plaque with echolucent (*short arrow*) and echogenic properties (*long arrow*). (*C*) ICA velocity at 400 cm/s with blurring of the spectral window (*arrow*). (*D*) CTA demonstrating proximal ICA stenosis (*dotted Arrow*).

varies based on the degree of ICA stenosis. DUS consensus criteria for carotid artery stenosis have been published and validated.[9,32,34] The recommended surveillance intervals are presented in **Table 2**.

CAROTID ARTERY ENDARTERECTOMY

The primary goal of optimal medical therapy, surveillance imaging, and operative management is to mitigate the risk of stroke associated with progressive carotid

Table 2 Current consensus criteria for follow-up surveillance and operative management of carotid artery stenosis	
Degree of Stenosis	**Surveillance Frequency**
0%–50% Stenosis	Every 1–2 y
50%–69%	Every 6–12 mo
>/ = 70%; less than near occlusion	Consideration for revascularization
Near occlusion	Consideration for revascularization

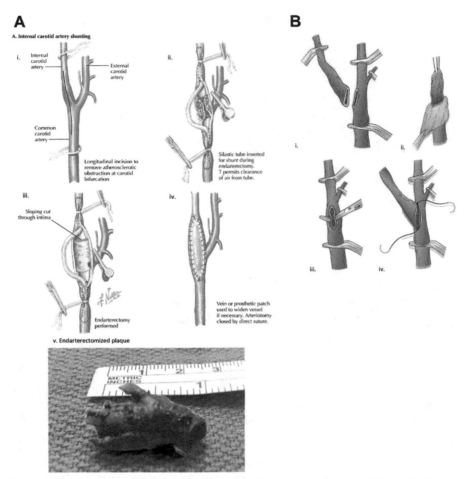

Fig. 5. (*A*) Representation of traditional CEA with shunt versus no shunt: (i) Longitudinal arteriotomy (ii) Shunt placement (iii) Endarterectomy performed (iv) Patch angioplasty with bovine pericardial patch or vein (v) Endarterectomized plaque from carotid bifurcation. (*B*) Eversion endarterectomy with oblique transection of ICA with primary reimplantation (i) Transection of the internal carotid artery from carotid bifurcation (ii) Eversion endarterectomy performed (iii) Completion endarterectomy (iv) Reimplantation of internal carotid artery to carotid bifurcation. ([*A*] *From* Hardy DM, Perry W. Carotid Endarterectomy. In: Delaney CP. Netter's Surgical Anatomy and Approaches, Second Edition. Chapter 41, pp 431-440; and [*B*] Sidawy AN PB, ed. Rutherford's Vascular Surgery and Endovascular Therapy, 10th Edition. 10th Edition ed. Elsevier; 2023.)

atherosclerotic disease. The underlying mechanism of carotid-based CVA is understood to be embolic in nature and successful stroke prevention relies on successful exclusion of at-risk plaque and associated debris from the cerebral circulation. CEA is a well-established surgical technique and is considered the gold standard for operative management of carotid artery disease (**Fig. 5**). Many randomized controlled trials regarding CEA have been conducted over the last several decades with a primary focus on symptomatic versus asymptomatic disease.

Symptomatic Carotid Artery Stenosis

The European Carotid Surgery Trial (ECST) and NASCET are the foundational trials comparing optimal medical management (OMT) with CEA for symptomatic carotid artery disease with high-grade carotid artery stenosis.[30,31,35] OMT involved in the initiation of aspirin, antihypertensives, and smoking cessation. NASCET demonstrated an overall risk of recurrent ipsilateral stroke with OMT of 26% versus 9% in patients undergoing CEA and a 10.6% risk reduction in debilitating/fatal stroke at 2 years after CEA.[30] Results from NASCET demonstrate that CEA confers significant risk reduction of ipsilateral stroke at 3 years in patients with moderate (50%–69%) to severe stenosis (70%–99%) at 6.5% and 19.4%, respectively.[36] However, this benefit is not seen in patients with mild disease (<50% stenosis). Secondary analyses of NASCET have demonstrated that patients with increasing number of risk factors for stroke (>/ = 7 risk factors) experience a 39% risk of stroke at 2 years with OMT alone.[30] Although differences in experimental design exist, ECST revealed similar findings demonstrating a 14% risk reduction for ipsilateral stroke at 3 years in patient with severe carotid artery stenosis (70%–99%).[35] In their final analysis, ECST demonstrated long-term advantage of CEA compared with OMT with a 5.7% 5 year stroke/death reduction in moderate stenosis and 21.2% in severe stenosis.[37] Perioperative risk (30 days from CEA) of stroke/death ranged from 5.8% to 7.9% in moderate to severe stenosis.[30,36,37] Other studies investigating the long-term durability of CEA have revealed excellent results with 10-year ipsilateral stroke risk of 9.7% and restenosis rate (>70%) of 2.2% at 12 years (**Table 3**).[38,39]

The importance of CEA timing in symptomatic patients remains a matter of debate. Traditionally, CEA was reserved up to 6 weeks due to concerns for high perioperative risk and hemorrhagic conversion. However, emerging data have demonstrated no difference in perioperative stroke risk in patients undergoing CEA at 14 days versus 6 weeks.[40] Current recommendations are to consider patients for CEA within 14 days of acute event due to the recurrent stroke risk at 14 days of 20% and 37% at 1 year.[40] In fact, appropriate time interval to CEA within the 14-day window continues to be refined. In one study involving 8404 patients within the Vascular Quality Initiative (VQI), patients with CEA performed at 8 to 14 days experienced lower rates of in-hospital stroke or mortality compared with earlier or later time intervals.[41] Other studies advocate for earlier CEA (3–7 days) in acutely symptomatic patients due to improved neurologic deficit at discharge, perioperative stroke rate of 2.74% to 3.4%, myocardial infarction (MI) rate of 1.3% and 1-year stroke rate of 5%.[42,43] Urgent CEA (<24 hours) is indicated In patients presenting with crescendo transient ischemic attacks or ischemic stroke in evolution to prevent propagation of neurologic deficit.[9,40] Urgent CEA in patients with unstable neurologic status or unstable atherosclerotic plaque has been performed with perioperative stroke ranging from 2.2% to 10%.[40,44] However, even in the most contemporary studies, the highest risk for perioperative complication exists in patients undergoing CEA less than 24 hours from onset of neurologic deficit. As such, this should be reserved only for those with compounding neurologic deficits as described above. Based on these data, our practice has shifted to offering CEA to post-CVA patients at greater than 48 hours from initial neurologic deficit but before hospital discharge.

One caveat to these recommendations is assessment for potential hemorrhagic conversion in those with large volume ischemic parenchyma within the cerebrum. Pini and colleagues[45] demonstrated that patients experiencing debilitating strokes with findings of large volume cerebral ischemia (>4000 mm^3) and profound neurologic deficit may benefit from a delayed CEA to 4 weeks due to decreased perioperative

Table 3
Important randomized controlled trials comparing carotid endarterectomy to optimal medical management and transfemoral carotid artery stenting as well as early transcarotid artery revascularization trials

Study	Study Size	Purpose	Stroke (>30 D)	Mortality (>30 D)	CNI	Myocardial Infarction (>30 D)	Long-Term Stroke
NASCET[30]	N = 1415	OMT vs CEA (symptomatic)	CEA 5.5% OMT 3.3%	CEA 0.6% OMT 0.3%	CEA 7.6%	CEA 0.9%	2 y: CEA 9% OMT 26%
ECST[35]	N = 3018	OMT vs CEA (symptomatic)	CEA 7.5%	CEA 1.0%	—	—	5 y: CEA reduces stroke risk by 21.2% (70%–99% stenosis) and 5.7% (50%–69%)
VACS-1[108]	N = 309	OMT vs CEA (symptomatic)	CEA 2.2% OMT 6%	CEA 3.3%	CEA 5%	CEA 2%	1 y: CEA 7.7% 1 y OMT 19.4% (P = 0.01)
VACS-2[109]	N = 444	OMT vs CEA (asymptomatic)	CEA 8.0% OMT 20.6% (P < 0.001)	CEA 1.9% OMT 1.3%	CEA 3.8%	CEA 3.8%	—
ACAS[33]	N = 1662	OMT vs CEA (asymptomatic)	CEA 2.3% OMT 0.4% (P = 0.004)	**	—	CEA 0.1%	5 y: CEA 5.1% OMT 11%

	N	Comparison					
ACST[46,47]	N = 3120	OMT vs CEA (asymptomatic)	CEA 3.1%	CEA 0.6% OMT 0.1%	—	CEA 0.6%	5 y: CEA 3.8% OMT 11% (P < 0.001) 10 y: CEA 13.4% OMT 1 7.9%
SAPPHIRE[110,111]	N = 334	CEA vs TFCAS (symptomatic; asymptomatic)	TFCAS 3.1% CEA 3.3% (P = 0.94)	TFCAS 0.6% CEA 2.0%	TFCAS 0% CEA 5.3% (P = 0.003)	TFCAS 1.9% CEA 6.6% (P = 0.04)	3 y: TFCAS 10.1% CEA 1 0.7% (P = 0.99)
EVA-3S[65,112]	N = 527	CEA vs TFCAS (symptomatic)	TFCAS 8.8% CEA 2.7% (P = 0.004)	TFCAS 0.8% CEA 1.2% (P = 0.68)	TFCAS 1.1% CEA 7.7% (P < 0.001)	TFCAS 0.4% CEA 0.6% (P = 0.62)	4 y: TFCAS 11.1% CEA 6.2% (P = 0.03)
SPACE-1[113]	N = 1,200	CEA vs TFCAS (symptomatic)	TFCAS 6.84% CEA 6.34% (P = 0.09)	TFCAS 0.7% CEA 0.9%	—	None reported for TFCAS or CEA	2 y: TFCAS 9.5% CEA 8.8% (P = 0.62)
SPACE-2[114]	N = 513	CEA vs TFCAS vs OMT (asymptomatic)	TFCAS 2.5% CEA 2.5% OMT 0% (P = 0.24)	Zero deaths for any group	—	Zero reported for any group	1 y: TFCAS 4.1% CEA 3.9% OMT 0.9% (P = 0.26)
ICSS[70]	N = 1,713	CEA vs TFCAS (symptomatic)	TFCAS 7.4% CEA 4.0% (P = 0.003)	TFCAS 1.3% CEA 0.72% (P = 0.017)	TFCAS 0.1% CEA 0.1%	TFCAS 0.4% CEA 0.6%	120 d: TFCAS 7.7% CEA 5.2% (P = 0.006)

(continued on next page)

Table 3
(continued)

Study	Study Size	Purpose	Stroke (>30 D)	Mortality (>30 D)	CNI	Myocardial Infarction (>30 D)	Long-Term Stroke
ACT-1[71]	N = 1,453	CEA vs TFCAS (asymptomatic)	*TFCAS* 2.8% *CEA* 1.4% (P = 0.23)	*TFCAS* 0.1% *CEA* 0.3% (P = 0.43)	*TFCAS* 0.1% *CEA* 1.1% (P = 0.02)	*TFCAS* 0.5% *CEA* 0.9% (P = 0.41)	5 y: *TFCAS* 6.9% *CEA* 5.3% (P = 0.44)
ACST-2[72]	N = 3625	CEA vs TFCAS (asymptomatic)	*TFCAS* 3.6% *CEA* 2.4% (P = 0.06)	*TFCAS* 0.9% *CEA* 1.0% (P = 0.77)	*CEA* 5.4%	*TFCAS* 0.3% *CEA* 0.7% (P = 0.15)	5 y: *TFCAS* 5.3% *CEA* 4.5% (P = 0.33)
CREST-1[67,68]	N = 2,502	CEA vs TFCAS (asymptomatic, symptomatic)	*TFCAS* 4.1% *CEA* 2.3% (P = 0.01)	*TFCAS* 0.7% *CEA* 0.3% (P = 0.18)	*TFCAS* 0.3% *CEA* 4.7% (P = 0.07)	*TFCAS* 1.1% *CEA* 2.3% (P = 0.03)	10 y: *TFCAS* 6.9% *CEA* 5.6% (P = 0.96)
ROADSTER-1[84]	N = 141	TCAR (symptomatic; asymptomatic)	1.4%	1.4%	0.7%	0.7%	–
ROADSTER-2[86]	N = 692	TCAR (symptomatic; asymptomatic)	0.6% (1.9% in non-protocol group)	0.2%	1.4%	0.9%	–

Abbreviations: ACAS, Asymptomatic Carotid Atherosclerosis Study; ACST, Asymptomatic Carotid Surgery Trial; ACT-1, Asymptomatic Carotid Trial; CEA, carotid endarterectomy; CREST, Carotid Revascularization Endarterectomy versus Stenting Trial; ECST, European Carotid Surgery Trial; EVA-3S, Endarterectomy Versus Angioplasty in Patients with Symptomatic Severe Carotid Stenosis; ICSS, International Carotid Stenting Study; NASCET, North American Symptomatic Carotid Endarterectomy Trial; ROADSTER, Reverse Flow Used During Carotid Stenting Procedure; SAPPHIRE, Stenting and Angioplasty with Protection in Patients at High Risk for Endarterectomy; SPACE, stent-protected angioplasty versus carotid endarterectomy; TCAR, transcarotid artery revascularization; TFCAS, transfemoral carotid artery stenting; VACS, Veterans Affairs Cooperative Study. **Perioperative stroke and mortality reported as composite outcome.

stroke rate from 13.9% to 1.7%.[45] Overall, timing of intervention in symptomatic patients requires further study to elucidate the optimal time interval for CEA.

Asymptomatic Carotid Artery Stenosis

The role of CEA as a prophylactic operation in asymptomatic carotid artery stenosis was established by the landmark RCTs Asymptomatic Carotid Atherosclerosis Study (ACAS) and Asymptomatic Carotid Surgery Trial (ACST-1).[33,46] These studies evaluated asymptomatic patients with carotid artery stenosis of 60% to 99% stenosis by arteriography. In 1662 patients, ACAS demonstrated that CEA plus aspirin conferred a risk reduction of 6% at 2.7-year follow-up when compared with OMT alone (11% vs 5%).[33] ACST demonstrated similar results at 5 years with lower ipsilateral stroke rate in CEA group (6.9%) compared with OMT alone (10.9%).[46,47] This advantage in CEA group was demonstrated again at 10 years with 13.4% stroke rate in CEA group compared with 17.9% in OMT group.[47] Patients experienced a perioperative stroke risk of 2.3% in ACAS and 3.1% in ACST. In addition, annual stroke risk was 1% to 1.1% in patients undergoing CEA compared with 2% to 3% annual risk in OMT patients in these RCTs (see **Table 3**).[33,46]

Much criticism is lavished on those advocating for aggressive treatment of asymptomatic disease with the main critique being that OMT in historical papers did not incorporate modern anti-lipid and antiplatelet agents. However, a small study consisting of 55 patients receiving modern OMT including statin therapy further demonstrated a benefit in patients undergoing CEA with the risk reduction of 17.6%.[48]

Modern OMT consists of high-intensity statin, antihypertensives, antiplatelet medications, and modification of other risk factors such as DM and smoking cessation. Multidisciplinary approaches and the consistent implementation of modern OMT have decreased significantly with annual stroke risk in patients with carotid artery stenosis of 50% to 99% estimated at 1% in 2005.[49] As the OMT for asymptomatic carotid artery disease evolves, further studies will be required to elucidate a true benefit in OMT alone. Although revascularization for asymptomatic carotid artery disease remains under investigation, the current recommendations are for consideration of revascularization in patients with greater than 80% stenosis on DUS, a life expectancy greater than 5 years, and a surgeon with operative mortality/stroke risk of less than 3%.[9]

Operative Techniques

Conventional CEA (CCEA) is a well-established technique (see **Fig. 5**). Closure technique (primary closure vs patch angioplasty) has been investigated in multiple RCTs and meta-analyses. Patch angioplasty is favored due to the decreased risk of restenosis rate greater than 50% stenosis (1.1%–11.9% vs 3.1%–33%, respectively), decreased rate of perioperative stroke/death (1.5%–1.6% vs 4.5%), and decreased in long-term stroke (1.6% vs 4.8%).[50,51] In addition, options for patch material include synthetic (Polytetrafluoroethylene or Dacron), autogenous vein (saphenous or neck vein), or bovine pericardium.[9] One meta-analysis demonstrated no difference between synthetic or autogenous patch in perioperative stroke, restenosis, or wound infection rates.[50]

A smaller subset of surgeons uses the eversion CEA (ECEA). This technique involves transection of the ICA with endarterectomy of the distal CCA/bifurcation with reflection of the ICA adventitia and media for completion endarterectomy (see **Fig. 5**).[9] The ICA is then primarily reimplanted. This technique has demonstrated utility in short-segment lesions at the bifurcation, tortuous or redundant ICAs, or high bifurcations.[9] Proponents of this technique point to the decreased risk of suture line for bleeding and shorter clamp times for cerebral ischemia. However, multiple RCTs including EVEREST (EVERsion CEA vs Standard Trial), meta-analyses, and VQI data have demonstrated no difference between patched CCEA and ECEA regarding perioperative stroke/death or postoperative complications.[52–54] In fact, recent VQI data set has shown that the single strongest determinant of prevention of postoperative bleeding and return to operating room (OR) for hematoma was protamine administration and it is now recommended at case conclusion unless significant adverse reaction to protamine or allergy is expected.[55]

Neuromonitoring and Intraoperative Shunting

There are multiple modalities for neuromonitoring in patients undergoing carotid surgery, including operation with regional anesthesia, electroencephalogram (EEG), somatosensory evoked potential monitoring (SSEP), transcranial Doppler (TCD), or cerebral oximetry. These methods along with the measurement of intraoperative distal CCA stump pressure (SP) are used to determine the requirement for intraoperative shunting to reduce cerebral ischemia.[10] No data have determined superior modality of neuromonitoring under general anesthesia (GA).[56] However, performing CEA under local anesthesia mitigates the inherent risk of GA and provides the most accurate assessment of neurologic changes indicating need for intraoperative shunting.[10,57] However, local anesthesia has been associated with increase in patient anxiety and difficulty maintaining operative positioning, limiting its application.[56] Based on VQI analysis, only 16% of surgeons perform CEA under local anesthesia in the modern era.[58] The most used criteria for selective shunting in various methods of neuromonitoring are presented in **Table 4**.

The practice of intraoperative shunting during CEA has remained controversial and is used at variable rates nationally.[59] It is understood that cross-clamping during CEA is associated with cerebral hypoperfusion and can result in neurologic injury.[9] Intraoperative shunting during CEA is primarily divided into routine shunting, routine non-shunting, and selective shunting. Within the VQI, approximately 6% of surgeons never shunt, 44% selectively shunt, and 50% routinely shunt.[58] Preoperatively, the decision to shunt is primarily based on preoperative anatomy and assessment of the adequacy of collateral cerebral perfusion and contralateral disease burden as well as availability of neuromonitoring devices and patient symptom status. Intraoperatively, the decision is based on neurologic deficits in local anesthesia or changes in neuromonitoring (see **Table 4**).[59,60] This is balanced against the risk of intraoperative embolic event, dissection, and nerve injury related to shunt placement as well as decreased visualization of the lesion and increased operative times.[59,60] In the literature, approximately 10% to 15% of patients undergoing CEA will require shunting secondary to poor collateral perfusion.[56] One prospective study comparing outcomes after selective shunting based on SP and routine shunting in 102 patients revealed a perioperative stroke rate of 0% and 2%, respectively ($P = 0.498$).[61] In addition, a systematic review revealed similar findings with a stroke rate in routine shunting of 1.4% compared with 2% in no shunting.[56] This study also demonstrated no significant difference in perioperative stroke rate based on the method of neuromonitoring used (1.6% EEG, 4.8% TCD, 1.6% SP, and 1.8% SSEP).[56] These results were further corroborated by a Cochrane review including 1270 patients and a VQI study of greater than 28,000 patients that demonstrated no significant difference in perioperative stroke or death between routine shunting and not shunting regardless of method of neuromonitoring. However, neither study could provide recommendations or against routine shunting.[58,62] Other studies have revealed selective shunting subjects patients to a higher risk of stroke when compared with routine shunting or non-shunting.[58,59,63] These findings are similar in asymptomatic and symptomatic patients.[59,63] Overall, the decision to shunt remains by surgeon preference and perceived risk of stroke to the patient.

Table 4
Different modalities for neuromonitoring and accepted criteria for selective shunting

Method	Utility	Description	Selective Shunting	Perioperative Stroke Risk	Shunt Rate
EEG	49% of surgeons	• Provides continuous preoperative and intraoperative monitoring • Sensitivity 70% • Specificity 96% • Can be negatively affected by anesthesia and change in body temperature • Requires specialist for interpretation	• 50% slowing of waveforms, increase frequency of theta waves at test clamp	0%–5.2%	7.5%–24%
TCD	<13% of surgeons	• Measures MCA velocities by Doppler • Sensitivity 81% • Specificity 92% • No temporal window in 20% of patients • Only 60% predictive of ischemia	• Decrease in MCA velocities, detection of embolic events, and restoration of velocity after clamp removal	3.0%–6.1%	10%–19%
Regional anesthesia	16% of surgeons	• Regional anesthesia, procedure performed awake	• Direct observation of neurological changes with test clamp	0.5%–3.0%	4.5%–11.5%
SSEP	<13% of surgeons	• Cerebral reaction to peripheral stimuli • Sensitivity 100% • Specificity 94%	• 50% decrease in amplitude or 10% delayed response in evoked potentials • Limited only to somatosensory pathways	0.3%–5.0%	4.5%–17%
Stump pressure	18% of surgeons	• Measurement of back-bleeding pressure by inserting 21-gauge needle into distal CCA • Sensitivity 75% • Specificity 88%	• Decreased stump pressure >50 mm Hg	0.3%–8.0%	7%–21%
Cerebral oximetry	<13% of surgeons	• Spectroscopy-detecting oxygen saturation of hemoglobin in cerebral capillaries • Straight-forward interpretation • Sensitivity 30%–80% • Specificity 77%–98%	• Decrease 10%–25% of cerebral oximetry	2.1%	11%

Abbreviations: EEG, electroencephalogram; MCA, middle cerebral artery; SSEP, somatosensory evoked potentials; TCD, transcranial Doppler.

Wiske 2018[58]; AbuRahma 2011[34]; Li 2017[116]; Sihotsky 2018[115]

TRANSFEMORAL CAROTID ARTERY STENTING

Although implemented with great success, CEA is limited in high operative risk patients. The risk of CEA to the patient is best considered in terms of either medical risk of surgery or anatomic risk of carotid exposure. High medical risk is typically attributed to factors exacerbated by the stress of surgery (even under local) such as active coronary ischemia; fluid shifts with GA especially congestive heart failure (CHF); and pulmonary embarrassment. Anatomic risk is attributed to the difficulty of exposure in prior operative or radiated fields leading to increase the incidence of cranial nerve injury (CNI) and/or bleeding, high carotid lesions making distal clamping to plaque difficult, or contralateral vocal cord palsy which could infer permanent airway deficit with a second insult. The combination of anatomic and medical high-risk features confers greater incidence of perioperative stroke and MI.[10] Specifically, in patients with prior neck irradiation, the risk of CNI during CEA has been reported as high as 9.2%.[64] To mitigate these risks and extend carotid artery revascularization to high operative risk patients, transfemoral carotid artery stenting (TFCAS) was developed as an alternative, less invasive method more reasonably performed under local anesthesia.

Generally, TFCAS requires navigation of the aortic arch, selective cannulation of the effected carotid artery, traversing of the lesion, pre-dilation angioplasty followed by stent deployment, and post-stent angioplasty. Navigating a tortuous aortic arch, traversing the carotid lesion, and angioplasty led to the concern for iatrogenic embolic events. This led to the development of embolic protection devices (EPDs) that are deployed proximally or distally before pre-dilation angioplasty in attempt to mitigate embolic events. There are multiple commercially available EPDs, but none have proven superior to others.[10] EPDs demonstrated significant 17.1% reduction in perioperative stroke rates in the Endarterectomy Versus Angioplasty in Patients with Symptomatic Severe Carotid Stenosis trial.[65] Although EPDs decrease the risk of intraoperative embolic events, navigation of a diseased aortic arch and tortuous target vessel is required in TFCAS. Thus, extensive operative planning through preoperative imaging is imperative to improve technical success and prevent adverse events.[66]

Multiple RCTs have been conducted comparing outcomes of CEA with TFCAS (see **Table 3**). The Carotid Revascularization Endarterectomy versus Stenting Trial (CREST-1) is the largest and most prominent RCT including 2502 asymptomatic and symptomatic patients that demonstrated a decreased rate of perioperative stroke in CEA (2.3%) compared with TFCAS (4.1%) with an increased rate of MI after CEA (2.3% vs 1.1%).[67] At 10 years, rates of ipsilateral stroke and significant restenosis were similar between the two techniques.[67–69] These results were corroborated by the International Carotid Stenting Study Trial (ICSS) with a near twofold increase in perioperative stroke in TFCAS patients.[70] In another RCT focusing on asymptomatic patients meeting criteria for carotid revascularization (ACT-1), TFCAS trended toward increased perioperative stroke at 2.9% compared with 1.7% in CEA.[71] However, there were no significant differences between perioperative or 5-year outcomes between the two groups.[71] The recently completed ACST-2 RCT demonstrated a trend toward increased rate of perioperative stroke in TFCAS at 3.6% compared with 2.4% ($P = 0.06$) with similar stroke rates at 5 years (5.3% TFCAS vs 4.5% CEA).[72] A large Cochrane review analyzing 22 RCTs and 9753 patients revealed an increased risk of perioperative stroke or death in TFCAS compared with CEA in symptomatic patients (OR1.70; 95% CI; 1.31–2.19 $P < 0.001$). This study also demonstrated a trend toward increased perioperative stroke risk in asymptomatic patients, but this did not reach statistical significance.[73]

More recent data from large databases seem to confirm the findings of clinical trial in a "real world" application to patients. VQI data demonstrated a significant 4.1% risk of perioperative stroke or death in high-risk, symptomatic patients undergoing TFCAS.[74] Further, a retrospective study of 58,840 patients in the VQI-VISION database demonstrated an increased risk of stroke and death at 1 and 5 years in patients undergoing TFCAS compared with CEA suggesting superior durability after CEA.[75] The CREST-2 trial investigating modern OMT with OMT + CEA and OMT + TFCAS is currently underway with estimated conclusion date of February 2026.

Anatomical limitations of TFCAS involve tortuosity and atherosclerotic disease burden of the aortic arch, carotid lesion characteristics, and angulation of the carotid artery. Redundancy and tortuosity of the CCA, aortic arch elongation, and calcification have been postulated as the explanation for higher risk of perioperative stroke or death in older patients (>70 years).[76,77] Older patients, specifically octogenarians, have more complex aortic arch anatomy and atherosclerotic disease.[78] Studies have demonstrated an up to 1.5-fold increased risk of perioperative stroke in patients greater than 70 years undergoing TFCAS when compared with CEA,[77] and these patients were of the highest risk of neurologic event in CREST-1. Patients with aberrant aortic arch anatomy, specifically Type II and III arch configurations, are at higher risk of adverse events during TFCAS.[9,79]

Secondary analysis of the CREST-1 cohort demonstrated a near 3.5-fold increased risk of stroke or death in patients undergoing TFCAS with long (>10–12 mm) more complex carotid lesions.[80,81] In addition, carotid artery angulation of greater than 60° limits technical success and has been associated with three to fourfold increase in cerebral ischemia when compared with CEA for similar lesions.[81,82] Carotid tortuosity can also prevent the successful deployment of EPDs, thus increasing perioperative stroke risk.[79] Last, severely calcified lesions place patients undergoing TFCAS at an increased risk of perioperative stroke by 4.1%.[83] Relative and absolute contraindications to TFCAS are listed in **Table 5**. These limitations highlight the necessity of preoperative imaging and careful patient selection. Overall, it is clear that the increased risk of neurologic injury associated with TFCAS is procedural in nature owing to the consistently doubling of risk at 30 days but then stability in long-term risk of stroke after successful procedure.

TRANSCAROTID ARTERY REVASCULARIZATION

Transcarotid artery revascularization (TCAR) is a novel hybrid technique in the treatment of carotid artery stenosis. This approach provides threefold embolic protection by combining (1) dynamic cerebral flow reversal with CCA clamping while simultaneous (2) avoidance of aortic arch navigation, and (3) elimination of carotid lesion traversal before the initiation of embolic protection measures. Dynamic flow reversal is created by establishing an arteriovenous gradient between the CCA and femoral

Table 5	
Absolute and relative contraindications to carotid artery stenting	
Absolute Contraindications	**Relative Contraindications**
Thrombus within carotid lesion	Heavily calcified aortic arch or aberrant anatomy such as Type III aortic arch
Lack of peripheral access (iliac occlusion)	Failure of embolic protection device
Recent stroke with possible hemorrhage	Tortuous carotid artery (>60°)
Evolving stroke within 24 hours	Near occlusion, string sign

vein. A filter within the circuit removes particulate and debris from the channel. The key operative steps with angiographic images are presented in **Fig. 6.**[10]

The Safety and Efficacy Study for Reverse Flow Used During Carotid Artery Stenting Procedure (ROADSTER-1) pivotal trial consisted of 208 patients at multiple centers from 2012 to 2014. Approximately one-quarter of the patients were symptomatic. Patients included in the study were considered high risk for CEA with 60% of patients experiencing at least one anatomic factor and physiologic factor.[84] The average length and degree of stenosis were 17.8 ± 12.51 mm and 85.9 ± 8.7%.[84] Most of the cases (53%) were performed under local anesthesia. Overall, the perioperative stroke and death rate were 1.4% with perioperative risk of MI at 0.7%.[84] This trial demonstrated comparable perioperative outcomes to CREST with superior operative time at 73.6 minutes compared with 171 minutes in TFCAS.[84] Despite 36% of patients having hostile cervical anatomy, only 0.7% experienced CNI compared with 4.7% in CEA within CREST.[67,84] This landmark trial led to the United States Food and Drug Administration approval of TCAR in 2015. The results of this study were followed to 1 year demonstrating a rate of ipsilateral at 0.6% and 4.2% mortality.[85] This was followed by the post-market approval study, ROADSTER-2. A large cohort of 632 patients was selected with similar high-risk qualities and demographics to ROADSTER-1. This study reinforced the previous findings with excellent technical success and a perioperative stroke rate of 0.6%.[86] Including patients who violated protocol due to noncompliance with preoperative antiplatelet regimen, perioperative stroke rate was 1.9%. Perioperative MI and CNI rates were 0.9% and 1.3%, respectively.[86]

The utility and outcomes of TCAR have been further analyzed within the VQI with the development of the TCAR Surveillance Project (TCAR-SP).[87] This allowed for real-world evaluation and comparison with other techniques. In a study consisting of nearly 12,000 patients (1182 TCAR) within the VQI, Schermerhorn and colleagues demonstrated similar perioperative outcomes regarding stroke rate (1.4% TCAR vs 1.2%

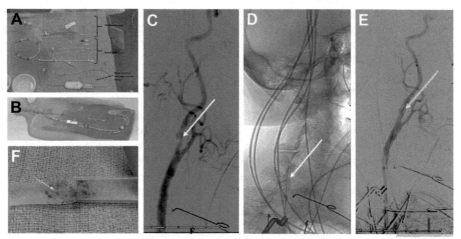

Fig. 6. TCAR components and angiographic images. (*A, B*). Operative setup with dynamic flow circuit in place. (*C*) ICA lesion on initial angiography (*arrow*). (*D*). Lesion traversed only by wire (*arrow*) after initiation of flow reversal. (*E*) Completion angiogram with stent in place (*arrow*). (*F*) Filtered embolic debris (*arrow*). (Hicks CW, Malas MB. Cerebrovascular Disease: Carotid Artery Stenting. In: Sidawy AN, Perler BA. Rutherford's Vascular Surgery and Endovascular Therapy, Ninth Edition. Chapter 92, 1215-1233.e4; and [*E*] Firnhaber JM, Powell CS. Arterial Atherosclerosis: Vascular Surgery Interventions. Am Fam Physician. 2022;105(1):65-72; with permissions.)

CEA; $P = 0.68$), MI (1.1% TCAR vs 0.6% CEA; $P = 0.11$), and 30-day mortality (0.9% TCAR vs 0.4% CEA; $P = 0.06$). TCAR was superior to CEA regarding perioperative hemodynamic instability, CNI, and operative time.[87] It is important to understand that patients undergoing TCAR in this study were significantly comorbid compared with CEA group.[87] An additional VQI study, Malas and colleagues used propensity-matched groups to compare TCAR ($n = 6348$) and CEA ($n = 6348$). Their study produced similar results with perioperative stroke/death rates of 1.6% for both groups.[88] However, they indicated significant increase in risk of MI (0.9% vs 0.5%), CNI (2.7% vs 0.4%), hemodynamic instability, and longer length of stay in the CEA group.[89] In a VQI study, TCAR demonstrated superior perioperative stroke rates at 1.9% TCAR vs 3.3% TFCAS ($P =< 0.001$).[74] These findings have been corroborated by other VQI propensity-matched studies demonstrating the in-hospital stroke/death rate of 1.6% in TCAR versus 3.1% in TFCAS.[90] At 1 year, there are no significant differences in outcomes when comparing TCAR with TFCAS or CEA in propensity-matched studies.[74] In systematic review of 12 studies by comparing TCAR with TFCAS and CEA, Wu and colleagues superior outcomes in TCAR and CEA compared with TFCAS regarding perioperative stroke. This study also revealed that TCAR is approximately twice the cost compared with CEA ($\sim$\$10,000 vs $\sim$\$5000).[91]

Although patients selected for TCAR are considered medically high-risk, multiple anatomical and pharmacologic requirements must be met to be included within current studies. Preoperatively, pharmacologic regimen includes 3 to 5 days of DAPT (aspirin and clopidogrel) as well as high-intensity statin. The DAPT regimen is to be continued at least for 30 days. This is primarily based on prior studies evaluating DAPT following percutaneous coronary intervention.[9] Anatomical requirements for TCAR include 5 cm of CCA proximal to the lesion, CCA diameter of greater than 6 mm, ICA diameter of 4 to 9 mm, CCA access site is free of disease within 1 cm. Severely calcified lesions are also a contraindication to TCAR. However, one VQI study revealed that TCAR maintains similar performance and superiority to TFCAS in patients with greater than 50% calcification compared with those with less than 50% stenosis.[92] Despite the anatomical restrictions within the instructions for use (IFU) for TCAR, the anatomical feasibility remains robust. Two large studies consisting of 702 patients examining anatomical applicability of TCAR revealed a 68% to 86% TCAR eligibility rate by IFU.[93,94] The requirements for IFU in TCAR are tabulated in **Table 6**.

Initial studies investigating the feasibility of TCAR only included patients considered high risk for CEA. A recent study using the TCAR-SP consisting of 14,979 CEAs and 4993 TCARs demonstrated similar perioperative outcomes between with

Table 6
Anatomical, medical, intraoperative management for transcarotid artery revascularization

Anatomical	Medical	Intraoperative
Greater than 5 cm between common carotid access site and lesion	Dual antiplatelet therapy (DAPT) 3–5 days before operation	Maintain systolic blood pressure 140–160 mm Hg
Common carotid artery diameter of >6 mm	Statin therapy	Maintain heart rate >70
Internal carotid diameter of 4–9 mm	Continue DAPT for 30 d before transition to monotherapy	Maintain activated clotting time > 250 after heparinization
Access site free from disease within 1 cm		

perioperative stroke rate of 1.4% TCAR and 1.3% CEA ($P = 0.75$) and 30-day mortality of 0.3% in both groups. At 1 year, ipsilateral stroke rates and all-cause mortality were similar.[95] This study prompted the expansion of TCAR as a consideration in standard risk patients and was approved in May of 2022. The ROADSTER-3 post-market approval trial to further determine the efficacy of TCAR in standard risk patients was initiated in September of 2022 with estimated completion by May 2025. Overall, TCAR provides a minimally invasive method that affords excellent embolic protection while limiting morbidity and mortality. Although long-term outcomes are still needed, this novel technique has changed the landscape of carotid artery interventions.

SUMMARY

Surgical management of the carotid artery atherosclerosis to prevent stroke remains one of the most elegant and well-studied procedures within vascular surgery. Perhaps no other prophylactic intervention has done more to prevent subsequent death and disability. The impact of loss of function and independence after CVA cannot be overstated. Further, carotid artery revascularization remains a hallmark of the accomplished vascular specialist given that the majority of interventional morbidity can be attributed to the conduct of the procedure itself.

Given the imperative for precise operative conduct, it is critical to maximize the perioperative variables associated with success. Fortunately, modern vascular care has equipped the vascular specialist with several modalities to provide optimal care including more precise imaging, improved medical management, and well-studied interventions. A careful understanding of patient risk, life expectancy, anatomic risk, and medical risk can lead the surgeon toward the correct choice for the individual patient, be it medical therapy, minimally invasive therapy, or open surgical revascularization.

CLINICS CARE POINTS

- Carotid endarterectomy remains the gold standard operative approach in patients with symptomatic carotid artery disease or asymptomatic patients with >80% stenosis without prohibitive comorbidities as demonstrated in the ACAS, NASCET, and CREST-1 trials.
- Diligent patient selection is required when considering surgical intervention for carotid artery stenosis and preoperative cardiac work-up is imperative.
- Detailed cross-sectional imaging should be strongly considered prior to proceeding with carotid endarterectomy to further characterize the patient's cerebral vasculature and extent of carotid disease.
- The utilization of cerebral monitoring during any carotid artery intervention is critical when performed under general anesthesia. No modality has proven superior, but provides real-time feedback and informs the decision to perform intraoperative shunting.
- Intraoperative shunting should be performed in patients with any neurological deficits or neuromonitoring changes when carotid artery is clamped. Preoperative factors such as a vertebral artery terminating in posterior inferior cerebellar artery or contralateral carotid artery occlusion predisposing the patient to cerebral hypoperfusion with clamping.
- Transfemoral carotid artery stenting carries a higher burden of perioperative stroke compared to carotid endarterectomy or TCAR and should be reserved for cases in which open surgery or hybrid operations are not feasible.
- TCAR presents a novel hybrid operation that can be performed with excellent technical success with a low perioperative stroke rate. Abiding by the IFU and ensuring patients are initiated on the appropriate preoperative medications are critical when utilizing TCAR.

DISCLOSURES

C.A. Banks is funded by the VA Quality Scholars Program, Birmingham Veterans Affairs Medical Center, Birmingham, Alabama, 35322.

REFERENCES

1. Robicsek F, Roush TS, Cook JW, et al. From Hippocrates to palmaz-schatz, the history of carotid surgery. Eur J Vasc Endovasc Surg 2004;27(4):389–97.
2. Stevanovic K, Sabljak V, Kukic B, et al. A brief history of carotid artery surgery and anesthesia. J Anesth Hist 2016;2(4):147–50.
3. Debakey ME, Crawford ES, Cooley DA, et al. Cerebral arterial insufficiency: one to 11-year results following arterial reconstructive operation. Ann Surg 1965; 161(6):921–45.
4. Cooley DA, Al-Naaman YD, Carton CA. Surgical treatment of arteriosclerotic occlusion of common carotid artery. J Neurosurg 1956;13(5):500–6.
5. Feigin VL, Krishnamurthi RV, Parmar P, et al. Update on the global burden of ischemic and hemorrhagic stroke in 1990-2013: the GBD 2013 study. Neuroepidemiology 2015;45(3):161–76.
6. Benjamin EJ, Blaha MJ, Chiuve SE, et al. Heart disease and stroke statistics-2017 update: a report from the American heart association. Circulation 2017; 135(10):e146–603.
7. Grysiewicz RA, Thomas K, Pandey DK. Epidemiology of ischemic and hemorrhagic stroke: incidence, prevalence, mortality, and risk factors. Neurol Clin 2008;26(4):871–95, vii.
8. Virani SS, Alonso A, Aparicio HJ, et al. Heart disease and stroke statistics-2021 update: a report from the American heart association. Circulation 2021;143(8): e254–743.
9. AbuRahma AF, Avgerinos ED, Chang RW, et al. The Society for Vascular Surgery implementation document for management of extracranial cerebrovascular disease. J Vasc Surg 2022;75(1S):26S–98S.
10. Moacdieh MP, Khan MA, Layman P, et al. Innovation in the open and endovascular treatment of carotid artery stenosis. Semin Vasc Surg 2021;34(4):163–71.
11. Dossabhoy S, Arya S. Epidemiology of atherosclerotic carotid artery disease. Semin Vasc Surg 2021;34(1):3–9.
12. Rockman CB, Hoang H, Guo Y, et al. The prevalence of carotid artery stenosis varies significantly by race. J Vasc Surg 2013;57(2):327–37.
13. Lawes CM, Bennett DA, Feigin VL, et al. Blood pressure and stroke: an overview of published reviews. Stroke 2004;35(4):1024.
14. Banerjee C, Moon YP, Paik MC, et al. Duration of diabetes and risk of ischemic stroke: the Northern Manhattan Study. Stroke 2012;43(5):1212–7.
15. Smith NL, Barzilay JI, Shaffer D, et al. Fasting and 2-hour postchallenge serum glucose measures and risk of incident cardiovascular events in the elderly: the Cardiovascular Health Study. Arch Intern Med 2002;162(2):209–16.
16. Goldstein LB, Adams R, Alberts MJ, et al. Primary prevention of ischemic stroke: a guideline from the American heart association/American stroke association stroke council: cosponsored by the atherosclerotic peripheral vascular disease interdisciplinary working group; cardiovascular nursing council; clinical cardiology council; nutrition, physical activity, and metabolism council; and the quality of care and outcomes research interdisciplinary working Group. Circulation 2006;113(24):e873–923.

17. Herder M, Arntzen KA, Johnsen SH, et al. The metabolic syndrome and progression of carotid atherosclerosis over 13 years. The Tromso study. Cardiovasc Diabetol 2012;11:77.

18. Group AS, Cushman WC, Evans GW, et al. Effects of intensive blood-pressure control in type 2 diabetes mellitus. N Engl J Med 2010;362(17):1575–85.

19. Wang JG, Staessen JA, Li Y, et al. Carotid intima-media thickness and antihypertensive treatment: a meta-analysis of randomized controlled trials. Stroke 2006; 37(7):1933–40.

20. Baigent C, Keech A, Kearney PM, et al. Efficacy and safety of cholesterol-lowering treatment: prospective meta-analysis of data from 90,056 participants in 14 randomised trials of statins. Lancet 2005;366(9493):1267–78.

21. Ironside N, Brenner D, Heyer E, et al. Systematic review and meta-analysis of perioperative and long-term outcomes in patients receiving statin therapy before carotid endarterectomy. Acta Neurochir 2018;160(9):1761–71.

22. Taylor AJ, Kent SM, Flaherty PJ, et al. ARBITER: Arterial Biology for the Investigation of the Treatment Effects of Reducing Cholesterol: a randomized trial comparing the effects of atorvastatin and pravastatin on carotid intima medial thickness. Circulation 2002;106(16):2055–60.

23. Sillesen H, Amarenco P, Hennerici MG, et al. Atorvastatin reduces the risk of cardiovascular events in patients with carotid atherosclerosis: a secondary analysis of the Stroke Prevention by Aggressive Reduction in Cholesterol Levels (SPARCL) trial. Stroke 2008;39(12):3297–302.

24. Rothwell PM, Algra A, Chen Z, et al. Effects of aspirin on risk and severity of early recurrent stroke after transient ischaemic attack and ischaemic stroke: time-course analysis of randomised trials. Lancet 2016;388(10042):365–75.

25. Kennedy J, Quan H, Buchan AM, et al. Statins are associated with better outcomes after carotid endarterectomy in symptomatic patients. Stroke 2005; 36(10):2072–6.

26. Wang Y, Wang Y, Zhao X, et al. Clopidogrel with aspirin in acute minor stroke or transient ischemic attack. N Engl J Med 2013;369(1):11–9.

27. Zhang Q, Wang C, Zheng M, et al. Aspirin plus clopidogrel as secondary prevention after stroke or transient ischemic attack: a systematic review and meta-analysis. Cerebrovasc Dis 2015;39(1):13–22.

28. Naylor AR, McCabe DJH. New data and the Covid-19 pandemic mandate a rethink of antiplatelet strategies in patients with TIA or minor stroke associated with atherosclerotic carotid stenosis. Eur J Vasc Endovasc Surg 2020;59(6):861–5.

29. King A, Shipley M, Markus H, et al. The effect of medical treatments on stroke risk in asymptomatic carotid stenosis. Stroke 2013;44(2):542–6.

30. North American Symptomatic Carotid Endarterectomy Trial C, Barnett HJM, Taylor DW, et al. Beneficial effect of carotid endarterectomy in symptomatic patients with high-grade carotid stenosis. N Engl J Med 1991;325(7):445–53.

31. Ferguson GG, Eliasziw M, Barr HW, et al. The North American symptomatic carotid endarterectomy trial : surgical results in 1415 patients. Stroke 1999;30(9): 1751–8.

32. Grant EG, Benson CB, Moneta GL, et al. Carotid artery stenosis: gray-scale and Doppler US diagnosis–Society of Radiologists in Ultrasound Consensus Conference. Radiology 2003;229(2):340–6.

33. Irvine CD, Baird RN, Lamont PM, et al. Endarterectomy for asymptomatic carotid artery stenosis. BMJ 1995;311(7013):1113–4.

34. AbuRahma AF, Srivastava M, Stone PA, et al. Critical appraisal of the Carotid Duplex Consensus criteria in the diagnosis of carotid artery stenosis. J Vasc Surg 2011;53(1):53–9 [discussion: 59-60].
35. MRC European Carotid Surgery Trial: interim results for symptomatic patients with severe (70-99%) or with mild (0-29%) carotid stenosis. European Carotid Surgery Trialists' Collaborative Group. Lancet 1991;337(8752):1235–43.
36. Naylor AR, Rothwell PM, Bell PR. Overview of the principal results and secondary analyses from the European and North American randomised trials of endarterectomy for symptomatic carotid stenosis. Eur J Vasc Endovasc Surg 2003; 26(2):115–29.
37. Rothwell PM, Gutnikov SA, Warlow CP. European Carotid Surgery Trialist's C. Reanalysis of the final results of the European Carotid Surgery Trial. Stroke 2003;34(2):514–23.
38. Ballotta E, Da Giau G, Piccoli A, et al. Durability of carotid endarterectomy for treatment of symptomatic and asymptomatic stenoses. J Vasc Surg 2004; 40(2):270–8.
39. Cunningham EJ, Bond R, Mehta Z, et al. Long-term durability of carotid endarterectomy for symptomatic stenosis and risk factors for late postoperative stroke. Stroke 2002;33(11):2658–63.
40. Berek PKI, Sihotsky V, Kubikova M, et al. Carotid endarterectomy during the acute period of ischemic stroke. Cor Vasa 2018;60:169–73.
41. Tanious A, Pothof AB, Boitano LT, et al. Timing of carotid endarterectomy after stroke: retrospective review of prospectively collected national database. Ann Surg 2018;268(3):449–56.
42. Blay E Jr, Balogun Y, Nooromid MJ, et al. Early carotid endarterectomy after acute stroke yields excellent outcomes: an analysis of the procedure-targeted ACS-NSQIP. Ann Vasc Surg 2019;57:194–200.
43. Chisci E, Lazzeri E, Masciello F, et al. Timing to carotid endarterectomy affects early and long term outcomes of symptomatic carotid stenosis. Ann Vasc Surg 2022;82:314–24.
44. Gunka I, Krajickova D, Lesko M, et al. Outcomes of urgent carotid endarterectomy for crescendo transient ischemic attacks and stroke in evolution. Ann Vasc Surg 2019;61:185–92.
45. Pini R, Faggioli G, Vacirca A, et al. The benefit of deferred carotid revascularization in patients with moderate-severe disabling cerebral ischemic stroke. J Vasc Surg 2021;73(1):117–24.
46. Halliday A, Mansfield A, Marro J, et al. Prevention of disabling and fatal strokes by successful carotid endarterectomy in patients without recent neurological symptoms: randomised controlled trial. Lancet 2004;363(9420):1491–502.
47. Halliday A, Harrison M, Hayter E, et al. 10-year stroke prevention after successful carotid endarterectomy for asymptomatic stenosis (ACST-1): a multicentre randomised trial. Lancet 2010;376(9746):1074–84.
48. Kolos I, Troitskiy A, Balakhonova T, et al. Modern medical treatment with or without carotid endarterectomy for severe asymptomatic carotid atherosclerosis. J Vasc Surg 2015;62(4):914–22.
49. Abbott AL. Medical (nonsurgical) intervention alone is now best for prevention of stroke associated with asymptomatic severe carotid stenosis: results of a systematic review and analysis. Stroke 2009;40(10):e573–83.
50. Bond R, Rerkasem K, Naylor AR, et al. Systematic review of randomized controlled trials of patch angioplasty versus primary closure and different types of patch materials during carotid endarterectomy. J Vasc Surg 2004;40(6):1126–35.

51. Malas M, Glebova NO, Hughes SE, et al. Effect of patching on reducing restenosis in the carotid revascularization endarterectomy versus stenting trial. Stroke 2015;46(3):757–61.

52. Cao P, Giordano G, De Rango P, et al. Eversion versus conventional carotid endarterectomy: late results of a prospective multicenter randomized trial. J Vasc Surg 2000;31(1 Pt 1):19–30.

53. Schneider JR, Helenowski IB, Jackson CR, et al. A comparison of results with eversion versus conventional carotid endarterectomy from the vascular quality initiative and the mid-America vascular study group. J Vasc Surg 2015;61(5): 1216–22.

54. Paraskevas KI, Robertson V, Saratzis AN, et al. Editor's choice - an updated systematic review and meta-analysis of outcomes following eversion vs. Conventional carotid endarterectomy in randomised controlled trials and observational studies. Eur J Vasc Endovasc Surg 2018;55(4):465–73.

55. Stone DH, Giles KA, Kubilis P, et al. Editor's choice - protamine reduces serious bleeding complications associated with carotid endarterectomy in asymptomatic patients without increasing the risk of stroke, myocardial infarction, or death in a large national analysis. Eur J Vasc Endovasc Surg 2020;60(6):800–7.

56. Aburahma AF, Mousa AY, Stone PA. Shunting during carotid endarterectomy. J Vasc Surg 2011;54(5):1502–10.

57. Pasin L, Nardelli P, Landoni G, et al. Examination of regional anesthesia for carotid endarterectomy. J Vasc Surg 2015;62(3):631–634 e631.

58. Wiske C, Arhuidese I, Malas M, et al. Comparing the efficacy of shunting approaches and cerebral monitoring during carotid endarterectomy using a national database. J Vasc Surg 2018;68(2):416–25.

59. Stewart LM, Spangler EL, Sutzko DC, et al. Carotid endarterectomy with concomitant distal endovascular intervention is associated with increased rates of stroke and death. J Vasc Surg 2021;73(3):960–967 e961.

60. Jamil M, Usman R, Ghaffar S. Advantages of selective use of intraluminal shunt in carotid endarterectomy: a study of 122 cases. Ann Vasc Dis 2016;9(4):285–8.

61. Aburahma AF, Stone PA, Hass SM, et al. Prospective randomized trial of routine versus selective shunting in carotid endarterectomy based on stump pressure. J Vasc Surg 2010;51(5):1133–8.

62. Chongruksut W, Vaniyapong T, Rerkasem K. Routine or selective carotid artery shunting for carotid endarterectomy (and different methods of monitoring in selective shunting). Cochrane Database Syst Rev 2014;2014(6):CD000190.

63. Levin SR, Farber A, Goodney PP, et al. Shunt intention during carotid endarterectomy in the early symptomatic period and perioperative stroke risk. J Vasc Surg 2020;72(4):1385–1394 e1382.

64. Fokkema M, den Hartog AG, Bots ML, et al. Stenting versus surgery in patients with carotid stenosis after previous cervical radiation therapy: systematic review and meta-analysis. Stroke 2012;43(3):793–801.

65. Mas JL, Chatellier G, Beyssen B, et al. Endarterectomy versus stenting in patients with symptomatic severe carotid stenosis. N Engl J Med 2006;355(16): 1660–71.

66. Wyers MC, Powell RJ, Fillinger MF, et al. The value of 3D-CT angiographic assessment prior to carotid stenting. J Vasc Surg 2009;49(3):614–22.

67. Brott TG, Hobson RW 2nd, Howard G, et al. Stenting versus endarterectomy for treatment of carotid-artery stenosis. N Engl J Med 2010;363(1):11–23.

68. Brott TG, Howard G, Roubin GS, et al. Long-Term Results of Stenting versus Endarterectomy for Carotid-Artery Stenosis. N Engl J Med 2016;374(11): 1021–31.
69. Lal BK, Brott TG. Restenosis after carotid endarterectomy and stenting–authors' reply. Lancet Neurol 2013;12(2):130–1.
70. International Carotid Stenting Study I, Ederle J, Dobson J, et al. Carotid artery stenting compared with endarterectomy in patients with symptomatic carotid stenosis (International Carotid Stenting Study): an interim analysis of a randomised controlled trial. Lancet 2010;375(9719):985–97.
71. Rosenfield K, Matsumura JS, Chaturvedi S, et al. Randomized trial of stent versus surgery for asymptomatic carotid stenosis. N Engl J Med 2016; 374(11):1011–20.
72. Halliday A, Bulbulia R, Bonati LH, et al. Second asymptomatic carotid surgery trial (ACST-2): a randomised comparison of carotid artery stenting versus carotid endarterectomy. Lancet 2021;398(10305):1065–73.
73. Muller MD, Lyrer P, Brown MM, et al. Carotid artery stenting versus endarterectomy for treatment of carotid artery stenosis. Cochrane Database Syst Rev 2020;2(2):CD000515.
74. Malas MB, Dakour-Aridi H, Wang GJ, et al. Transcarotid artery revascularization versus transfemoral carotid artery stenting in the Society for Vascular Surgery Vascular Quality Initiative. J Vasc Surg 2019;69(1):92–103 e102.
75. Yei KS, Elsayed N, Mathlouthi A, et al. Long-term outcomes of carotid endarterectomy versus transfemoral carotid artery stenting in the VQI-VISION database. J Vasc Surg 2020;74 (3).
76. Voeks JH, Howard G, Roubin GS, et al. Age and outcomes after carotid stenting and endarterectomy: the carotid revascularization endarterectomy versus stenting trial. Stroke 2011;42(12):3484–90.
77. Nejim B, Alshwaily W, Dakour-Aridi H, et al. Age modifies the efficacy and safety of carotid artery revascularization procedures. J Vasc Surg 2019;69(5): 1490–1503 e1493.
78. Lam RC, Lin SC, DeRubertis B, et al. The impact of increasing age on anatomic factors affecting carotid angioplasty and stenting. J Vasc Surg 2007;45(5): 875–80.
79. Fanous AA, Jowdy PK, Morr S, et al. Vascular anatomy and not age is responsible for increased risk of complications in symptomatic elderly patients undergoing carotid artery stenting. World Neurosurg 2019;128:e513–21.
80. Moore WS, Popma JJ, Roubin GS, et al. Carotid angiographic characteristics in the CREST trial were major contributors to periprocedural stroke and death differences between carotid artery stenting and carotid endarterectomy. J Vasc Surg 2016;63(4):851–7, 858 e851.
81. Naggara O, Touze E, Beyssen B, et al. Anatomical and technical factors associated with stroke or death during carotid angioplasty and stenting: results from the endarterectomy versus angioplasty in patients with symptomatic severe carotid stenosis (EVA-3S) trial and systematic review. Stroke 2011;42(2):380–8.
82. Muller MD, Ahlhelm FJ, von Hessling A, et al. Vascular anatomy predicts the risk of cerebral ischemia in patients randomized to carotid stenting versus endarterectomy. Stroke 2017;48(5):1285–92.
83. AbuRahma AF, DerDerian T, Hariri N, et al. Anatomical and technical predictors of perioperative clinical outcomes after carotid artery stenting. J Vasc Surg 2017;66(2):423–32.

84. Kwolek CJ, Jaff MR, Leal JI, et al. Results of the ROADSTER multicenter trial of transcarotid stenting with dynamic flow reversal. J Vasc Surg 2015;62(5): 1227–34.

85. Malas MB, Leal Lorenzo JI, Nejim B, et al. Analysis of the ROADSTER pivotal and extended-access cohorts shows excellent 1-year durability of transcarotid stenting with dynamic flow reversal. J Vasc Surg 2019;69(6):1786–96.

86. Kashyap VS, Schneider PA, Foteh M, et al. Early outcomes in the ROADSTER 2 study of transcarotid artery revascularization in patients with significant carotid artery disease. Stroke 2020;51(9):2620–9.

87. Schermerhorn ML, Liang P, Dakour-Aridi H, et al. In-hospital outcomes of transcarotid artery revascularization and carotid endarterectomy in the Society for Vascular Surgery Vascular Quality Initiative. J Vasc Surg 2020;71(1):87–95.

88. Malas MB, Elsayed N, Naazie I, et al. Propensity score-matched analysis of 1-year outcomes of transcarotid revascularization with dynamic flow reversal, carotid endarterectomy, and transfemoral carotid artery stenting. J Vasc Surg 2022;75(1):213–222 e211.

89. Malas MB, Dakour-Aridi H, Kashyap VS, et al. Transcarotid revascularization with dynamic flow reversal versus carotid endarterectomy in the vascular quality initiative surveillance project. Ann Surg 2022;276(2):398–403.

90. Schermerhorn ML, Liang P, Eldrup-Jorgensen J, et al. Association of transcarotid artery revascularization vs transfemoral carotid artery stenting with stroke or death among patients with carotid artery stenosis. JAMA 2019;322(23): 2313–22.

91. Wu H, Wang Z, Li M, et al. Outcomes of transcarotid artery revascularization: a systematic review. Interv Neuroradiol 2022. 15910199221123283.

92. Elsayed N, Yei KS, Naazie I, et al. The impact of carotid lesion calcification on outcomes of carotid artery stenting. J Vasc Surg 2022;75(3):921–9.

93. Wu WW, Liang P, O'Donnell TFX, et al. Anatomic eligibility for transcarotid artery revascularization and transfemoral carotid artery stenting. J Vasc Surg 2019; 69(5):1452–60.

94. Kumins NH, King AH, Ambani RN, et al. Anatomic criteria in the selection of treatment modality for atherosclerotic carotid artery disease. J Vasc Surg 2020;72(4):1395–404.

95. Liang P, Cronenwett J, Secemsky E, et al. Expansion of transcarotid artery revascularization to standard risk patients for treatment of carotid artery stenosis, J Vasc Surg, 74(3), E27–28.

96. Obeid T, Arhuidese I, Gaidry A, et al. Beta-blocker use is associated with lower stroke and death after carotid artery stenting. J Vasc Surg 2016;63(2):363–9.

97. Whelton PK, Carey RM, Aronow WS, et al. 2017 ACC/AHA/AAPA/ABC/ACPM/AGS/APhA/ASH/ASPC/NMA/PCNA guideline for the prevention, detection, evaluation, and management of high blood pressure in adults: executive summary: a report of the American college of cardiology/American heart association task force on clinical practice guidelines. Circulation 2018;138(17):e426–83.

98. Johnson ES, Lanes SF, Wentworth CE 3rd, et al. A metaregression analysis of the dose-response effect of aspirin on stroke. Arch Intern Med 1999;159(11): 1248–53.

99. De Schryver EL, Algra A, Kappelle LJ, et al. Vitamin K antagonists versus antiplatelet therapy after transient ischaemic attack or minor ischaemic stroke of presumed arterial origin. Cochrane Database Syst Rev 2012;(9):CD001342.

100. Levi CR, Stork JL, Chambers BR, et al. Dextran reduces embolic signals after carotid endarterectomy. Ann Neurol 2001;50(4):544–7.

101. Bucher HC, Griffith LE, Guyatt GH. Effect of HMGcoA reductase inhibitors on stroke. A meta-analysis of randomized, controlled trials. Ann Intern Med 1998; 128(2):89–95.
102. van den Bogaard B, van den Born BJ, Fayyad R, et al. On-treatment lipoprotein components and risk of cerebrovascular events in the Treating to New Targets study. Eur J Clin Invest 2011;41(2):134–42.
103. McGirt MJ, Perler BA, Brooke BS, et al. 3-hydroxy-3-methylglutaryl coenzyme A reductase inhibitors reduce the risk of perioperative stroke and mortality after carotid endarterectomy. J Vasc Surg 2005;42(5):829–36 [discussion: 836-827].
104. Verzini F, De Rango P, Parlani G, et al. Effects of statins on early and late results of carotid stenting. J Vasc Surg 2011;53(1):71–9 [discussion: 79].
105. de Weerd M, Greving JP, Hedblad B, et al. Prevalence of asymptomatic carotid artery stenosis in the general population: an individual participant data meta-analysis. Stroke 2010;41(6):1294–7.
106. Hogberg DK,B, Bjorck M, Tjarnstrom J, et al. Carotid artery atherosclerosis among 65-year-old Swedish men - a population-based screening study. Eur J Vasc Endovasc Surg 2014;48:5–10.
107. Zhang C, Zhou YH, Xu CL, et al. Efficacy of intensive control of glucose in stroke prevention: a meta-analysis of data from 59,197 participants in 9 randomized controlled trials. PLoS One 2013;8(1):e54465.
108. Mayberg MR, Wilson SE, Yatsu F, et al. Carotid endarterectomy and prevention of cerebral ischemia in symptomatic carotid stenosis. Veterans Affairs Cooperative Studies Program 309 Trialist Group. JAMA 1991;266(23):3289–94.
109. Hobson RW 2nd, Weiss DG, Fields WS, et al. Efficacy of carotid endarterectomy for asymptomatic carotid stenosis. The Veterans Affairs Cooperative Study Group. N Engl J Med 1993;328(4):221–7.
110. Yadav JS, Wholey MH, Kuntz RE, et al. Protected carotid-artery stenting versus endarterectomy in high-risk patients. N Engl J Med 2004;351(15):1493–501.
111. Gurm HS, Yadav JS, Fayad P, et al. Long-term results of carotid stenting versus endarterectomy in high-risk patients. N Engl J Med 2008;358(15):1572–9.
112. Mas JL, Trinquart L, Leys D, et al. Endarterectomy versus angioplasty in patients with symptomatic severe carotid stenosis (EVA-3S) trial: results up to 4 years from a randomised, multicentre trial. Lancet Neurol 2008;7(10):885–92.
113. Group SC, Ringleb PA, Allenberg J, et al. 30 day results from the SPACE trial of stent-protected angioplasty versus carotid endarterectomy in symptomatic patients: a randomised non-inferiority trial. Lancet 2006;368(9543):1239–47.
114. Reiff T, Eckstein HH, Mansmann U, et al. Angioplasty in asymptomatic carotid artery stenosis vs. endarterectomy compared to best medical treatment: One-year interim results of SPACE-2. Int J Stroke 2019;15(6). 1747493019833017.
115. Sihotsky V., Frankovicova M., Kubikova M., et al., Transcranial cerebral oximetry as neuromonitoring during carotid endarterectomy, J Vasc Surg, 68, 2018, e131.
116. Li J, Shalabi A, Ji F, et al. Monitoring cerebral ischemia during carotid endarterectomy and stenting. J Biomed Res 2017;31(1):11–6.

Options for Dialysis and Vascular Access Creation

Yana Etkin, MD[a,1], Karen Woo, MD, PhD[b,*], London Guidry, MD[c,2]

KEYWORDS

- Dialysis access • HD • Peritoneal dialysis • Arteriovenous fistula
- Arteriovenous graft • Tunneled dialysis catheter

KEY POINTS

- All patient with CKD and end-stage kidney disease (ESKD) should have a Life-Plan in place.
- The primary principle of the Life-Plan is to create "the right access, for the right patient, at the right time, for the right reasons."
- Although general principles of arteriovenous access include starting as distally as possible in the nondominant arm and autogenous fistulas are preferred, these may not be appropriate in all patients, and the final decision should be individualized to the characteristics and preferences of each patient.
- Peritoneal dialysis catheters can be placed via open surgical, laparoscopic, or percutaneous approach with similar outcomes.
- Shared decision-making and palliative care evaluation should be performed for each patient with CKD and ESKD.

BACKGROUND

End-stage kidney disease (ESKD) requiring chronic renal replacement affects nearly 800,000 patients in the United States with 126,000 new patients starting dialysis annually.[1] In the United States, the overwhelming majority (84%) of patients with ESKD use hemodialysis (HD), 13% undergo peritoneal dialysis (PD), and 3% receive a kidney transplant annually.[1] Patients may undergo a range of vascular surgery procedures to establish and maintain HD vascular access. Since the arteriovenous fistula (AVF) was introduced more than 60 years ago,[2] it has been considered to be the "gold

[a] Division of Vascular and Endovascular Surgery, Department of Surgery, Zucker School of Medicine at Hofstra/Northwell, Hempstead, NY, USA; [b] Division of Vascular Surgery, Department of Surgery, David Geffen School of Medicine at UCLA, 200 UCLA Medical Plaza Suite 526, Los Angeles, CA 90095, USA; [c] Division of Vascular and Endovascular Surgery, Department of Surgery, Louisiana State University Health and Science Center, New Orleans, LA, USA
[1] Present address: 1999 Marcus Avenue, Suite 106B, Lake Success, NY 11042.
[2] Present address: 8585 Picardy Suite 310, Baton Rouge, LA 70809.
* Corresponding author.
E-mail address: kwoo@mednet.ucla.edu

Surg Clin N Am 103 (2023) 673–684
https://doi.org/10.1016/j.suc.2023.05.006
0039-6109/23/© 2023 Elsevier Inc. All rights reserved.

surgical.theclinics.com

standard" for access, and along with arteriovenous graft (AVG), it is superior to tunneled dialysis catheters (TDCs) in most clinical scenarios. However, the decision-making regarding the choice of HD access is complex.

In 2019, "Advancing American Kidney Health" was signed as an executive order.[3] This initiative established 3 goals: (1) by 2030, reduce the incidence of kidney failure in the United States by 25%; (2) by 2025, ensure 80% of patient have HD at home or receive a kidney transplant; and (3) by 2030, double the number of kidneys available for transplantation. These are lofty goals that will require coordination by numerous providers who engage in care of these patients.[3]

Types of Kidney Replacement Therapy

Patients with ESKD need life-long kidney replacement therapy; the available options are HD and PD. HD is most commonly used in the United States and can be delivered in-center or at home. In-center HD is delivered 3 times a week for 3 to 4 hours per session. Disadvantages include fatigue after treatment, cramping in the lower extremities during HD, the need to limit liquid intake, and strict dietary restrictions to limit the intake of potassium and phosphorous. Home HD is administered 3 to 7 days a week with varying session duration. Home HD offers a more flexible schedule and increased patient autonomy, with fewer dietary restrictions and more liberal liquid intake. Longer treatment sessions may also reduce symptoms of fatigue and leg cramps while on HD. Both in-center and home HD have a risk of access complications including bleeding, infection, and thrombosis. There is an increased need for assistance at home or family support with at-home dialysis. A systematic review that looked at effectiveness of home-based HD versus in-center dialysis demonstrated lower cost for in home dialysis although the variables analyzed in each study were different.[4]

PD is typically performed in the patient's own home, which can increase patient autonomy. PD can be performed as continuous ambulatory peritoneal dialysis (CAPD) and automated PD. CAPD is done by hand with multiple exchanges per day. Automated PD is done via a machine throughout the night and allows for the daytime hours to be free. PD is associated with lower incidence of anemia, reduced blood stream infections, and more hemodynamic stability compared with HD. Disadvantages are risk of peritonitis, encapsulating peritoneal sclerosis, malnutrition, and hernias.[5] In reported series, hernias occurred in 12% to 37% of patients on PD.[6] To give a historical perspective, 50 years ago PD patients averaged 6 episodes of peritonitis per year. The International Society for Peritoneal Dialysis now proposes a benchmark of 0.5 episode per year or 1 episode of peritonitis in a 2-year span. This is imperative because there is a 5% mortality associated with each episode of peritonitis.[7]

LIFE PLAN

The 2019 National Kidney Foundation Kidney Dialysis Outcomes Quality Initiative guidelines focus on the ESKD Life-Plan.[8] This paradigm calls for collaborative decision-making between the patient and their interdisciplinary kidney care team when formulating a plan for kidney replacement therapy. The Life-Plan includes determining the preferred modality of renal replacement, setting (home vs in-center) and access type (AVF, AVG, TDC) and should be based on patient's medical comorbidities, anatomic limitations, and preferences. The primary principle of the Life-Plan is to create "the right access, for the right patient, at the right time, for the right reasons."

PATIENT SELECTION FOR HEMODIALYSIS VERSUS PERITONEAL DIALYSIS

When choosing PD versus HD, the initial decision typically occurs between the nephrologist and the patient. The primary factor in the decision should be patient preference. There are a number of barriers for PD. From a surgical perspective, a hostile abdomen is the most common contraindication to PD catheter placement. Other barriers include obesity, ileostomy/colostomy, and prior transplant.[9] Additional factors that may make a patient a less ideal candidate for PD are advanced age, diabetes, heart failure, and hearing loss.[10] Measures that can ameliorate the barriers include the parasternal PD catheter placement, the use of low-volume dialysate, and the use of vibration or light alarms for the hearing impaired. Communication and education between the nephrologist, surgeon, and patient is critical to formulate a plan for patients who are interested in PD.

If a patient chooses HD, the decision tree must consider if the patient has viable options for arteriovenous (AV) access. For patients in whom viable vascular access options for HD have been exhausted, PD should be considered as an alternative. However, patients who cannot tolerate PD due to access complications, poor clearance, or inability to perform treatments on their own can be transitioned to HD.

HEMODIALYSIS ACCESS SELECTION

Vascular access options for HD include AV access (fistula or graft) and TDC. Patients who will receive HD should be referred to a vascular access surgeon at least 6 months before they are anticipated to start.[8] Early referral allows adequate time for an AVF to mature and possibly undergo any required maturation procedures or for a second AV access to be created if the initial fails. The decision-making around placing an AVF or AVG is evolving. Previously, an AVF was considered to be superior to AVG in nearly all circumstances, leading to the dictum "Fistula First."[11] In general, an AVF should be considered before an AVG, particularly in predialysis patients. However, there is increasing evidence that AVF may not have superior patency and function compared with AVG in all patients. In particular, the elderly may be more appropriate for AVG based on evidence that they may have inferior patency and maturation of AVFs.[12,13] Some authors have suggested that AVGs and AVFs have equivalent patency and function for the first 18 months after creation.[14] Thus, patients with limited life expectancy may not get the long-term benefits of an AVF. Further, a number of demographic characteristics and comorbidities may negatively affect AVF maturation and patency, including female sex, coronary artery disease, diabetes, and obesity.[13,15] However, this evidence is not conclusive and the decision regarding AVG versus AVF must be made on an individualized basis considering demographics, comorbidities, patient and family preferences, and the patient's vascular access Life-Plan.[8]

For predialysis patients for whom the Life-Plan suggests AVG, the AVG creation should be performed as close to the start of HD as possible because AVGs have a higher risk of infection and generally lower patency than AVFs. Patients already HD dependent have more urgent need for functional long-term vascular access and AVG may be preferred in select circumstances because it is associated with earlier catheter removal and fewer catheter days than AVF.[16]

Patients that present with urgent need for HD should undergo TDC placement and be evaluated for AV access after being medically optimized. Patients with short life expectancy (less than 9 months) may not be good candidates for AV access and chronic TDC should be considered. Patients with chronic hypotension and/or depressed cardiac output are also poor candidates for an AV access, due to low patency rates.[17] Finally, some patients find frequent cannulation and possible infiltration events to be unacceptably painful, rendering TDC the only option. TDC is associated with significant longer term complications, including infection, catheter dysfunction, and central venous stenosis and should be reserved as long-term access option for only a minority of patients.[8]

PATIENT EVALUATION FOR ARTERIOVENOUS ACCESS CREATION

When counseling a patient regarding vascular access type, the surgeon is subject to multiple constraints, including patient anatomy, physiology, and need to minimize catheter dwell time. Before creation of an AV access, a thorough history should be obtained, and physical examination performed on all patients. The evaluation should focus on arterial inflow, superficial veins that can be used for an AVF, possible recipient outflow veins for an AVG, and central venous outflow. Review of previous operative reports, chest radiographs, venograms, and CT scans can also assist in characterizing possible impediments such as indwelling vascular stents or devices, central venous stenotic lesions, or previous AV access attempts.

The nondominant arm is preferred for AV access placement. However, the dominant arm should be selected if the anatomic requirements for durable access are not present in the nondominant arm.

Arterial Inflow Evaluation and Treatment

All upper extremity pulses should be examined, and blood pressure should be measured in both arms. An upper extremity arterial duplex ultrasound (DUS) to assess brachial, radial, and ulnar arteries is advisable to confirm normal arterial inflow. The waveform in the intended inflow artery should be triphasic and the blood pressure should be equal in both arms. On DUS, the artery should have no more than a moderate degree of calcification. The brachial artery should be at least 3 mm in diameter and the radial and ulnar arteries should at least 2 mm. Emerging evidence suggests that smaller arterial diameter may be an independent risk factor for AVF nonmaturation, suggesting that larger arteries should be used when possible.[18] An intact palmar arch and adequate ulnar inflow, as demonstrated by an Allen test, should be ensured before creating AV access using the radial artery inflow.

If neither arm has adequate arterial inflow at baseline, then the inflow of the nondominant arm should be treated, if possible, to establish an access site. Endovascular revascularization can usually be performed to correct arterial inflow in at least one arm. Rarely, open bypass may be needed.

Central Venous Outflow Evaluation and Treatment

A thorough history should include a detailed inventory of any central venous devices that the patient may have in place currently or in the past. Physical examination may reveal dilated chest wall veins and/or arm swelling suggestive of central venous stenosis/obstruction. If there is any suspicion of compromised venous outflow, a CT venogram and/or catheter-based venogram should be performed.

If neither arm has adequate venous outflow at baseline, the venous outflow of the optimal arm should be treated, if possible. The preferred treatment of central venous stenosis is endovascular balloon venoplasty. A stent may be required if significant recoil occurs. Unfortunately, patency of bare-metal stents to improve venous outflow is poor, with 1-year primary patency of 30% to 40%.[19,20] There is some evidence to suggest that the patency of stent grafts is superior to bare metal stents.[20] In patients who have no other options for access and have a central occlusion on the ipsilateral side, open surgical options such as jugular venous turndown or bypass around the occlusion, if possible, may be considered.[21]

Vein Assessment for Arteriovenous Fistula Creation

The veins for the AVF creation need to be in a convenient location for puncture, reasonably straight, and not deeper than 6 mm under the skin. Ideally, the cephalic vein is used due to its location and typically shallow course. If the basilic vein in the upper arm is used, transposition is required. The likelihood of functional maturity after AVF creation has been associated with increasing vein diameter,[22] and a 4 mm veins are associated with excellent maturation rates. However, many HD patients have poor quality superficial veins due to repeated blood draws and intravenous catheter placements. Thus, if the only vein that is available has a diameter of less than 3 mm, it may be considered for AVF creation. No exact vein diameter criteria have been established. In the literature, vein diameters resulting in successful AVF vary widely, with diameters as low as 2 mm have been reported.[23] Measurement of vein diameter by DUS also varies depending on hydration status, room temperature, and use of a tourniquet. Vascular surgeons should be familiar with ultrasound techniques and have DUS available in the operating room to examine the veins immediately before the operation.[24]

Evaluation of Arteriovenous Graft Recipient Vessels

A brachial or superficial vein in the antecubital fossa may be used for venous outflow of a forearm AVG if patent on DUS. The other option is use of the axillary vein for upper arm AVG. In all cases, a venous diameter of 4 mm or greater is required.[25]

ARTERIOVENOUS FISTULA CREATION

To determine the appropriate site for AVF creation, a distal-to-proximal and superficial veins first approach is recommended. Creation of initial AVF distally preserves more proximal vessels for future access sites. AVF using cephalic (superficial) veins is preferred over basilic (deep) veins because it is technically less challenging, require less revisions and may be easier to cannulate on HD.[26,27]

Based on this approach, radiocephalic AVF should be considered first if adequate arterial inflow and venous outflow is available. Radiocephalic access has been shown to have lower patency and maturation when compared with upper arm access in patients aged older than 65 years, women, and patients with diabetes.[12,28] Although the evidence regarding any one of these characteristics is not conclusive, patients with increasing numbers of these adverse characteristics are not ideal candidates for radial artery-based AVF, and as such a more proximal site should be considered.

The forearm basilic AVF is another option for distal access and can be created using either the radial or the ulnar arteries.[29] Depending on the individual patient's anatomy, the distal segment of the basilic vein may need to be mobilized and transposed in order for it to be anastomosed to the artery. The outcomes of forearm basilic AVF are relatively poor, with 60% maturation rates and 50% primary and 70% secondary 1-year patency.[29-31] However, the complication rates of access-related hand ischemia and infection are very low. This is a particularly attractive option in younger patients with long life expectancies who may need numerous permanent vascular access sites over their life span.

When forearm AVF is not an option, upper arm cephalic fistula is typically considered as another option. Utilizing proximal radial artery as in inflow is preferred over the brachial artery because it is associated with lower rates of access-related hand ischemia. One prospective study demonstrated no difference in the 1-year patency rate of proximal radiocephalic AVFs with significantly lower incidence of steal, arm swelling, and pseudoaneurysm as compared with brachiocephalic fistulas.[32] Upper arm fistulas utilizing cephalic vein as an outflow may require transposition in some patients due to depth. This can be done at the index operation or as a secondary procedure. Although there is a paucity of data on this topic, there is a large single institutional review of basilic vein transposition (BVT) and cephalic vein transposition (CVT), which demonstrated a 5-year primary and secondary patency of 52% and 62%, respectively, for the BVT compared with 40% and 46% for the CVT. Both are significantly better than AVG.[33]

If cephalic vein is not suitable, upper arm brachial artery to basilic vein AVF is another option. It can be created in a single-stage or 2-stage manner. The basilic vein is not anatomically located in an immediate subcutaneous position needed for access, and it must be transposed to a more superficial and anterolateral position. In the single-stage procedure, the entire basilic vein is dissected out, transposed to a superficial position, and anastomosed to the brachial artery. In the 2-stage procedure, the basilic vein is anastomosed to the brachial artery in the first operation, and at the second operation, the fistula is superficialized. Typically, 4 to 6 weeks elapse between the first and second stages to allow for maturation of the fistula.

The basilic vein can be superficialized by passing it through a superficial tunnel or placing the vein in a superficial pocket by creating a skin flap that is no more than 5 mm thick. If tunneling is used in a 2-stage approach, the fistula is divided near the anastomosis, passed through the tunnel, and reanastomosed to itself or to the brachial artery higher up in the arm. Using a superficial pocket in the 2-stage approach obviates a new anastomosis but it does create a larger tissue flap that may lead to a wound complication.

There is some evidence that the 2-stage approach may be more durable and cost-effective than is the 1-stage procedure.[34] One meta-analysis demonstrated no difference in 1-year primary and secondary patency rates between the 1-stage and 2-stage approaches, despite the veins in the 2-stage group being smaller in diameter. Three of the 8 studies included in the meta-analysis preferentially reserved 2-stage transpositions for patients with smaller veins. There was no difference in primary failure rate in patients with 1-stage transpositions (15%–45%) and in patients with 2-stage transpositions (10%–42%, $P = .46$). Similarly, there was no difference in 1-year primary and secondary patency.[35] This suggests that for smaller basilic veins, the 2-stage approach may be preferred.

As of 2020, there are 2 percutaneous AVF creation technologies available in the United States: Ellipsys (Avenu Medical, San Juan Capistrano, CA) and WavelinQ (Bard Peripheral Vascular Inc, Tempe, AZ). Both technologies rely on a perforator vein that connects the deep and the superficial venous systems in the antecubital fossa. In patients who have are candidates for radiocephalic AVF, percutaneous fistula should not be a first choice because it creates upper arm fistula and bypasses the distal first approach. The Ellipsys system is performed under ultrasound and uses transvenous sharp needle access to the proximal radial artery; a 6F sheath is placed over a wire into the radial artery, and a single catheter with an integrated heating element is passed. The AVF is created using pressure and heat. The connection is then dilated open using balloon angioplasty. The perforator must be in close proximity to the proximal artery (<1.5 mm), and both the perforator vein and the artery must be at least 2 mm in diameter.

The WavelinQ system creates a fistula near the venous perforator between either the proximal radial or the ulnar artery and a corresponding deep vein. Two catheters are used: arterial and venous. Access to the creation site requires adequately sized vessels for passage of 4F sheaths. Once the catheters are in position, a radiofrequency electrode is used to create the AVF.

Unlike surgical AVF, there is no surgical scar, and the anastomosis is relatively distal in the antecubital fossa. As such, "side-by-side" cannulation at the antecubital fossa, with 1 needle in the median basilic vein and 1 needle in the median cephalic vein is possible, as is 2-needle cannulation in the median basilic vein. This geometry may enable patients to avoid BVT.

Although early results are promising, secondary procedures are frequently necessary to obtain functional maturity.[36,37] As such, further studies will be required in order to more clearly define the role of percutaneous AVF versus surgical AVF.

ARTERIOVENOUS GRAFT CREATION

A number of types of prosthetic grafts are available and can be used for AVG construction. However, none has been shown to have superior patency or lower complication rates. The most commonly used is the expanded polytetrafluoroethylene (ePTFE) graft. Other available materials are heparin-bonded ePTFE and multilayer early-access grafts. EPTFE grafts are available as a conventional single-diameter tube and tapered versions that include a 4 to 7-mm taper and a 6 to 8-mm taper. Randomized comparisons of tapered grafts compared with conventional grafts have not demonstrated differences in access-related hand ischemia or patency.[38,39] Heparin-bonded ePTFE has not been shown to improve patency over conventional ePTFE grafts.[40,41]

Standard grafts require 2 to 3 weeks of tissue ingrowth after creation before it can be accessed without access site extravasation. Early-cannulation grafts can be accessed within 24 hours after creation and can be used to decrease catheter dwell-time. There are 3 commercially available grafts in the United States; 3-layer ePTFE graft (Flixene), 3-layer graft composed of polyetherurethaneurea and a siloxane-containing surface-modifying additive (Vectra), and a 3-layer graft with the inner and outer layer being ePTFE and a low-bleed elastomeric middle layer (Acuseal). The 12-month primary patency of all the early cannulation grafts ranges from 43% to 63% and the secondary patency ranges from 70% to 86%.[42] Early cannulation does not seem to adversely affect graft patency,[33] although the risk of ischemic steal requiring treatment may be as high as 11%.[43]

The infection rate of upper extremity AVG has been reported to be anywhere from 3.5% to 19.7%.[44] Patients who are immunocompromised, those with a chronic infection, or who have had vascular access infections in the past are at an increased risk of AVG infection and biologic rather than prosthetic conduit can be considered. A number of biologic grafts are available including bovine carotid artery, bovine ureter, bovine mesenteric vein, cryopreserved human vein, and cryopreserved human artery. Of the bovine conduits, the bovine carotid artery is the most commonly used. In a randomized trial of bovine carotid artery and ePTFE AVGs, the bovine carotid artery had higher 1-year primary (60.5% vs 10.1%, $P = .0062$) and primary-assisted patency (60.5% vs 20.8%, $P = .012$), with fewer interventions to maintain patency (1.3 vs 2.5 per patient-year, $P = .014$). EPTFE AVGs also had higher rates of infection (0.3 vs 0 per patient-year compared, $P = .008$).[45]

CHALLENGING SITUATIONS

For patients in whom the aforementioned access options are not possible, other, less commonly used options can be considered. The brachial artery to brachial vein AVF is a technically challenging operation, with high rates of maturation failure (up to 50%) and various 1-year primary patency (24%–77%).[46,47] The brachial vein is a thin-walled and deep with numerous tributaries that require careful dissection. The median nerve runs close to the vein and must be carefully preserved. The brachial–brachial

AVF can be created in 1 stage or in 2 stages, in the same manner as the brachial–basilic AVF. The limited evidence supports better outcomes with the 2-stage approach.[46,47] Although brachial–brachial AVF maturation and patency rates are inferior to brachiocephalic and brachiobasilic AVF, it offers an autogenous alternative for patients who do not have adequate superficial veins and may be preferable to an AVG in certain otherwise robust patients.

In patients without any available options for arm access, a chest wall AVG may be considered. It requires normal axillary artery inflow and axillary vein outflow. The graft can be performed in a looped manner between the ipsilateral axillary artery and vein or in a "necklace" configuration between the axillary artery and the contralateral axillary vein. Both configurations are comparable with approximately 80% 1-year secondary patency.[48,49]

For patients with central venous stenosis/occlusion that cannot be successfully treated but can be crossed using endovascular techniques, the HD Reliable Outflow (HeRO) Graft (Merit Medical, South Jordan, UT) is an option for upper extremity access. The HeRO is a composite of a prosthetic graft and a catheter that is completely subcutaneous. The graft is anastomosed to arterial inflow in the arm, tunneled subcutaneously, and connected to the central catheter at the deltopectoral groove. One-year primary patency rate is only 22% but secondary patency is 60%. On average, 1.5 to 3 interventions per year are required to maintain patency and the device-related bacteremia rates are between 0.13 and 0.7 episodes per 1000 days.[50] A HeRO may be preferred to preserve lower extremity options for future access or in patients who do not have lower extremity access options.[50]

If no arm access is possible, thigh access can be considered. In evaluating a patient for a lower extremity access, screening for lower extremity PAD is imperative. Placement of a thigh access in patients with significant PAD can result in ischemic steal, leading to limb-threatening ischemia, gangrene, and amputation. Inflow can be from the comon femoral artery (CFA), profunda, or superfical femoral artery (SFA) with outflow into the common femoral, femoral, or great saphenous vein (GSV) vein.

AVF in the thigh is preferentially constructed using the transposed femoral-popliteal vein, which is a technically demanding operation involving a complex dissection and, as such, is reserved for good-risk patients. Femoral vein AVFs have been associated with 18% major complication rate; however, high maturation (82%) and patency rates (56% at 9 years) were described in one large series.[51] Thigh AVF using the saphenous vein is less technically demanding; however, results are not satisfactory because of the lack of dilation of the GSV over time.[52] Prosthetic thigh AVGs are associated with a higher rate of infection than are arm AVGs. In one series of 125 thigh AVGs, 41% developed infection, requiring an intervention at 20 months of mean follow-up.[53] In a recent meta-analysis, approximately 18% of thigh AVGs was abandoned because of infection compared with less than 2% of fistulas. However, thigh AVGs had a lower incidence of ischemic complications compared with fistulas (21% vs 7%).[54] In a comparison of thigh AVG with long-term TDCs, despite a relatively high rate of thigh graft infection (21% at 1 year), grafts were associated with significantly higher infection-free survival rates.[55]

ACCESS FOR PERITONEAL DIALYSIS

PD catheter can be placed via open, laparoscopic, or percutaneous surgical approaches. The literature describes a 10% to 35% catheter malfunction rate when using the open technique and 2.8% to 13% catheter failures for the laparoscopic insertion technique.[56] Based on a metanalysis comparing open versus laparoscopic PD catheter placement, laparoscopic approach was associated with decreased migration rate and increased 1-year catheter survival. There was no difference in incidence of peritonitis.[56] Perceived benefits of laparoscopic would be better visualization during the procedure and increased patient satisfaction.

Another meta-analysis compared percutaneous versus surgical placement (open and laparoscopic). Significantly lower rates of exit-site infections and peritonitis were observed in percutaneous group at 30 days without any difference in mechanical complications.[57]

PALLIATIVE CARE DISCUSSION

Based on Renal Physician Association practice guidelines,[58] the shared decision-making for initiation and withdrawal of dialysis should be made by physician, patient, and family. Patient and family should be fully informed about the diagnosis, prognosis, and all treatment options. Consideration to forgo dialysis should be considered for patients who have a very poor prognosis or for whom dialysis cannot be provided safely. A time-limited trial of dialysis can be considered for patients who have an uncertain prognosis, or for whom a consensus cannot be reached about providing dialysis. To improve patient-centered outcomes, physicians should offer palliative care services to all patients with ESKD who suffer from burdens of their disease. Goals of care discussions are critical in these situations.

CLINICS CARE POINTS

- Contemporary selection of optimal renal replacement modality and vascular access type should be guided by the principles of the ESKD Life-Plan, which including shared decision-making between the patient and the multidisciplinary care team.

- Although general principles of AV access include starting as distally as possible in the nondominant arm and autogenous fistulas are preferred, general principles may not apply equally in all patients and the final decision should be individualized to the characteristics and preferences of each patient.

- Patients who are dependent on dialysis require timely functional access and efforts to minimize percutaneous catheter dependence should be considered.

- Patients who are not yet dependent on dialysis (predialysis) should not have a prosthetic AV graft created more than 4 weeks before the anticipated start of dialysis dependence.

- A small percentage of patients, such as those of advanced age with multiple comorbidities or those with limited life expectancy are appropriate candidates for long-term HD through a tunneled catheter.

- PD catheters can be placed via open surgical, laparoscopic, or percutaneous approach with similar outcomes.

DISCLOSURE

The authors have nothing to disclose.

REFERENCES

1. System USRD. 2022 USRDS annual data report: epidemiology of kidney disease in the United States. Bethesda (MD): National Institutes of Health, National Institute of Diabetes and Digestive and Kidney Diseases; 2022.

2. Brescia MJ, Cimino JE, Appel K, et al. Chronic HD using venipuncture and a surgically created arteriovenous fistula. N Engl J Med 1966;275:1089–92.
3. Pearson J, Turenne M, Leichtman A. The Executive Order on Kidney Care: An Opportunity to Improve Outcomes for Individuals With Kidney Disease. Kidney Int Rep 2019 Sep 18;4:1519–22.
4. Ishani A, Slinin Y, Greer N, et al. Comparative effectiveness of home-based kidney dialysis versus in-center or other outpatient kidney dialysis locations- a systematic review. Washington (DC): Department of Veterans Affairs (US); 2015.
5. Eroglu E, Heimbürger O, Lindholm B. Peritoneal dialysis patient selection from a comorbidity perspective. Semin Dial 2022;35:25–39.
6. Balda S, Power A, Papalois V, et al. Impact of hernias on peritoneal dialysis technique, survival and residula renal function. Perit Dial Int 2013;33:629–34.
7. Slazer WL. Peritoneal dialysis-related peritonitis: challenges an dsolutions. Int J Nephrol Renovasc Dis 2018;11:173–86.
8. Lok CE, Huber TS, Lee T, et al. KDOQI Clinical Practice Guideline for Vascular Access: 2019 Update. Am J Kidney Dis 2020;75:S1–164.
9. Sinnakirouchenan R, Holley JL. Peritoneal dialysis versus HD: risks, benefits, and access issues. Adv Chronic Kidney Dis 2011;18:428–32.
10. Eroglu E, Heimbürger O, Lindholm B. Peritoneal dialysis patient selection from a comorbidity perspective. Semin Dial 2022;35:25–39.
11. Neumann ME. "Fistula first" initiative pushes for new standards in access care. Nephrol News Issues 2004;18:43, 47-48.
12. Misskey J, Faulds J, Sidhu R, et al. An age-based comparison of fistula location, patency, and maturation for elderly renal failure patients. J Vasc Surg 2018;67: 1491–500.
13. Woo K, Ulloa J, Allon M, et al. Establishing patient-specific criteria for selecting the optimal upper extremity vascular access procedure. J Vasc Surg 2017;65: 1089–103.
14. Lee T, Qian J, Thamer M, et al. Tradeoffs in Vascular Access Selection in Elderly Patients Initiating HD With a Catheter. Am J Kidney Dis 2018;72:509–18.
15. Wilmink T, Corte-Real Houlihan M. Diameter Criteria Have Limited Value for Prediction of Functional Dialysis Use of Arteriovenous Fistulas. Eur J Vasc Endovasc Surg 2018;56:572–81.
16. Leake AE, Yuo TH, Wu T, et al. Arteriovenous grafts are associated with earlier catheter removal and fewer catheter days in the United States Renal Data System population. J Vasc Surg 2015;62:123–7.
17. Chang TI, Paik J, Greene T, et al. Intradialytic hypotension and vascular access thrombosis. J Am Soc Nephrol 2011;22:1526–33.
18. Farrington CA, Robbin ML, Lee T, et al. Early Predictors of Arteriovenous Fistula Maturation: A Novel Perspective on an Enduring Problem. J Am Soc Nephrol 2020;31:1617–27.
19. Kundu S. Review of central venous disease in HD patients. J Vasc Interv Radiol 2010;21:963–8.
20. Ginsburg M, Lorenz JM, Zivin SP, et al. A practical review of the use of stents for the maintenance of HD access. Semin Intervent Radiol 2015;32:217–24.
21. Wooster M, Fernandez B, Summers KL, et al. Surgical and endovascular central venous reconstruction combined with thoracic outlet decompression in highly symptomatic patients. J Vasc Surg Venous Lymphat Disord 2019;7:106–12.
22. Lauvao LS, Ihnat DM, Goshima KR, et al. Vein diameter is the major predictor of fistula maturation. J Vasc Surg 2009;49:1499–504.

23. Wang B, Rao A, Pappas K, et al. Maturation Rates of Arteriovenous Fistulas Using Small Veins in the Era of Endovascular Interventions. Ann Vasc Surg 2021;71: 208–14.
24. Taubenfeld E, Minjoo Kim YH, Hoffstaetter T, et al. Intraoperative vascular mapping improves patient eligibility for arteriovenous fistula creation. Am J Surg 2022;22:S0002–9610.
25. Silva MB Jr, Hobson RW, Pappas PJ, et al. A strategy for increasing use of autogenous HD access procedures: impact of preoperative noninvasive evaluation. J Vasc Surg 1998;27:302–7.
26. Ramanathan AK, Nader ND, Dryjski ML, et al. A retrospective review of basilic and cephalic vein-based fistulas. Vascular 2011;19:97–104.
27. Quencer KB, Arici M. Arteriovenous Fistulas and Their Characteristic Sites of Stenosis. AJR Am J Roentgenol 2015;205:726–34.
28. Mousa AY, Dearing DD, Aburahma AF. Radiocephalic fistula: review and update. Ann Vasc Surg 2013;27:370–8.
29. Schwein A, Georg Y, Lejay A, et al. Promising Results of the Forearm Basilic Fistula Reveal a Worthwhile Option between Radial Cephalic and Brachial Fistula. Ann Vasc Surg 2016;32:5–8.
30. Al Shakarchi J, Khawaja A, Cassidy D, et al. Efficacy of the Ulnar-Basilic Arteriovenous Fistula for HD: A Systematic Review. Ann Vasc Surg 2016;32:1–4.
31. Glowinski J, Glowinska I, Malyszko J, et al. Basilic vein transposition in the forearm for secondary arteriovenous fistula. Angiology 2014;65:330–2.
32. Arnaoutakis DJ, Deroo EP, McGlynn P, et al. Improved outcomes with proximal radial-cephalic arteriovenous fistulas compared with brachial-cephalic arteriovenous fistulas. J Vasc Surg 2017;66:1497–503.
33. Woo K, Farber A, Doros G, et al. Evaluation fo the efficacy of the transposed upper arm arteriovenous fistula: A single institutionl review of 190 basilic and cephalic vein transposition procedures. J Vasc Surg 2007;46:94–9.
34. Ghaffarian AA, Griffin CL, Kraiss LW, et al. Comparative effectiveness of one-stage versus two-stage basilic vein transposition arteriovenous fistulas. J Vasc Surg 2018;67:529–35.
35. Cooper J, Power AH, DeRose G, et al. Similar failure and patency rates when comparing one- and two-stage basilic vein transposition. J Vasc Surg 2015;61: 809–16.
36. Lok CE, Rajan DK, Clement J, et al. Endovascular Proximal Forearm Arteriovenous Fistula for HD Access: Results of the Prospective, Multicenter Novel Endovascular Access Trial (NEAT). Am J Kidney Dis 2017;70:486–97.
37. Hull JE, Jennings WC, Cooper RI, et al. The Pivotal Multicenter Trial of Ultrasound-Guided Percutaneous Arteriovenous Fistula Creation for HD Access. J Vasc Interv Radiol 2018;29:149–58.
38. Polo JR, Ligero JM, Diaz-Cartelle J, et al. Randomized comparison of 6-mm straight grafts versus 6- to 8-mm tapered grafts for brachial-axillary dialysis access. J Vasc Surg 2004;40:319–24.
39. Han S, Seo PW, Ryu JW. Surgical Outcomes of Forearm Loop Arteriovenous Fistula Formation Using Tapered versus Non-Tapered Polytetrafluoroethylene Grafts. Korean J Thorac Cardiovasc Surg 2017;50:30–5.
40. Allemang MT, Schmotzer B, Wong VL, et al. Heparin bonding does not improve patency of polytetrafluoroethylene arteriovenous grafts. Ann Vasc Surg 2014; 28:28–34.
41. Zea N, Menard G, Le L, et al. Heparin-Bonded Polytetrafluorethylene Does Not Improve HD Arteriovenous Graft Function. Ann Vasc Surg 2016;30:28–33.

42. Al Shakarchi J, Inston N. Early cannulation grafts for haemodialysis: An updated systematic review. J Vasc Access 2019;20:123–7.
43. Glickman MH, Burgess J, Cull D, et al. Prospective multicenter study with a 1-year analysis of a new vascular graft used for early cannulation in patients undergoing HD. J Vasc Surg 2015;6:434–41.
44. Akoh JA. Prosthetic arteriovenous grafts for HD. J Vasc Access 2009;10:137–47.
45. Kennealey PT, Elias N, Hertl M, et al. A prospective, randomized comparison of bovine carotid artery and expanded polytetrafluoroethylene for permanent HD vascular access. J Vasc Surg 2011;53:1640–8.
46. Kotsis T, Moulakakis KG, Mylonas SN, et al. Brachial Artery-Brachial Vein Fistula for HD: One- or Two-Stage Procedure-A Review. Journal of Angiology 2016; 25:14–9.
47. Jennings WC, Sideman MJ, Taubman KE, et al. Brachial vein transposition arteriovenous fistulas for HD access. J Vasc Surg 2009;50:1121–5.
48. Gale-Grant O, Chemla ES. Single-center results of a series of prosthetic axillary-axillary arteriovenous access grafts for HD. J Vasc Surg 2016;64:1741–6.
49. Hunter JP, Nicholson ML. Midterm experience of ipsilateral axillary-axillary arteriovenous loop graft as tertiary access for haemodialysis. J Transplant 2014; 2014:908738.
50. Steerman SN, Wagner J, Higgins JA, et al. Outcomes comparison of HeRO and lower extremity arteriovenous grafts in patients with long-standing renal failure. J Vasc Surg 2013;57:776–83.
51. Bourquelot P, Rawa M, Van Laere O, et al. Long-term results of femoral vein transposition for autogenous arteriovenous HD access. J Vasc Surg 2012;56:440–5.
52. Pierre-Paul D, Williams S, Lee T, et al. Saphenous vein loop to femoral artery arteriovenous fistula: a practical alternative. Ann Vasc Surg 2004;18:223–7.
53. Cull JD, Cull DL, Taylor SM, et al. Prosthetic thigh arteriovenous access: outcome with SVS/AAVS reporting standards. J Vasc Surg 2004;39:381–6.
54. Antoniou GA, Lazarides MK, Georgiadis GS, et al. Lower-extremity arteriovenous access for haemodialysis: a systematic review. Eur J Vasc Endovasc Surg 2009; 38:365–72.
55. Ong S, Barker-Finkel J, Allon M. Long-term outcomes of arteriovenous thigh grafts in HD patients: a comparison with tunneled dialysis catheters. Clin J Am Soc Nephrol 2013;8:804–9.
56. Hagen SM, Lafranca JA, Steyerberg EW, et al. Laparoscopic versus open peritoneal dialysis catheter insertion: a meta-analysis. PLoS One 2013;8(2):e56351.
57. Agarwal A, Whitlock RH, Bamforth RJ, et al. Percutaneous Versus Surgical Insertion of Peritoneal Dialysis Catheters: A Systematic Review and Meta-Analysis. Can J Kidney Health Dis 2021;8. https://doi.org/10.1177/20543581211052731.
58. Renal Physicians Association. Shared decision-making in the appropriate initiation of and withdrawal from dialysis. Clinical practice guideline. 2nd edition. Rockville (MD): Renal Physicians Association; 2010.

Maintenance and Salvage of Hemodialysis Access

John Iguidbashian, MD[a], Rabbia Imran, MS[b],
Jeniann A. Yi, MD, MS[a],*

KEYWORDS

- Hemodialysis access • Salvage • Arteriovenous • Fistula • Graft • Maintenance

KEY POINTS

- Endovascular and open techniques are both critical to maintaining and salvaging hemodialysis access sites.
- The most common issue resulting in hemodialysis access failure is stenosis, usually related to a prior surgical anastomosis.
- Open revision may be necessary for recurrent/recalcitrant stenosis, aneurysmal and pseudoaneurysmal degeneration, hemodialysis access-induced digital ischemia, and infection.

INTRODUCTION

Chronic kidney disease affects an estimated 37 million Americans, of which nearly 786,000 are living with end-stage kidney disease (ESKD).[1,2] Individuals living with ESKD typically rely on renal replacement therapy such as hemodialysis (HD) as a life-sustaining treatment while awaiting kidney transplantation. Unfortunately, the median waitlist time for kidney transplant has been reported up to 49.2 months.[1,3] Thus, the need for reliable and sustainable HD access is of great importance. Herein we discuss the evaluation of HD access sites, mechanisms of HD access failure, and the approach to maintenance and salvage of failing HD access sites.

BACKGROUND

The goal of HD access is to provide simple and reproducible access to the patient's circulatory system, while minimizing complications. There are three main options to achieve this: arteriovenous fistula (AVF) creation, arteriovenous graft (AVG) creation, and placement of temporary hemodialysis catheters. Any patient with a suspected

a Department of Surgery, University of Colorado Anschutz School of Medicine, 457 South Kingston Cir, Aurora, CO 80012, USA; b University of Colorado Anschutz School of Medicine, 13001 East 17th Place, Aurora, CO 80045, USA
* Corresponding author. Division of Vascular Surgery and Endovascular Therapy, 12631 E. 17th Avenue, MC C312, Aurora, CO 80045.
E-mail address: jeniann.yi@cuanschutz.edu

Surg Clin N Am 103 (2023) 685–701
https://doi.org/10.1016/j.suc.2023.05.004
0039-6109/23/© 2023 Elsevier Inc. All rights reserved.
surgical.theclinics.com

need for HD within 1 year should begin discussions regarding long-term HD access planning.[4] Furthermore, a detailed End-Stage Kidney Disease Life Plan has many demonstrated benefits for patient quality of life and can help guide decision-making regarding maintenance and salvage of HD access.[5]

The rates of short- and long-term access-associated complications in addition to the inherent risk of primary failure remain high.[6-8] AVFs and AVGs have a considerable risk of both early and late complications leading to significant morbidity, health care costs, and unusable HD access if unaddressed. One study found that only 54% of AVFs were successfully used for HD in the first year after creation.[6] Additionally, approximately one-third of patients require intervention to achieve maturation and nearly 50% will require reintervention to maintain patency of the HD access.[9] The culmination of surveillance and interventions results in an average cost of $7,871 per patient/year for AVFs that maintained primary patency in contrast to $13,282 per patient/year for AVFs that experienced patency loss at 1 year.[10,11] AVGs have similar patency rates of 49.4% at 1 year, 31.6% at 2 years, and 20.2% at 3 years.[12] These statistics clearly highlight the need for effective strategies to maintain and salvage HD access once established.

ASSESSMENT OF HEMODIALYSIS ACCESS
Clinical Exam Findings

Surveillance of mature AVFs is a critical component of postoperative care. Nearly all complications have an associated underlying pathology that can frequently be detected and intervened upon prior to loss of functionality. Thus, surveillance should include clinical monitoring with the physical examination via inspection, palpation, and auscultation of access sites at each dialysis session.[4,13]

Notable signs on physical exam that should raise suspicion for an underlying problem include distal extremity edema, changes in thrill, alterations in the bruit on auscultation, or neurologic deficits in the extremity. Specific signs of stenosis include the collapse of the AVF with abduction, increased pulsatility with either no thrill or a short systolic thrill felt in the pulsatile portion with a more continuous thrill beyond the stenosis, or a high-pitched systolic bruit distal to the stenosis.

Pain, enlargement, and skin erosions may be associated with aneurysmal degeneration, requiring further investigation and potential intervention. Pseudoaneurysms may also present as skin erosions, and often necessitate urgent intervention due to bleeding and/or infectious risk. During dialysis, concerning signs and symptoms include the aspiration of clots, high pressure in lines, prolonged bleeding from the insertion site, or difficulty with cannulation. Further imaging decisions and interventions are determined based on these initial findings.

Surveillance Imaging

Concerns raised by physical exam should be investigated utilizing diagnostic imaging modalities including duplex ultrasound, computed tomographic angiography (CTA)/ magnetic resonance angiography (MRA), static dialysis venous pressure, and intra-access flow rate measurements. CTA/MRA can be utilized to visualize anatomic abnormalities but lacks dynamic flow measurement capabilities; thus, duplex ultrasound is the gold standard for the initial evaluation of failing HD access. Studies should include measurements of flow volume, velocities, direction, waveforms, and anatomic characteristics such as vessel diameter.[14] Flow volumes <600 mL/minute, >50% diameter narrowing, waveforms indicative of high resistance and a large discrepancy of peak systolic velocities across a visualized stenosis should raise suspicion for a clinically significant lesion. These findings should prompt the use of more invasive imaging such as a diagnostic fistulogram with potential for intervention as well.[15]

DEFINING HEMODIALYSIS ACCESS FAILURE

Primary failure is defined as HD access that is never usable or fails within three months of creation.[7,8] The cause of primary HD access failure is typically an anatomic etiology resulting in a lack of adequate flow volumes and subsequent dysfunctional maturation (**Box 1**). Failure rates have been reported up to 50%, with the highest failure rate occurring in radiocephalic AVFs.[7,8] Risk factors for primary failure include obesity, older age, female sex, cardiovascular disease, diabetes, and thrombophilia.[6]

Secondary failure is defined as the inability to use a matured AV fistula or graft after at least three months of normal usage. Functional success and maturation are indicated by the ability to use the access site for dialysis. Secondary failure following successful maturation is typically due to the occurrence or re-occurrence of stenotic lesions, late thrombosis formation, or development of aneurysm or pseudoaneurysmal dilation. Risk factors for delayed access failure are similar to primary failure with the addition of increased risk in access sites that required intervention to achieve maturation initially.

CASE STUDY

A 54-year-old female on HD underwent brachiocephalic AVF creation in her non-dominant left arm with an existing right tunneled dialysis catheter in place. Initial concerns

Box 1	
Common etiologies of access failure	
Venous hypertension	• Associated with central stenosis and prior central venous catheters.
	• Identified in approximately 5–10% of patients with failing HD access[16]
High-flow HD access	• Defined as a flow rate >1500 mL/min
	• Leads to aneurysmal enlargement, accelerated development of central venous stenosis, pulmonary hypertension, and cardiac overload, with potential for hemodialysis access-induced distal ischemia
Stenosis	• 85–90% of thrombosed AV grafts are caused by an anatomic stenosis.[17]
	• Most common stenosis = anastomotic (eg, venous (60%) in AVGs, arteriovenous (60–67%) in AVFs[18])
	• Alternate sites for stenosis = cephalic arch (45%), peripheral draining veins (37.1%), cannulation zone (38.4%), central veins (3.2%), and feeding artery (5%)[18]
Inadequate vasculature	• Appropriate vessel selection should avoid any extremity with increased risk of impaired outflow (eg, prior surgery, radiation, pacemaker, or central catheter placement)
	• Preoperative imaging evaluating both arteries and veins is highly recommended to ensure adequate vessel size[19]
Infection	• Incidence as high as 2.18 per 100 patient-months for all types of vascular access, with lower incidence of infection with AVFs vs AVGs (0.2–0.4 per 1000 days vs. 1–2 per 1000 days)[19,20]
	• Access-related infectious complications account for approximately 20% of HD access loss[20]

with maturation prompted angiography, but no issues were identified and the AVF was successfully used (**Fig. 1**). Development of high pressures resulting in difficulty completing HD prompted a subsequent fistulogram at 6 months, demonstrating filling of a large collateral system in the upper arm and stenoses of the cephalic arch. This lesion was treated with balloon angioplasty with subsequent improvement (**Fig. 2**). The AVF was again used for 3 months until recurrent issues developed. Repeat fistulography demonstrated recurrent cephalic arch stenosis with occlusion, which was traversed endovascularly but failed to dilate adequately post-angioplasty (**Fig. 3**). Based on this, open revision with cephalic vein turndown was recommended to improve venous outflow (**Fig. 4**).

TREATMENT

Failing HD access sites should undergo intervention when a stenotic lesion narrows the vascular lumen greater than 50% and is associated with symptoms, abnormal physical exam findings, and/or abnormal flow measurements. These often coincide with issues successfully completing HD, prompting further evaluation and the need for intervention as well.

Endovascular Intervention

Angiography with potential intervention is the preferred initial approach, allowing for both the evaluation and treatment of failing HD access. Post-intervention results can be judged as anatomic and/or clinical success. Whereas anatomic success can be defined intraoperatively based on the amount of residual stenosis seen on completion angiogram, clinical or physiologic success is determined postoperatively by relief of symptoms and the ability to use the access for dialysis.

Percutaneous transluminal balloon angioplasty
Technical success is reliant on the physical disruption of the stenotic vessel's layers to allow for re-expansion. Failure to create mechanical change results in immediate vessel recoil and the need for repeat intervention. One technique to ensure adequate angioplasty is performing intravenous ultrasound (IVUS) intraoperatively to confirm adequate vessel expansion. Providers may also consider modification to a larger balloon size and/or higher-pressure balloons to limit recurrence.

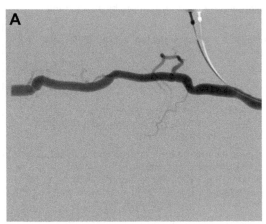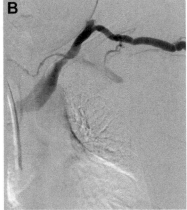

Fig. 1. Initial angiography of the matured brachiocephalic AVF demonstrating patent (*A*) upper arm and (*B*) central portions.

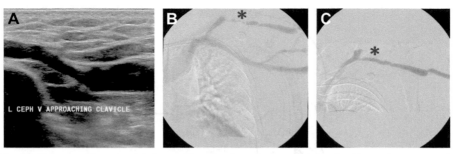

Fig. 2. Ultrasound imaging of the malfunctioning AVF at 6 months demonstrating a stenotic portion of the cephalic vein as it approaches the clavicle (*A*), with corresponding angiography of the cephalic arch (*B*) and its response post-angioplasty (*C*). *Note: red asterisk denotes cephalic arch on angiogram.*

- Traditional balloon angioplasty: conventionally used as a first-line treatment of stenoses, often utilizing a high-compliance balloon. However, there are high recurrence rates with primary assisted patency rate <24% at 3 years and 23% restenosis rate within 6 months of intervention.[21] Thus, alternative angioplasty techniques have been explored in recent years.
- Cutting balloon angioplasty: utilizes mounted external elements that can score the intima upon inflation and often utilized for recurrent stenoses and elastic lesions. A meta-analysis by Agarwal and colleagues[22] found that although the immediate procedural success rate was unchanged, 6-month patency was significantly higher with cutting balloon (67.2% vs 55.6%, p < 0.05) as compared to traditional balloon angioplasty.
- Drug-eluting balloon angioplasty (DEA): disseminates an anti-proliferative agent (commonly paclitaxel) during insufflation via direct contact with the intima to limit neointimal hyperplasia and recurrence. Initial studies showed no difference in primary patency at 6 months (OR 2.03, 95% CI 0.64–6.45) compared to traditional balloon angioplasty; however, there was superior 12-month patency overall (OR 3.66, 95% CI 1.32–10.14)[21,23,24] with further confirmation of the utility of DEA via multiple clinical trials.[25,26] Newer iterations have included additional

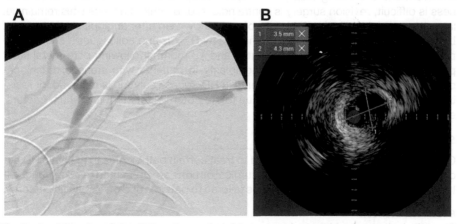

Fig. 3. Angiography of the AVF at 9 months with recurrent stenosis and occlusion of the cephalic arch (*A*), with inadequate response post-angioplasty on intravascular ultrasound (*B*).

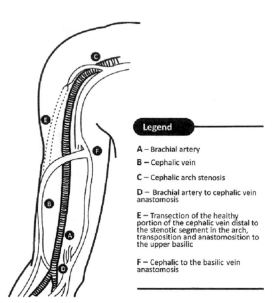

Legend

A – Brachial artery

B – Cephalic vein

C – Cephalic arch stenosis

D – Brachial artery to cephalic vein anastomosis

E – Transection of the healthy portion of the cephalic vein distal to the stenotic segment in the arch, transposition and anastomosition to the upper basilic

F – Cephalic to the basilic vein anastomosis

Fig. 4. Diagram of cephalic vein turndown procedure, where the cephalic vein is transected proximal to the arch stenosis and reimplanted onto a larger vein (eg, the basilic vein) for improved venous outflow. (*From* Cândido C, Viegas M, Sobrinho G, et al. Transposition of the cephalic vein in therapeutic rescue of cephalic arch stenosis. Clin Kidney J. 2014;7(5):501–503; with permission.)

anti-proliferative agents; the MATILDA, IMPRESSION, and ISABELLA trials studied sirolimus-coated balloons with promising early patency rates and decreased reintervention rates at 6 months, though long-term results are yet to be published.[27–29]

Transcatheter stenting

Indications for AVF stenting, over balloon angioplasty alone, include: (1) a stenotic lesion that is elastic with immediate intraoperative recoil; (2) early recurrent stenosis within 3 months following initially successful angioplasty in an area where surgical access is difficult, revision surgery is contraindicated, or limited access sites remain (ie, late stage salvage), and/or (3) rupture of an outflow vein after angioplasty that cannot be managed conservatively. A meta-analysis by D'Cruz and colleagues[30] showed superior primary patency rates at 6 months and 12 months following bare-metal stent placement over traditional balloon angioplasty in patients with stenotic brachiocephalic fistulas. However, the use of stents in HD access salvage is reserved for resistant lesions and/or high-risk patients due to the potential for stent migration, fracture, erosion, infection, or thrombosis.

Surgical Revision

Open surgical revision may be required to treat certain pathologies to maintain HD access. Several potential scenarios with surgical options are presented herein, though ultimately the surgical approach should be tailored to patients and their specific anatomy.

Recurrent stenosis

Stenotic lesions requiring endovascular intervention multiple times within a three-month period should be considered for open surgical revision if clinically feasible.[30,31]

Anastomotic stenoses may require the creation of a novel anastomosis and moving the site elsewhere, or revision using patch angioplasty to broaden the existing anastomosis. Furthermore, HD access sites with proximal patency but distal stenosis can be potentially salvaged using transposition or turndown procedures, where the access is revised to redirect venous outflow into a patent channel. Described examples include direct anastomosis of the arterialized cephalic vein to the brachial, axillary, or basilic vein for cephalic arch stenoses and internal jugular turndown to bypass subclavian vein stenosis/occlusion.[31–34]

Aneurysm/pseudoaneurysm management

The presence of aneurysm or pseudoaneurysm with associated flow disruption, dialysis dysfunction, or overlying skin changes often requires surgical revision. The incidence of AV access-related fatal hemorrhage due to aneurysms of all etiologies is 1 per 1000 patient years and likely occurs every decade in a dialysis unit.[33] Risk of rupture associated with pseudoaneurysms is not well-defined but due to the underlying etiology is considered to be higher than true aneurysms of comparable size (0.3–1% rate of rupture per year) and thereby mandate more urgent intervention.[35–37] Risk factors for pseudoaneurysm formation include anticoagulation, repeated buttonhole punctures, blind venipuncture, and venous hypertension.[35,38] If infection is a concern, removal of the affected segment at minimum is recommended with the reconfiguration of the HD access into healthy, uninvolved tissue.

Treatment of all exposed pseudoaneurysms and aneurysms involves excision and primary repair if able, or patch vs. interposition graft repair when necessary.[35,39–42] Surgical options depend on the morphology of the aneurysm and integrity of the compromised surrounding tissue, with variable reported outcomes limited to observational studies.[35] Several described techniques include aneurysmorraphy, which involves plication or partial resection of the aneurysmal wall and primary closure of the remaining vessel to preserve an autogenous AVF.[35,36] **(Fig. 5)** A systematic review of surgical management of AVF aneurysms found a pooled primary patency of 82% at 12 months with this method.[36] The primary patency rates were similar for aneurysmorrhaphy with an external prosthetic reinforcement at 85%.[36] Aneurysmectomy is another described technique, where aneurysmal portions are completely excised and the remaining vessel ends are anastomosed back together with mobilization. This method has a reported 3-year secondary patency of 95% for AVF revisions and a 1-year secondary patency of 96% for AVG revisions.[37] More extensive resections may require autologous or prosthetic interposition graft repair to reestablish the dialysis access in order to completely excise the aneurysmal portion.[35,38,39] The advantage of this technique is its ability to treat all types of access aneurysms, with the disadvantage that it increases the chance of infection and thrombosis.[38,39] In comparison to aneurysmorrhaphy, interposition graft repair has a lower primary patency rate at 1-year (72% vs 92%) and increased access abandonment at 2 years (adjusted hazards ratio = 3.07; 95% CI = 1.61–5.87).[39]

Hemodialysis reliable outflow graft

The HeRO graft can be considered in the setting of venous hypertension when all upper extremity options have been exhausted, provided that suitable patient anatomy exists. The HeRO graft involves anastomosis of a prosthetic graft onto an adequate inflow artery (eg, the brachial artery) and connection of this graft to a proprietary tunneled catheter that crosses the central venous stenosis. The utility of the HeRO graft is to provide a definitive access solution for dialysis patients with no further upper extremity access options, and who wish to avoid lower extremity access for quality of

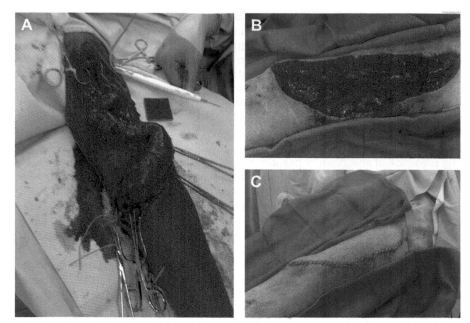

Fig. 5. Surgical revision of an aneurysmal brachiocephalic fistula causing pain. (*A*) Exposure of the fistula with the circumferential dissection and ligation of any feeding branches. (*B*) Modified fistula following the resection of the greatest aneurysmal portions to reduce overall length and aneurysmorrhaphy of remaining fistula to decrease overall diameter. (*C*) Final appearance following excision of excess skin and skin closure. (Courtesy of Omid Jazaeri, MD, Aurora, CO.)

life. Though associated with poor primary patency rates of 21.9% and secondary patency rates of 59.4% at 1-year,[43] the infection rate is low at 0.13-0.7 events per 1000 days and the overall complication rate is minimal.[43,44] This option can be used to convert an existing tunneled dialysis catheter into a more permanent method of access with less infectious risk but is only considered in select cases often as a last resort. Nonetheless, it has important clinical implications as central stenosis is common and the success of angioplasty in this region is limited.[45]

Accessory veins leading to arteriovenous fistula failure
Accessory veins are branching vessels between superficial veins and are common variations of normal anatomy. These can become problematic as competitive outflow during AVF maturation and when present proximal to a stenosis associated with an existing HD access. Treatment can include accessory vein ligation that divert significant flow and detected early including at the time of access creation. Endovascular treatment via embolization is also a reliable and less invasive option to treat accessory veins.[46,47] Unfortunately, there is limited data evaluating the success of accessory vein obliteration and improving AVF maturation.[48,49] In fact, a large meta-analysis by Purwono and colleagues[50] found no benefit when adding accessory vein obliteration to PTA for assisted AVF maturation, with the authors concluding that angioplasty alone was sufficient.

Hemodialysis access-induced distal ischemia
Hemodialysis access-induced distal ischemia (HAIDI), also called dialysis access-associated steal syndrome, is a rare complication and occurs in 6% of all patients

dialyzing via AVF/AVGs (**Box 2**).[51] Clinical sequelae manifest secondary to distal ischemia and can range from mild symptoms (pain, numbness) manifested only with HD to severe symptoms including tissue loss and limb threat that present independent of HD. The salvage techniques discussed later in discussion can improve symptoms of HAIDI while preserving the access site. Unfortunately, patients with advanced HAIDI and irreversible ischemic changes may benefit only from HD access ligation and/or amputation of the impacted extremity.

Management of HAIDI has multiple potential approaches depending on the etiology of ischemia and the clinical disease severity. Proximal arterial disease can be addressed via endovascular techniques such as angioplasty and possible stenting to increase inflow. Ischemia related to high flows should be addressed via flow reduction techniques. Plication or banding techniques create intentional stenosis of the HD access to limit flow while maintaining patency. The MILLER banding technique (minimally invasive limited ligation endoluminal assisted revision) as described by Miller and colleagues achieved symptomatic relief was achieved in 109/183 patients with primary patency rates of 85% at 6 months. Numerous studies have since been published concluding that the MILLER procedure appears to be an effective and durable option for treating HAIDI.[52–55] Proximal radial artery ligation can be utilized in high-flow distal radiocephalic fistulas, where proximal ligation improves direct flow into the hand and redirects inflow to the fistula via the palmar arch.[56] More recently, the effects of this technique on heart function have shown immediate regression of heart failure symptoms.[57]

In advanced HAIDI, more complex surgical revision may be necessary (**Fig. 6**). Proximalization of the arterial inflow (PAI) converts the arterial inflow of the HD access to a more proximal site utilizing a conduit such as PTFE. Flow is reduced due to higher resistance from the elongated dialysis circuit and can be further reduced using a small caliber graft. A series by Zanow and colleagues[58] demonstrated complete resolution in 84% and symptomatic improvement in 16% of patients following PAI. Revision using distal inflow (RUDI) includes the ligation of the access proximal to the arterial anastomosis with the reestablishment of inflow via the proximal radial or ulnar arteries through an autogenous or prosthetic bypass.[59] Several retrospective studies have shown RUDI to be a safe and effective therapy.[60–64] Finally, the distal revascularization and interval ligation (DRIL) procedure was first described in 1988 and was considered the preferred treatment for HAIDI for over two decades. This involves the ligation of the artery distal to the arterial anastomosis followed by bypass from the artery proximal to the anastomosis to the artery distal to the ligation using PTFE or vein conduit such as a reversed greater saphenous.[64] DRIL procedures have become less common with the

Box 2	
Classification of hemodialysis access-induced distal ischemia	
Grade 0	• No clinical symptoms
Grade 1	• Mild symptoms (ie, cool extremity) and demonstrable flow augmentation with access occlusion
	• No intervention indicated, but close monitoring is warranted
Grade 2	• Moderate symptoms (ie, pain) present with dialysis or increased effort
	• Intervention typically warranted to alleviate symptoms and prevent progression to tissue loss
Grade 3	• Severe symptoms (ie, rest pain and/or tissue loss)
	• Intervention mandatory, but may entail salvage procedures such as access ligation or amputation

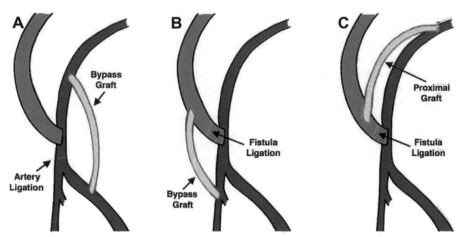

Fig. 6. Diagrammatic representation of dialysis access revision techniques for hemodialysis access-induced distal ischemia. (*A*) Distal revascularization and interval ligation. (*B*) Revascularization using distal inflow. (*C*) Proximalization of the arterial inflow. (*Modified from* Axley J, Novak Z, Blakeslee-Carter J, et al. Long-Term Trends in Preoperative Cardiac Evaluation and Myocardial Infarction after Elective Vascular Procedures. Ann Vasc Surg. 2021;71:19–28; with permission.)

improving efficacy of less invasive endovascular techniques.[63] However, the DRIL procedure remains the most effective method with superior access preservation and lower rates of reintervention if the patient is a suitable candidate for a major operation.[65] Though greater saphenous vein is the preferred autogenous conduit,[66] arm vein may be considered to avoid general anesthesia. In their comparative study, Weaver and colleagues[66] reported similar functional outcomes but significantly fewer wound complications with arm vein conduits.

TREATMENT OF THROMBOSED HEMODIALYSIS ACCESS

AVG thrombosis occurs 0.5-2 times per patient year and AVF thrombosis occurs 0.1-0.5 times per patient year post-creation. Thrombosed HD access can lead to inpatient admissions, urgent procedures, missed dialysis sessions, and prolonged need for temporary dialysis catheters. Moreover, it is the leading cause of permanent HD access loss (65–85%).[67]

Early Thrombosis

Thrombosis of a newly created HD access presents a challenging clinical decision due to the risk of exacerbating neointimal hyperplasia with invasive manipulation. Patients with early thrombosis should undergo initial endovascular thrombectomy and angioplasty if any culprit lesions are identified with close post-procedure surveillance as the risk of restenosis and access failure increases significantly. Initial clinical success rates for endovascular thrombectomy are consistently high and reported as 76-96% for AVF and 79-100% for AVG.[68–70] Miller and colleagues[71] found that among 140 patients with thrombosed immature fistula, thrombectomy was performed successfully in 85% of patients with hemodialysis adequacy achieved in 79%. A concordant cost analysis found that endovascular salvage of thrombosed immature fistulas costs $4-15,000 less than abandonment with new access creation. Thus, aggressive endovascular intervention on early HD access thrombosis is recommended despite its limitations in addressing resistant lesions and technical challenges in patients with anatomy less conducive to endovascular devices.

Late Thrombosis

Recurrent or late HD access thrombosis is typically due to recurrent stenosis and is the most common cause of mature access failure. Treatment should begin with endovascular thrombolysis and repeat angioplasty. Early consideration of an open surgical approach in the setting of recurrent thrombosis is recommended to prevent irreversible damage to the access site. Open surgical revision should be considered after 3 failed endovascular treatments or if a stenotic lesion recurs within 3 months of intervention. Nassar and colleagues reported results from a large cohort of patients with thrombosed AVFs who underwent endovascular thrombectomy. The mean duration of primary patency was 227 days and the mean assisted duration of primary patency was 677 days following intervention.[68] Open surgical thrombectomy has similar clinical success rates as endovascular techniques. However, patency rates are higher with open thrombectomy, likely due to coinciding operative revision of an underlying stenosis.[72] Regardless of technique, the most important factor in post-thrombosis salvage rates is the timeliness of intervention from diagnosis. Several authors have[69,73] reported significantly higher reintervention rates and lower primary patency rates if thrombectomy was completed >24 hours after diagnosis.

High-risk patients with thrombosis within 3 months of access site creation should be considered for antithrombotic therapy such as dual antiplatelet therapy to prevent recurrent thrombosis.[45,46] In patients who experience recurrent graft thrombosis without a culprit lesion, a hypercoagulable work-up should be initiated. Select patients may require systemic anticoagulation until a definitive etiology is determined, or in the absence of a correctable anatomic problem (**Box 3**).

CONTROVERSIES

Endovascular vs. open surgical correction of juxta-anastomotic stenosis is a commonly debated topic that is difficult to study given the significant variability related

---

Box 3
Complications of treatment for failing hemodlalysls access

Recurrent stenosis: following PTA alone, patency rates are 24-65% at 3 months, 3-46% at 6 months, and 9-22% at one year due to recurrence of stenotic lesion.[74]

Venous rupture: complication of PTA with greater occurrence in fistulas than grafts. Incidence ranges widely from 1.7 to 14.9% and increases with lesion complexity and high-pressure balloon application.[75,76] Rupture can be managed by balloon tamponade, and stent placement with a cumulative salvage rate ranging from 60 to 100%.[75,77]

Infection: highest risk after AVG placement and/or revision and primarily occurs during first postoperative month. Partial excision can successfully manage infection in 60-80% of patients but with higher risk of re-infection compared to total graft excision (26.6% vs. 4.8%).[78,79]

Temporary dialysis catheter: occasionally needed as a bridge for slow/failed access maturation and following surgical revision. Catheter-associated infection incidence is 3.8-6.5/1000 catheter days; thus, recommended use is limited to <2 weeks.[80]

Thromboembolic event: can occur following thrombectomy and affect both the venous and arterial systems. Reported rates of clinically relevant pulmonary embolism following endovascular thrombectomy are 0-5%.[81] Thrombectomy is further contraindicated in patients with right-to-left shunt given potential for embolism to distal arterial vasculature and infected HD access in case of septic embolism.

to surgeon preference, experience, and patient selection criteria. Though studies suggest higher primary patency rates with surgical revision, the overall cumulative patency is fairly comparable. As such, endovascular treatment is the preferred initial approach as the less invasive option for HD salvage. Regardless, the management of complex HD patients requires a multidisciplinary approach to provide the highest level of care.

Additionally, the need for routine access surveillance is under debate. Routine surveillance can enable earlier detection with timely intervention of access issues, thereby improving overall patency. However, the potential for an increased number of interventions with unclear clinical utility raises concerns regarding cost and value. Thus, standardized diagnostic thresholds and management guidelines are requisite to avoid unnecessary procedures because of increased surveillance.

FUTURE DIRECTIONS

Thus far, the clinical focus has been on treating HD access failure once present. However, the underlying factors leading to stenosis and access failure are poorly understood. Xiao and colleagues[82] recently demonstrated an association between postoperative medial fibrosis and intimal hyperplasia with the upregulation of pro-inflammatory cytokine platelet factor 4. A study evaluating the transcriptome of native veins also found the upregulation of several pro-inflammatory genes in non-maturing AVFs localized to the smooth muscle cells. Such studies may identify targets for potential therapeutic intervention to improve access maturation rates and prevent stenosis, thereby diminishing the need for HD salvage interventions in the future.

SUMMARY

Maintenance and salvage of HD access require a thoughtful and individualized approach. While difficult, any salvage is better than abandonment given the limited options for ESKD patients. Treatment focuses on addressing the underlying etiology, which is often a stenotic lesion. Endovascular techniques are well-established as the preferred initial approach. Though surgical revision may ultimately be required, it is reserved for recalcitrant lesions or specific mechanisms of failure. Current treatment regimens can vary significantly between providers and institutions, and standardized algorithms for HD access maintenance and salvage are critical for improved outcomes and overall value of care.

CLINICS CARE POINTS

- Stenosis is the most common cause of HD access failure requiring intervention (approximately 60% of all AVFs and AVGs).
- Stenosis >50% with associated symptoms, abnormal physical exam findings, and/or abnormal flow measurements should prompt intervention.
- Plain balloon angioplasty has a recurrence rate of >20% within 6 months and thus may require adjunct techniques to improve outcomes.
- Endovascular techniques are highly effective in HD access salvage and are often the preferred initial approach; however, open revision may be necessary for certain scenarios including recalcitrant stenosis, hemodialysis access-induced distal ischemia, and infection.

DISCLOSURE

The authors have nothing to disclose.

REFERENCES

1. Johansen K, Chertrow G, Wetmore J. USRDS annual data report: epidemiology of kidney disease in the United States. National Institute of Diabetes and Digestive and Kidney Diseases; 2020. https://doi.org/10.1053/j.ajkd.2021.01.002. United States Renal Data System.
2. CDC. Centers for Disease Control and Prevention. Chronic Kidney Disease in the United States. Published September 2021. Available at: https://www.cdc.gov/kidneydisease/publications-resources/ckd-national-facts.html. Accessed December 3, 2022.
3. USRDS. End Stage Renal Disease -Annual Data Report. Published 2021. Available at: https://usrds-adr.niddk.nih.gov/2020/end-stage-renal-disease/5-mortality. Accessed December 3, 2022.
4. Lok CE, Huber TS, Lee T, et al. KDOQI Clinical Practice Guideline for Vascular Access: 2019 Update. Am J Kidney Dis 2020;75(4 Suppl 2):S1–164.
5. Lok CE, Rajan DK. KDOQI 2019 Vascular Access Guidelines: What Is New. Semin Intervent Radiol 2022;39(1):3–8.
6. Field M, MacNamara K, Bailey G, et al. Primary patency rates of AV fistulas and the effect of patient variables. J Vasc Access 2008;9(1):45–50.
7. Polkinghorne KR. Arteriovenous fistula patency: some answers but questions remain. Am J Kidney Dis 2014;63(3):384–6.
8. Al-Jaishi AA, Oliver MJ, Thomas SM, et al. Patency rates of the arteriovenous fistula for hemodialysis: a systematic review and meta-analysis. Am J Kidney Dis 2014;63(3):464–78.
9. Huber TS, Berceli SA, Scali ST, et al. Arteriovenous fistula maturation, functional patency, and intervention rates. JAMA Surg 2021;156(12):1111.
10. Nordyke RJ, Reichert H, Bylsma LC, et al. Costs attributable to arteriovenous fistula and arteriovenous graft placements in hemodialysis patients with medicare coverage. Am J Nephrol 2019;50(4):320–8.
11. Thamer M, Lee TC, Wasse H, et al. Medicare costs associated with arteriovenous fistulas among US hemodialysis patients. Am J Kidney Dis 2018;72(1):10–8.
12. Hung YN, Ko PJ, Ng YY, et al. The longevity of arteriovenous graft for hemodialysis patients—externally supported or nonsupported. Clin J Am Soc Nephrol 2010;5(6):1029–35.
13. Abreo K, Amin BM, Abreo AP. Physical examination of the hemodialysis arteriovenous fistula to detect early dysfunction. J Vasc Access 2019;20(1):7–11.
14. Zamboli P, Fiorini F, D'Amelio A, et al. Color Doppler ultrasound and arteriovenous fistulas for hemodialysis. J Ultrasound 2014;17(4):253–63.
15. Behera MR, John EE, Thomas A, et al. Difficult cannulation of hemodialysis arteriovenous fistula – role of imaging in access management (DICAF STUDY). J Vasc Access 2022;23(6):877–84.
16. Mcgill RL, Marcus RJ, Healy DA, et al. AV fistula rates: changing the culture of vascular access. J Vasc Access 2005;6(1):13–7.
17. Schild AF, Prieto J, Glenn M, et al. Maturation and failure rates in a large series of arteriovenous dialysis access fistulas. Vasc Endovascular Surg 2004;38(5):449–53.
18. Clark TWI, Cohen RA, Kwak A, et al. Salvage of nonmaturing native fistulas by using angioplasty. Radiology 2007;242(1):286–92.

19. Fysaraki M, Samonis G, Valachis A, et al. Incidence, clinical, microbiological features and outcome of bloodstream infections in patients undergoing hemodialysis. Int J Med Sci 2013;10(12):1632–8.

20. MacRae JM, Dipchand C, Oliver M, et al. Arteriovenous access failure, stenosis, and thrombosis. Can J Kidney Health Dis 2016;3. 205435811666912.

21. Rokoszak V, Syed MH, Salata K, et al. A systematic review and meta-analysis of plain versus drug-eluting balloon angioplasty in the treatment of juxta-anastomotic hemodialysis arteriovenous fistula stenosis. J Vasc Surg 2020; 71(3):1046–54.e1.

22. Agarwal SK, Nadkarni GN, Yacoub R, et al. Comparison of cutting balloon angioplasty and percutaneous balloon angioplasty of arteriovenous fistula stenosis: a meta-analysis and systematic review of randomized clinical trials. J Interv Cardiol 2015;28(3):288–95.

23. Kitrou PM, Katsanos K, Spiliopoulos S, et al. Drug-eluting versus plain balloon angioplasty for the treatment of failing dialysis access: final results and cost-effectiveness analysis from a prospective randomized controlled trial (NCT01174472). Eur J Radiol 2015;84(3):418–23.

24. Lai CC, Fang HC, Tseng CJ, et al. Percutaneous angioplasty using a paclitaxel-coated balloon improves target lesion restenosis on inflow lesions of autogenous radiocephalic fistulas: a pilot study. J Vasc Interv Radiol 2014;25(4):535–41.

25. Trerotola SO, Lawson J, Roy-Chaudhury P, et al, Clinical Trial Investigators. Drug coated balloon angioplasty in failing AV fistulas: a randomized controlled trial. Clin J Am Soc Nephrol 2018;13(8):1215–24.

26. Lookstein RA, Haruguchi H, Ouriel K, et al. Drug-coated balloons for dysfunctional dialysis arteriovenous fistulas. N Engl J Med 2020;383(8):733–42.

27. Pang SC, Tan RY, Choke E, et al. SIroliMus coated angioPlasty versus plain balloon angioplasty in the tREatment of dialySis acceSs dysfunctION (IMPRESSION): study protocol for a randomized controlled trial. Trials 2021;22(1):945.

28. Tang TY, Soon SXY, Yap CJQ, et al. Early (6 months) results of a pilot prospective study to investigate the efficacy and safety of sirolimus coated balloon angioplasty for dysfunctional arterio-venous fistulas: MAgicTouch Intervention Leap for Dialysis Access (MATILDA) Trial. PLoS One 2020;15(10):e0241321.

29. Tang TY, Soon SX, Yap CJ, et al. Endovascular salvage of failing arterio-venous fistulas utilising sirolimus eluting balloons: six months results from the ISABELLA trial. J Vasc Access 2021. https://doi.org/10.1177/11297298211067059. 112972 982110670.

30. D'cruz RT, Leong SW, Syn N, et al. Endovascular treatment of cephalic arch stenosis in brachiocephalic arteriovenous fistulas: a systematic review and meta-analysis. J Vasc Access 2019;20(4):345–55.

31. Davies MG, Hicks TD, Haidar GM, et al. Outcomes of intervention for cephalic arch stenosis in brachiocephalic arteriovenous fistulas. J Vasc Surg 2017;66(5): 1504–10.

32. Kim SM, Yoon KW, Woo SY, et al. Treatment strategies for cephalic arch stenosis in patients with brachiocephalic arteriovenous fistula. Ann Vasc Surg 2019;54: 248–53.

33. Suliman A, Greenberg JI, Angle N. Surgical bypass of symptomatic central venous obstruction for arteriovenous fistula salvage in hemodialysis patients. Ann Vasc Surg 2008;22(2):203–9.

34. Lew SQ, Nguyen BN, Ing TS. Hemodialysis vascular access construction in the upper extremity: a review. J Vasc Access 2015;16(2):87–92.

35. Meola M, Marciello A, di Salle G, et al. Ultrasound evaluation of access complications: thrombosis, aneurysms, pseudoaneurysms and infections. J Vasc Access 2021;22(1_suppl):71–83.
36. Vasanthamohan L, Gopee-Ramanan P, Athreya S. The management of cephalic arch stenosis in arteriovenous fistulas for hemodialysis: a systematic review. Cardiovasc Intervent Radiol 2015;38(5):1179–85.
37. Jose MD, Marshall MR, Read G, et al. Fatal dialysis vascular access hemorrhage. Am J Kidney Dis 2017;70(4):570–5.
38. di Nicolò P, Cornacchiari M, Mereghetti M, et al. Buttonhole cannulation of the AV fistula: a critical analysis of the technique. Semin Dial 2017;30(1):32–8.
39. Chang R, Alabi O, Mahajan A, et al. Arteriovenous fistula aneurysmorrhaphy is associated with improved patency and decreased vascular access abandonment. J Vasc Surg 2023;77(3):891–8.e1.
40. Inston N, Mistry H, Gilbert J, et al. Aneurysms in vascular access: state of the art and future developments. J Vasc Access 2017;18(6):464–72.
41. Wang S, Wang MS. Successful use of partial aneurysmectomy and repair approach for managing complications of arteriovenous fistulas and grafts. J Vasc Surg 2017;66(2):545–53.
42. Baláž P, Rokošný S, Bafrnec J, et al. Repair of aneurysmal arteriovenous fistulae: a systematic review and meta-analysis. Eur J Vasc Endovasc Surg 2020;59(4):614–23.
43. AL Shakarchi J, Houston JG, Jones RG, et al. A review on the hemodialysis reliable outflow (HeRO) graft for haemodialysis vascular access. Eur J Vasc Endovasc Surg 2015;50(1):108–13.
44. Glickman MH. HeRO graft versus lower extremity grafts in hemodialysis patients with long standing renal failure. J Vasc Access 2016;17(Suppl 1):S30–1.
45. Wang S, Almehmi A, Asif A. Surgical management of cephalic arch occlusive lesions: are there predictors for outcomes? Semin Dial 2013;26(4):E33–41.
46. Prasad R, Israrahmed A, Yadav R, et al. Endovascular embolization in problematic hemodialysis arteriovenous fistulas: A nonsurgical technique. Indian J Nephrol 2021;31(6):516.
47. Shelar A, Pol MM, Manohar M, et al. Accessory veins related hand ischemia: a case series. Ann Med Surg (Lond) 2021;68:102593.
48. Haq NU, Althaf MM, Lee T. Accessory vein obliteration for early fistula failure: a myth or reality? Adv Chron Kidney Dis 2015;22(6):438–45.
49. Dixon BS. Why don't fistulas mature? Kidney Int 2006;70(8):1413–22.
50. Purwono GY, Sultana R, Lee RE, et al. Accessory Vein Obliteration and Balloon-Assisted Maturation for Immature Arteriovenous Fistulas for Haemodialysis: A Systematic Review and Meta-Analysis. Cardiovasc Intervent Radiol 2022;45(10):1415–27.
51. Sidawy AN, Gray R, Besarab A, et al. Recommended standards for reports dealing with arteriovenous hemodialysis accesses. J Vasc Surg 2002;35(3):603–10.
52. Alqassieh A, Dennis PB, Mehta V, et al. MILLER Banding Procedure for Treatment of Dialysis Access–Related Steal Syndrome, Pulmonary Hypertension, and Heart Failure. Am Surg 2021. https://doi.org/10.1177/00031348211056259. 000313482 110562.
53. Sheaffer W, Hangge P, Chau A, et al. Minimally invasive limited ligation endoluminal-assisted revision (MILLER): a review of the available literature and brief overview of alternate therapies in dialysis associated steal syndrome. J Clin Med 2018;7(6):128.

54. Shukla PA, Kolber MK, Nwoke F, et al. The MILLER banding procedure as a treatment alternative for dialysis access steal syndrome: a single institutional experience. Clin Imaging 2016;40(3):569–72.

55. Miller GA, Goel N, Friedman A, et al. The MILLER banding procedure is an effective method for treating dialysis-associated steal syndrome. Kidney Int 2010; 77(4):359–66.

56. Bourquelot P, Gaudric J, Turmel-Rodrigues L, et al. Proximal radial artery ligation (PRAL) for reduction of flow in autogenous radial cephalic accesses for haemodialysis. Eur J Vasc Endovasc Surg 2010;40(1):94–9.

57. Maresca B, Filice FB, Orlando S, et al. Early echocardiographic modifications after flow reduction by proximal radial artery ligation in patients with high-output heart failure due to high-flow forearm arteriovenous fistula. J Vasc Access 2020;21(5):753–9.

58. Zanow J, Kruger U, Scholz H. Proximalization of the arterial inflow: a new technique to treat access-related ischemia. J Vasc Surg 2006;43(6):1216–21.

59. Callaghan CJ, Mallik M, Sivaprakasam R, et al. Treatment of dialysis access-associated steal syndrome with the "revision using distal inflow" technique. J Vasc Access 2011;12(1):52–6.

60. Kordzadeh A, Garzon LAN, Parsa AD. Revision using distal inflow for the treatment of dialysis access steal syndrome: a systematic review. Ann Vasc Dis 2018;11(4):473–8.

61. Minion DJ, Moore E, Endean E. Revision using distal inflow: a novel approach to dialysis-associated steal syndrome. Ann Vasc Surg 2005;19(5):625–8.

62. Loh TM, Bennett ME, Peden EK. Revision using distal inflow is a safe and effective treatment for ischemic steal syndrome and pathologic high flow after access creation. J Vasc Surg 2016;63(2):441–5.

63. Misskey J, Yang C, MacDonald S, et al. A comparison of revision using distal inflow and distal revascularization-interval ligation for the management of severe access-related hand ischemia. J Vasc Surg 2016;63(6):1574–81.

64. Davidson I, Beathard G, Gallieni M, et al. The DRIL procedure for arteriovenous access ischemic steal: a controversial approach. J Vasc Access 2017;18(1):1–2.

65. Leake AE, Winger DG, Leers SA, et al. Management and outcomes of dialysis access-associated steal syndrome. J Vasc Surg 2015;61(3):754–61.

66. Weaver ML, Holscher CM, Graham A, et al. Distal revascularization and interval ligation for dialysis access-related ischemia is best performed using arm vein conduit. J Vasc Surg 2021;73(4):1368–75.e1.

67. Quencer KB, Oklu R. Hemodialysis access thrombosis. Cardiovasc Diagn Ther 2017;7(Suppl 3):S299–308.

68. Nassar GM, Rhee E, Khan AJ, et al. Percutaneous Thrombectomy of AVF: Immediate Success and Long-term Patency Rates. Semin Dial 2015;28(2):E15–22.

69. Hsieh MY, Lin L, Chen TY, et al. Timely thrombectomy can improve patency of hemodialysis arteriovenous fistulas. J Vasc Surg 2018;67(4):1217–26.

70. Tordoir JHM, Bode AS, Peppelenbosch N, et al. Surgical or endovascular repair of thrombosed dialysis vascular access: is there any evidence? J Vasc Surg 2009;50(4):953–6.

71. Miller GA, Hwang W, Preddie D, et al. Percutaneous salvage of thrombosed immature arteriovenous fistulas. Semin Dial 2011;24(1):107–14.

72. Ghaffarian AA, Al-Dulaimi R, Kraiss LW, et al. Clinical effectiveness of open thrombectomy for thrombosed autogenous arteriovenous fistulas and grafts. J Vasc Surg 2018;68(1):189–96.

73. Sadaghianloo N, Jean-Baptiste E, Gaid H, et al. Early surgical thrombectomy improves salvage of thrombosed vascular accesses. J Vasc Surg 2014;59(5): 1377–84.e2.
74. Kouvelos GN, Spanos K, Antoniou GA, et al. Balloon angioplasty versus stenting for the treatment of failing arteriovenous grafts: a meta-analysis. Eur J Vasc Endovasc Surg 2018;55(2):249–56.
75. Liao MT, Luo CM, Hsieh MC, et al. Stent grafts improved patency of ruptured hemodialysis vascular accesses. Sci Rep 2022;12(1):51.
76. Kornfield ZN, Kwak A, Soulen MC, et al. Incidence and management of percutaneous transluminal angioplasty–induced venous rupture in the "fistula first" era. J Vasc Interv Radiol 2009;20(6):744–51.
77. Pappas JN, Vesely TM. Vascular rupture during angioplasty of hemodialysis graft-related stenoses. J Vasc Access 2002;3(3):120–6.
78. Tullavardhana T, Chartkitchareon A. Meta-analysis of total versus partial graft excision: which is the better choice to manage arteriovenous dialysis graft infection? Ann Saudi Med 2022;42(5):343–50.
79. Benrashid E, Youngwirth LM, Mureebe L, et al. Operative and perioperative management of infected arteriovenous grafts. J Vasc Access 2017;18(1):13–21.
80. Weijmer MC, Vervloet MG, ter Wee PM. Compared to tunnelled cuffed haemodialysis catheters, temporary untunnelled catheters are associated with more complications already within 2 weeks of use. Nephrol Dial Transplant 2004;19(3):670–7.
81. Arinze N, Ryan T, Pillai R, et al. Perioperative and long-term outcomes after percutaneous thrombectomy of arteriovenous dialysis access grafts. J Vasc Surg 2020;72(6):2107–12.
82. Xiao Y, Vazquez-Padron RI, Martinez L, et al. Role of platelet factor 4 in arteriovenous fistula maturation failure: what do we know so far? J Vasc Access 2022. https://doi.org/10.1177/11297298221085458. 112972982210854.

Current Approaches for Mesenteric Ischemia and Visceral Aneurysms

Oonagh H. Scallan, MD, FRCSC, Audra A. Duncan, MD, FACS, FRCSC*

KEYWORDS

- Mesenteric ischemia • Acute • Chronic • Visceral aneurysms • Treatment
- Endovascular

KEY POINTS

- A high clinical suspicion is required to make the diagnosis of acute mesenteric ischemia, and approach to revascularization should be individualized to each patient, with the consideration of assessment of bowel perfusion and requirement for bowel resection.
- Although endovascular therapy is generally recommended as the first line intervention for patients with chronic mesenteric ischemia and suitable lesions, the decision should be a shared decision-making process between the patient and provider, considering the risks and benefits of the various options and the patient's goals of care.
- Given the rarity of this entity, the natural history of many visceral aneurysms is unclear. It is prudent to treat these aneurysms according to the society for vascular surgery (SVS) guidelines to prevent rupture given the high rates of mortality.

ACUTE MESENTERIC ISCHEMIA

Introduction

Acute mesenteric ischemia (AMI) is an uncommon but highly complex clinical problem. The overall incidence is low, and has been shown to represent 0.09% to 0.2% of all acute admissions to emergency departments.[1–3] In a 1967 autopsy series, Ottinger and Austen reported a rate of 8.8 cases of acute mesenteric ischemia per 10,000 hospital admissions.[4] The incidence of AMI increases exponentially with age, the incidence in an 80-year-old is roughly 10-fold that of a 60-year-old.[5] Early recognition is crucial, as irreversible bowel necrosis develops in many patients by the time of abdominal exploration, and every 6-hour delay of the diagnosis doubles mortality.[4,6] Overall mortality rate averages 69%, and AMI remains a morbid condition with poor short-term and long-term survival rates.[4]

Division of Vascular and Endovascular Surgery, Western University, 800 Commissioners Road East, PO Box 5010, London, Ontario N6A 5W9, Canada
* Corresponding author. 800 Commissioners Road East, PO Box 5010, Victoria Hospital, E2-119, London, Ontario N6A 5W9, Canada.
E-mail address: audra.duncan@lhsc.on.ca

Surg Clin N Am 103 (2023) 703–731
https://doi.org/10.1016/j.suc.2023.04.017   surgical.theclinics.com
0039-6109/23/© 2023 Elsevier Inc. All rights reserved.

Pathophysiology

Embolism

Acute superior mesenteric artery (SMA) embolism historically accounted for approximately half of AMI cases, but more recent reports have shown this to have decreased to 25%, likely secondary to the increased use of anticoagulation for atrial fibrillation.[7–9] The embolus may originate from the left ventricle, left atrium, or, less frequently, from the thoracic or upper abdominal aorta.[4] Emboli typically lodge at points of normal anatomic artery narrowing, with most emboli lodging 3 to 10 cm distal to the origin of the SMA, therefore, sparing the proximal jejunum and colon, as seen in **Fig. 1**. More than 20% of emboli are associated with concurrent emboli to another arterial bed, such as the spleen or the kidney.[10]

Thrombosis

In situ thrombosis of the SMA now accounts for 40% of AMI cases, while it historically accounted for approximately 25% of cases.[8] This presentation is typically associated with pre-existing chronic atherosclerotic disease leading to stenosis, where the underlying plaque progresses resulting in a critical stenosis and the development and hypertrophy of collateral circulation. Many patients have a history of chronic mesenteric ischemia (CMI) symptoms including postprandial abdominal pain, weight loss, or sitophobia (**Fig. 2**). Thrombosis usually occurs at the origin of visceral arteries, and symptomatic SMA thrombosis most often accompanies celiac occlusion.[11] Other than atherosclerosis, other etiologies of thrombosis include vasculitis, mesenteric dissection, or mycotic aneurysm.[6]

Non-occlusive mesenteric ischemia

Non-occlusive mesenteric ischemia (NOMI) develops as a result of hypoperfusion caused by a low cardiac output or mesenteric arterial spasm and accounts for roughly 20% of AMI cases.[4] Patients with NOMI are typically critically ill with cardiac failure, renal failure, septic shock or have a recent history of cardiac surgery using cardiopulmonary bypass. GI perfusion is often impaired early in critical illness, major surgery, or trauma, all of which are characterized by increased demands on the circulation to

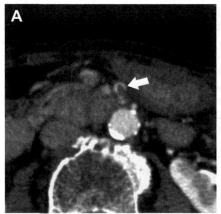
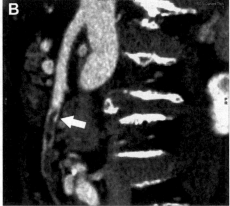

Fig. 1. Acute SMA embolus in a patient with atrial fibrillation, demonstrated in the axial (*A*) and saggital (*B*) curved planar reformatted images. (*From* Zhao YE, Wang ZJ, Zhou CS, Zhu FP, Zhang LJ, Lu GM. Multidetector computed tomography of superior mesenteric artery: anatomy and pathologies. Can Assoc Radiol J. 2014;65(3):267-274.; with permission.)

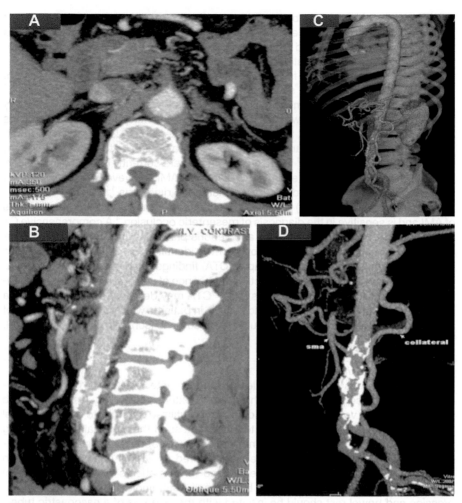

Fig. 2. A 74-year-old patient with recurrent post-prandial abdominal pain and weight loss, axial contrast-enhanced CT scan (*A*), sagittal reformatted image (*B*) and sagittal MIP (*C, D*) showed thrombosis and total occlusion of the proximal SMA with distal re-filling from collaterals, with advanced atherosclerotic changes of the SMA and aortoiliac arteries. (*From Amin MA, Nooman NA, Moussa GI. Acute and chronic mesenteric ischemia: Multidetector CT and CT angiographic findings. Egypt J Radiology Nucl Medicine. 2014;45(4):1063-1070.; with permission.*)

maintain tissue oxygen delivery.[12] Hypovolemia and the use of vasoconstrictive agents, such as norepinephrine and vasopressin, may precipitate NOMI.

Although mesenteric venous thrombosis can also cause mesenteric ischemia, this discussion is limited to arterial etiologies.

Patient Evaluation Overview

The diagnosis of AMI requires a high index of suspicion and a careful history to distinguish the pathophysiology of AMI. In a retrospective study by Park and colleagues, almost half of the patients with AMI had prior symptoms of CMI.[4] Nearly 50% of patients presenting with embolic AMI have atrial fibrillation and a third of patients have a prior history of arterial embolism with pre-existing peripheral vascular disease.[4] Gastrointestinal motility problems such as nausea, vomiting, and constipation are a frequent finding, and one-third of patients present with the triad of abdominal pain, fever, and hemoccult-positive stool.[4]

The classic physical exam finding is pain out of proportion to the physical exam. Pain is a frequent finding, but signs of frank peritonitis are frequently late or absent.[4] The ischemia starts from the mucosa and progresses toward the serosa, which is why there is initially severe pain without clinical findings. Other physical exam findings include abdominal distension, tachycardia, and hypotension.[13] Laboratory abnormalities are frequently present, particularly leukocytosis and high lactate levels. However, these are not specific to AMI.[4] There are no biomarkers currently identified in the literature specific enough to independently diagnose AMI, however, elevated lactate, leukocytosis, and elevated D-dimer may assist in the diagnosis.[14,15]

Computed tomography (CT) scanning continues to play a major role in the diagnosis of AMI and is sensitive in the diagnosis of mesenteric occlusion.[4] A comprehensive CT includes a pre-contrast scan, arterial, and venous phases.[16] Oral contrast is not indicated and is even harmful. CT also allows for the identification of nonvascular causes of acute abdominal pain. CT Angiography (CTA) findings of advanced AMI include intestinal dilatation and thickness, reduction or absence of visceral enhancement, pneumatosis intestinalis, and portal venous gas.[17] CTA may demonstrate bowel ischemia and free fluid despite patent mesenteric vessels in patients with NOMI. The absence of bowel abnormalities on CT does not rule out mesenteric ischemic or ischemic bowel.

Medical Treatment Options

Preoperative resuscitation
Fluid resuscitation is essential for patients with suspected AMI (**Box 1**). The fluid requirements in these patients may be high due to extensive capillary leakage, but the infusion of a large volume of crystalloid should be utilized carefully to optimize bowel perfusion.[18] Intestinal ischemia leads to the early loss of the mucosal barrier, putting the patient at risk for bacterial translocation and septic complications. Broad-spectrum antibiotic therapy should be administered early. Full-dose anticoagulation with unfractionated heparin should be initiated for all patients with the diagnosis of AMI before any surgical intervention, barring any contraindications. Gastric decompression and bowel rest should be initiated with the insertion of a nasogastric tube.

Non-occlusive mesenteric ischemia pharmacologic agents
NOMI management should be directed at treating the underlying cause with fluid resuscitation, optimization of cardiac output, and minimizing vasoconstricting medications.[6] Systemic anticoagulation with heparin may also be considered. Additional treatment with a catheter-directed infusion of vasodilatory and antispasmodic agents such as papaverine hydrochloride is also an option,[6] and direct SMA infusion with

---

Box 1
Initial management of acute mesenteric ischemia

- Fluid resuscitation
- Broad-spectrum parenteral antibiotics
- NG tube insertion and bowel rest
- Systemic anticoagulation

papaverine has been shown to reduce mortality.[19] Continuous intravenous prostaglandin E1 has also demonstrated mortality benefits in patients with early signs of NOMI.[20]

Surgical Treatment Options

The goal of surgical care in AMI is the assessment for and removal of non-salvageable bowel, prevention of further bowel infarction through urgent revascularization, and the preservation of small intestinal length.[4] A midline laparotomy is performed to assess bowel viability, and the location and extent of bowel necrosis (**Fig. 3**). Various methods for assessing bowel viability intraoperative are described in **Table 1**. Once revascularized, the bowel is reassessed and when areas of the bowel appear dusky but not clearly ischemic, a temporary abdominal closure with a negative pressure wound therapy device is applied and the patient is brought back to the operating room in 24 hours for a second look.

To revascularize the SMA in cases of AMI, there are two standard approaches which include an anterior and lateral approach. An anterior approach is suitable for performing SMA embolectomy, while a lateral approach may be used for retrograde bypasses from the infrarenal aorta.

To perform an embolectomy of the SMA, the anterior surface of the artery is exposed by reflecting the transverse colon and greater omentum cranially and mobilizing the small bowel to the right. The peritoneum is incised at the base of the transverse mesocolon, and the SMA is dissected from the autonomic nerve fibers, small lymphatics, and venous tributaries. The superior mesenteric vein lies to the right. The SMA is isolated between the middle and right colic branches, and jejunal

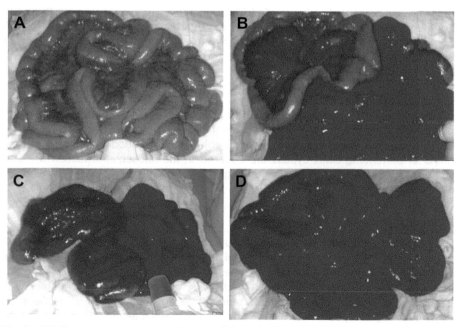

Fig. 3. ICG fluorescence imaging of the small bowel, demonstrating no gross signs of intestinal necrosis (*A*) and satisfactory emission at 3 to 4 minutes (*B–D*). (*From* Furusawa K, Yoshimitsu M, Matsukawa H, Oi K, Yunoki K, Tamura A. Precise diagnosis of acute mesenteric ischemia using indocyanine green imaging prevents small bowel resection: A case report. Int J Surg Case Rep. 2022 Aug;97:107463; with permission.)

Table 1
Techniques for assessing bowel viability

Technique	Description
Direct inspection	Visible and palpable pulsation in mesenteric arcade Normal color and appearance of bowel serosa Peristalsis Bleeding from cut surfaces
IV fluorescein	Administer 1 g IV sodium fluorescein and inspect bowel under ultraviolet (Wood's) lamp Viable bowel has smooth, uniform fluorescence
Doppler	Assessment of antimesenteric intestinal arterial flow
Indocyanine green (ICG) intraoperative laser angiography	25 mg of ICG diluted in 10 mL of distilled water, a minimum of 3 mL administered through a peripheral vein Using the SPY Intraoperative Perfusion Assessment System to obtain fluorescence images, ischemic segments may have no uptake or appear hypofluorescent or patchy compared to other segments

branches are preserved and controlled. Through a transverse arteriotomy, a 3- or 4-Fr Fogarty catheter is passed proximally to remove the embolus. A small 2- to 3-Fr Fogarty catheter may be passed distally if back-bleeding is poor, but this comes with the risk of dissecting the small ileocolic and jejunal branches. Once adequate embolectomy has been performed and inflow is confirmed, the SMA is closed primarily with interrupted sutures or with a vein patch if the artery is diminutive. Flow is reestablished and confirmed with Doppler.

The proximal SMA is exposed through a lateral approach by mobilizing the fourth part of the duodenum, dividing the ligament of Treitz and other peritoneal attachments. The SMA is isolated in the tissues cephalad to the duodenum. Technical aspects of performing SMA bypass are covered in the subsequent section on CMI. Options and considerations for performing an SMA bypass specifically for AMI are outlined in **Table 2**.

Endovascular Treatment Options

Endovascular techniques have become popular in the revascularization of the SMA, but there are no randomized controlled trial (RCT) comparing open and endovascular surgical approaches. Although some studies report a lesser need for laparotomy, less bowel resection, and lower mortality rate, there is controversy surrounding the use of endovascular techniques as the primary management of acute mesenteric ischemia.[21] The lack of capability to directly assess bowel viability is a major shortcoming of a total endovascular approach to AMI.[22,23]

Stenting

Percutaneous transluminal angioplasty and stenting may be appropriate for select patients with AMI, in combination with close observation or laparoscopic assessment of

Table 2
General considerations and potential options for revascularization in acute mesenteric ischemia

Consideration	Options
Inflow source	Supraceliac aorta
	Infrarenal aorta
	Iliac artery
Conduit	Great saphenous vein
	Rifampin-soaked Dacron
	Externally supported PTFE
Target vessels	Single vessel (celiac or SMA)
	Two vessel (celiac and SMA)

bowel ischemia. Patients presenting with acute on chronic symptoms, without peritonitis may be appropriate for percutaneous intervention. This technique is described in the CMI section.

Aspiration embolectomy

Aspiration thrombectomy, in which the embolus is removed by suction and mechanical thrombectomy, have been applied to treat SMA occlusion in AMI. After femoral or brachial access is obtained, the SMA is catheterized with a reverse-curve catheter and a hydrophilic 0.035 in guidewire. The wire is replaced with a stiffer wire, such as a Rosen wire, and is placed into an ileocolic branch of the SMA for stability. The tip of the wire should be visualized at all times. An over-the-wire aspiration catheter may be used to aspirate the embolus, which allows a stable position while performing the aspiration. In the absence of a reperfusion catheter, a 4 to 6 Fr guiding catheter may be introduced through a 7 Fr sheath with a removable hub or through an 8 Fr guiding catheter which is placed proximal to the SMA embolus.[24] Aspiration with a 20 mL syringe is manually applied to the smaller guiding catheter simultaneously with withdrawal, achieving aspiration of the embolus. Several passes are typically required and the sheath or larger guiding catheter should be back bled to remove any residual embolism.

Catheter-directed thrombolysis

Thrombolytic therapy as the sole revascularization procedure for AMI has been reported but it is rarely used. There is an increased risk of major bleeding from necrotic bowel and distal emboli and may hasten the need for open operation. In cases of incomplete aspiration embolectomy or distal embolization with residual clot, adjunctive local thrombolysis is sometimes used.[24] To perform thrombolysis, the sheath is left in the proximal SMA and a 10 cm long infusion catheter is placed. Local thrombolysis with recombinant tissue plasminogen activator is performed, at a rate of 0.5 to 1 mg/hour. Repeat angiography and reassessment of thrombolytics effect is completed every 12 hours or sooner if clinically indicated.

Hybrid Treatment Options

Retrograde open mesenteric stenting (ROMS) is a hybrid technique that may be appropriate for patients with suitable anatomy. The advantages of this approach compared to percutaneous stenting are the ability to directly assess bowel viability, have a short distance between the access site and the lesion, shorter operating time compared to bypass, and no exposed prosthetic. The patency rate of ROMS is similar to bypass (**Fig. 4**).[25] An overview of the ROMS technique is described in **Box 2**.[25]

Modifications of this technique may be required based on the anatomy of the visceral disease. In long, densely calcified occlusions in which it is not possible to pass the guidewire beyond the lesion, an antegrade brachial approach may be attempted. The celiac artery may also be stented using the ROMS technique, ensuring the median arcuate ligament is released to prevent compression of the stent. Other considerations for the ROMS technique include

- Position the patient to ensure the abdomen can be imaged fluoroscopically
- Prepare the left upper extremity and bilateral groins in the surgical field for potential brachial and/or femoral access
- Use a balloon-expandable stent for precise deployment and greater radial force
- Avoid covered stents in the setting of peritoneal contamination

Complications

A second-look laparotomy should be planned for patients with bowels of questionable viability, usually within 24 hours. The decision for a second look is made during the first operation and is independent of the clinical status of the patient during the two procedures.[4] Park and colleagues noted that 48% of patients who underwent second-look procedures required a bowel resection at the second operation.

Major postoperative complications remain excessive (25%–100%), and early and late mortality rates are high (16%–80%).[26] Factors associated with increased mortality include renal insufficiency, age, metabolic acidosis, symptom duration, and bowel

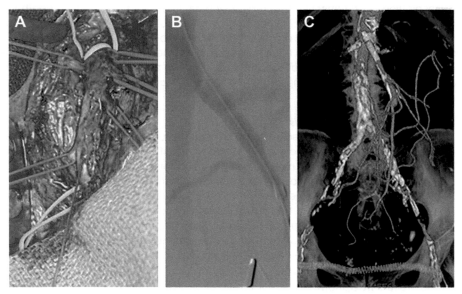

Fig. 4. Technique of hybrid retrograde SMA stenting. Infracolic exposure of the SMA (*A*). Completion angiography demonstrates a widely patent SMA post-stenting (*B*) and a post operative CT reveals a patent SMA stent and severe aortoiliac disease (*C*). (*From* Oderich GS, Gloviczki P, Bower TC. Open surgical treatment for chronic mesenteric ischemia in the endovascular era: when it is necessary and what is the preferred technique? *Semin Vasc Surg.* 2010;23(1):36-46; with permission.)

Box 2
Technique of retrograde open mesenteric stenting as described by Oderich and colleagues

1. Midline laparotomy performed under general anesthesia with endotracheal intubation

2. Abdominal exploration and control of frankly gangrenous or perforated bowel

3. Exposure of the SMA at the root of the mesentery

4. Control of the SMA and jejunal branches

5. Systemic heparinization (60–80 units/kg)

6. Retrograde access of the SMA using a 0.018 inch micropuncture kit

7. Placement of a 0.035 inch guidewire and a 45 cm 6 Fr or 7 Fr sheath

8. Angiography of the SMA through the sheath

9. Cross the SMA lesion and placement of a stiff guidewire into the aorta

10. Treatment of stenosis or occlusion with a balloon-expandable stent

11. Careful inspection of the arterial lumen after removal of the sheath for residual thrombus

12. Closure of the arteriotomy primarily or with patch angioplasty

---

resection.[4,27,28] After reperfusion of the ischemic bowel, an inflammatory response results in intestinal epithelial damage and cytokine release produces systemic effects on the lungs, liver, heart, and kidneys.[29] Postoperative complications of myocardial infarction, pneumonia, renal failure requiring dialysis, recurrent intestinal ischemia, postoperative ileus, renal insufficiency, and sepsis have all been reported.[29,30]

Long-Term Recommendations

Antiplatelet and/or anticoagulation therapy will be required after revascularization for AMI depending on the procedure performed and patient comorbidities. Dual antiplatelet therapy is typically administered for a minimum of 1 month after mesenteric stenting, followed by lifelong antiplatelet monotherapy. Anticoagulation may be indicated for patients with a diagnosis of atrial fibrillation or underlying hypercoagulability and should be considered for lifelong anticoagulation. Patients should be medically optimized according to their comorbidities.

Surveillance imaging for stent and graft stenosis is essential, as recurrent mesenteric ischemia is life-threatening. SVS guidelines for imaging surveillance are summarized in **Table 3**.[31]

Clinics Care Points

- A high clinical suspicion and prompt recognition of AMI is required to optimize patient outcomes, yet morbidity and mortality remain high for this diagnosis

- The goal of surgical care in AMI is the removal of non-salvageable bowel, the minimization and prevention of further bowel infarction, and the preservation of bowel length

- The approach to revascularize the bowel should be selected based on the patient's condition and visceral anatomy

- There is an increasing use of endovascular interventions to treat AMI. This approach may be appropriate in select patients yet the application is limited due to the lack of assessment of bowel viability

Table 3	
SVS imaging surveillance guidelines after mesenteric artery stenting or bypass	
Imaging Modality	**Recommendation**
Duplex ultrasound (DUS)	Within 1 mo for baseline
	At 6 mo, 12 mo, and annually
Contrast imaging	Symptoms of recurrent mesenteric ischemia
	DUS findings of
	1. Celiac axis: PSV > 370 cm/s or substantial increase from post-treatment baseline[a]
	2. SMA: PSV >420 cm/s or a substantial increase from post-treatment baseline[a]
	3. IMA: a substantial increase from post-treatment baseline[a]

[a] Substantial increase from baseline has not been defined.

CHRONIC MESENTERIC ISCHEMIA
Introduction

CMI is caused by inadequate postprandial intestinal blood flow, typically from atherosclerotic occlusive disease. In the fasting state, 20% of the cardiac output is directed through the mesenteric arteries.[32] After a meal, blood flow exceeds fasting values by 100% to 150% for 3 to 6 hours.[33] Vasodilation of the mesenteric vessels begins 3 to 5 minutes after ingestion and persists for 4 to 6 hours depending on the meal composition. In patients with CMI, the postprandial hyperemic response is reduced due to occluded or stenotic vessels resulting in a mismatch of oxygen supply and demand leading to pain, malabsorption, and bowel emptying. Revascularization techniques have evolved over the past six decades, with primary mesenteric stenting gaining widespread acceptance and becoming the most frequently utilized treatment of CMI. Open surgery is frequently reserved for patients who fail endovascular therapy or have complex lesions not amenable to endovascular intervention. This section provides an overview of the epidemiology, anatomy, clinical evaluation, and treatment options for patients with CMI.

Epidemiology

The presence of atherosclerotic disease in the visceral vessels is common. Wilson and colleagues reported that 17% of elderly adults had evidence of significant occlusive disease in the celiac artery (CA) or SMA on routine DUS screening.[34] Despite the frequency of visceral artery stenosis, CMI is significantly less so given the abundant collateral circulation. The incidence of CMI increases with age, consistent with atherosclerotic disease and associated risk factors, and is more common in women.[35]

Anatomy

Symptoms of CMI typically do not develop unless both the CA and SMA have hemodynamically significant lesions given the significant collateralization of mesenteric circulation.[36] **Fig. 5** shows a sagittal image and 3D reconstruction of a 54-year-old patient with chronic occlusion of the celiac and SMA, with significant collateralization from the inferior mesenteric artery (IMA).[37] This patient did not have any symptoms of mesenteric ischemia, demonstrating the impressive capability of mesenteric collateralization. However, it is possible to develop symptoms with significant occlusive disease in a single vessel, usually the SMA, if collateralization is insufficient.[36] The

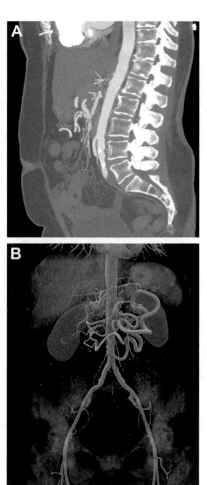

Fig. 5. Significant mesenteric collateralization in a patient with chronic occlusion of the celiac artery and SMA. (*From* Steiger K, Sandhu SJS, Veire AM, Erben Y. Collateralization in a patient with occluded celiac and superior mesenteric arteries without symptoms. *J Vasc Surg.* 2022;76(6):1733. https://doi.org/10.1016/j.jvs.2022.06.017; with permission.)

gastroduodenal and pancreaticoduodenal arteries provide collateralization between the CA and SMA. The marginal artery of Drummond and Arc of Riolan connect the IMA to the SMA, as demonstrated in **Fig. 6**.[38]

Oderich and colleagues described the arteriographic findings of over 200 patients with CMI; 98% had an occlusive disease of two vessels, and 92% had an occlusion or critical stenosis of the SMA.[36] SVS guidelines recommend making a diagnosis of CMI in patients with the appropriate clinical scenario and the presence of significant stenoses (>70%) within the celiac axis and SMA.[33] The diagnosis may also be made in patients with the appropriate clinical scenario and significant stenosis (>70%) in either the celiac axis or SMA alone.[33] Occlusive disease typically affects the orifice and the first few centimeters of the mesenteric vessels with relative sparing of the distal segment, and is usually associated with plaque within the aorta.[39]

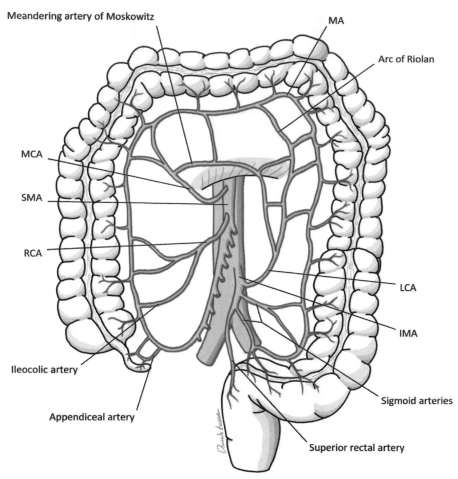

Meandering artery of Moskowitz

MA

Arc of Riolan

MCA

SMA

RCA

LCA

IMA

Ileocolic artery

Sigmoid arteries

Appendiceal artery

Superior rectal artery

Fig. 6. The anatomy of the mesenteric circulation and collateralization between the SMA and inferior mesenteric artery, through the meandering mesenteric artery (Moskowitz), marginal artery of Drummond (MA), and Arc of Riolan. (*From* Mann MR, Kawzowicz M, Komosa AJ, et al. The marginal artery of Drummond revisited: A systematic review. *Transl Res Anat.* 2021;24:100118.; with permission.)

Patient Evaluation Overview

There is no reliable functional test for CMI. The diagnosis is predicated on the clinical scenario and visceral occlusive disease. The typical triad of presenting symptoms includes postprandial abdominal pain, weight loss, and sitophobia. However, this triad is not always present and patients may present with nonspecific complaints of discomfort, nausea, vomiting, diarrhea, and constipation. Pain is usually described as mid-abdominal, crampy, or dull and occurs within 30 minutes of eating and can persist for up to 6 hours. Patients may avoid certain foods which exacerbate their symptoms. There is often a delay in diagnosis from the onset of symptoms and patients may present with significant malnutrition which impacts perioperative mortality and long-term survival.

There is a broad differential diagnosis for the clinical presentation and the diagnostic workup should include gastrointestinal causes including malignancy. In patients with abdominal pain, weight loss, and food fear, the SVS guidelines recommend an expedited workup including an esophagogastroduodenoscopy (EGD), a colonoscopy, an abdominal CT scan, and an abdominal ultrasound examination.[33] EGD findings of ischemic gastritis, duodenitis, or colitis are nonspecific but may be suggestive of CMI, as well as the presence of a gastric ulcer in the absence of malignancy. SVS guidelines recommend using the mesenteric duplex ultrasound (DUS) examination as the preferred screening test for mesenteric arterial occlusive disease (MAOD).[33] CTA is the preferred definitive imaging test for MAOD unless unusual anatomic features obscure the anatomy such that a catheter-based arteriogram may be required.[33]

Medical Treatment Options

CMI is a manifestation of a systemic process and patients typically present with atherosclerotic risk factors including smoking and hypertension. The SVS guidelines recommend that patients should be medically optimized before intervention although their perioperative evaluation should be expedited.[33] An antiplatelet agent and a cholesterol-lowering agent, preferably a statin, should be initiated.[33] Parenteral or enteral nutritional supplements may help replete the nutritional status of the malnourished CMI patient, but should not delay revascularization.[33] Bowel preparation should be avoided due to the theoretic risk of developing AMI.[33] Patients with asymptomatic severe MAOD should be medically optimized and undergo annual evaluation with mesenteric DUS.[33]

Surgical Treatment Options

The evidence supporting the diagnosis and treatment of CMI has been somewhat limited, despite the dramatic evolution in the care paradigms over the past decades. The supporting evidence is largely retrospective, single-center reports with heterogeneous patient populations in terms of comorbidities, distribution of occlusive disease, acuity of symptoms, and type of revascularization. The limitation of the evidence is compounded by the lack of widely accepted reporting standards.[33] The choice of treatment of patients with CMI should be a shared decision-making process between the patient and provider, considering the risks and benefits of the various options and the patient's goals of care. The SVS guidelines in **Box 3** recommend endovascular revascularization as the initial treatment of patients with CMI and suitable lesions, reserving open surgical revascularization for patients with CMI who have lesions that are not amenable to endovascular therapy, endovascular failures, and a select group of younger, healthier patients in which the long-term benefits may offset the increased perioperative risks.[33]

Open revascularization

There are several approaches to open surgical revascularization of the mesenteric vessels. The decision to proceed with a particular approach is based on the patient's anatomy and clinical risk assessment. Antegrade bypass requires a supraceliac clamp and is therefore typically reserved for patients who are a lower risk with no active cardiac disease, and no significant calcification or thrombus in the supraceliac aorta. The advantages of an antegrade bypass are that this segment of the aorta is often spared from atherosclerotic disease, improved hemodynamics, and the course of the graft avoids kinking. Elderly patients and those with a higher burden of comorbidities would be more suitably treated with a retrograde bypass using inflow from the infrarenal aorta or iliac arteries. Transaortic endarterectomy is a feasible option for patients

---

Box 3
SVS guidelines for visceral revascularization targets

We suggest that the SMA is the primary target for revascularization

We suggest that the celiac axis and IMA are secondary targets for revascularization and that revascularization may aid in symptom relief if the SMA is not suitable for intervention or the technical result is not acceptable

In patients with mesenteric artery occlusive disease and visceral aneurysms, we recommend revascularization at the time of treatment of their mesenteric artery aneurysms if the repair alone would disrupt the collateral network

A shared decision-making approach between the patient and provider to discuss revascularization as a treatment option is appropriate in the following circumstances:
• Symptoms of CMI and single-vessel disease
• Asymptomatic patients with severe mesenteric artery occlusive disease
• Patients undergoing aortic reconstruction with severe MAOD

---

with aortic and ostial disease and may be appropriate in the setting of gross contamination or when a retroperitoneal approach is preferred such as prior abdominal radiation or extensive abdominal wall hernias.

Antegrade bypass. Through a midline laparotomy or subcostal incision, the abdomen is explored for other pathology and the bowel is inspected for ischemia and perforations (**Fig. 7**). The lesser sac is entered by dividing the pars flaccida and the left triangular ligament is divided to enable retraction of the left lobe of the liver. The stomach is retracted caudally, and the esophagus is gently retracted to the patient's left. The crura of the diaphragm are divided to expose the supraceliac aorta, and the common hepatic artery, splenic artery, and left gastric artery are isolated. The left gastric artery can be divided to facilitate the anastomosis and tunneling of the graft. The hepatic artery proper may be a preferred target for the distal anastomosis in cases of extensive atherosclerosis. The transverse colon is then reflected cephalad and the SMA is exposed at the root of the small bowel mesentery. The SMA and jejunal branches are dissected free. Vessel loops may be placed at the time of clamping to avoid any unnecessary traction and potential avulsion. A retropancreatic tunnel is made anterior to the left renal vein from the celiac artery to the SMA. The patient is systemically heparinized and mannitol is administered before supraceliac clamping. A bifurcated knitted polyester graft is selected and the body is trimmed to a short, oblique length. The supraceliac aorta is clamped proximally and distally, or a side biting clamp is used such as a Satinsky (**Fig. 8**). An aortotomy is made and the main body of the graft is anastomosed end-to-side using a running Prolene suture. The left limb of the graft is brought through the retropancreatic tunnel to the SMA. The SMA and jejunal branches are controlled and clamped, and a longitudinal arteriotomy is made. In cases of extensive disease, the SMA may require endarterectomy and patch angioplasty before anastomosis of the graft limb. The limb is cut to length, taking care to avoid angulation or kinking, and is sewn end-to-side to the SMA. The celiac anastomosis is then performed end-to-end or often end-to-side to the common hepatic artery.

Retrograde bypass. Retrograde mesenteric bypass may be performed to revascularize the SMA, celiac artery, or both. The infrarenal aorta, prior aortic grafts, or the iliac arteries are sources of inflow. The iliac artery is preferred if anatomically suitable to avoid aortic cross-clamping. The graft tends to lay better from the right iliac artery. When the inflow source is the iliac artery, the proximal anastomosis is sewn first

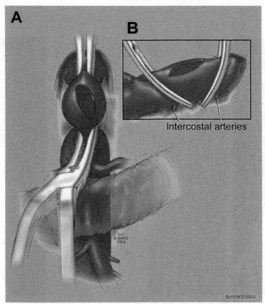

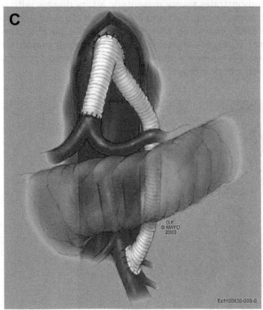

Fig. 7. Supraceliac clamping and antegrade two vessel mesenteric bypass, with the left limb of the graft tunneled behind the pancreas. (*From*: Oderich GS, Gloviczki P & Bower TC. Open Surgical Treatment for Chronic Mesenteric Ischemia in the Endovascular Era: When It is Necessary and What is the Preferred Technique? Semin Vasc Surg. 2010 Mar;23(1):36-46; used with permission of Mayo Foundation for Medical Education and Research, all rights reserved.)

end-to-side. The graft is then tunneled, in a lazy C shape to the SMA, and if performing two-vessel revascularization through a retropancreatic tunnel to the celiac artery, as described above. To avoid graft angulation or kinking, the SMA should be placed in its anatomic position by relaxing the retractors and the mesentery when cutting the graft (**Fig. 9**).

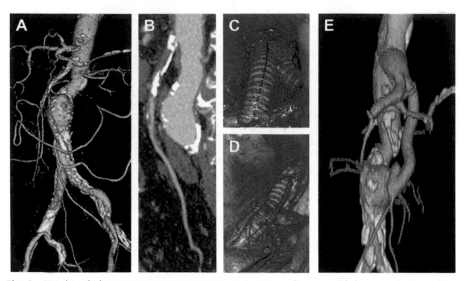

Fig. 8. CTA (*A, B*) demonstrates severe mesenteric artery disease with long occlusion of the SMA. A supraceliac aorta to celiac (*C*) and SMA bypass (*D*) with endarterectomy and patch angioplasty of the SMA. Follow-up CTA demonstrates a patent graft (*E*). (*From* Oderich GS, Gloviczki P, Bower TC. Open surgical treatment of chronic mesenteric ischemia in the endovascular era: when it is necessary and what is the preferred technique? *Semin Vasc Surg.* 2010;23(1):36-46; with permission.)

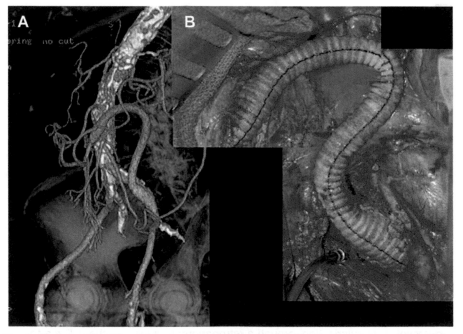

Fig. 9. Postoperative CT and intraoperative photo of a left iliac to SMA bypass. (*From* Oderich GS, Gloviczki P, Bower TC. Open surgical treatment of chronic mesenteric ischemia in the endovascular era: when it is necessary and what is the preferred technique? *Semin Vasc Surg.* 2010;23(1):36-46; with permission.)

Transaortic mesenteric endarterectomy. Access to the paravisceral aorta may be achieved through a midline laparotomy and left medial visceral rotation or from a retroperitoneal approach. The choice of exposure will determine patient positioning. The paravisceral aorta is exposed through a left medial visceral rotation or retroperitoneal approach, leaving the left kidney down and dissecting anterior to the left renal vein. Leaving the kidney down allows for access to a greater length of the SMA. The spleen is carefully dissected away from the diaphragm, mobilizing the lienophrenic ligament attaching the spleen to the diaphragm. The crus of the diaphragm is divided to expose the supraceliac aorta, celiac artery, and SMA. The SMA is dissected free for several centimeters. The infrarenal aorta or iliac arteries are exposed for distal control. The patient is systemically heparinized and mannitol is administered, and the supraceliac and infrarenal aorta are clamped. A longitudinal or trapdoor aortotomy is performed, from the origin of the celiac to the renal arteries, taking care to leave room around the orifice of each visceral vessel. Endarterectomy of the paravisceral aorta, celiac, SMA, and possibly, renal arteries is performed (**Fig. 10**). The aortotomy is closed longitudinally, occasionally requiring a patch. If the SMA has diffuse disease, a separate longitudinal SMA arteriotomy may be required and should be closed with a patch.

Endovascular treatment
Access. Visceral artery angioplasty and stenting may be approached through femoral access or upper extremity access. In cases where the angle of the SMA to the aorta is acute, upper extremity access is preferred. The advantage of femoral access is that it is commonly performed, clinicians are comfortable with the procedure and closure devices may be used.[40] The use of articulated sheaths has made treatment of the SMA from femoral access easier. Preoperative CTA should be used to help decide on the access, as the disease of the supraceliac or infrarenal aorta may influence this decision. Upper extremity access or a hybrid approach is preferred for flush occlusions.

Procedure. Access is obtained through upper extremity or femoral access and systemic anticoagulation is administered. A paravisceral aortogram is obtained with the

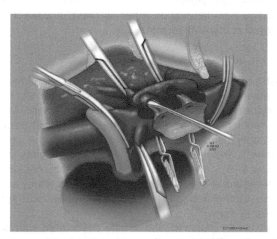

Fig. 10. Left medial visceral rotation and transaortic mesenteric endarterectomy. (*From:* Oderich GS, Gloviczki P & Bower TC. Open Surgical Treatment for Chronic Mesenteric Ischemia in the Endovascular Era: When It is Necessary and What is the Preferred Technique? Semin Vasc Surg. 2010 Mar;23(1):36-46; used with permission of Mayo Foundation for Medical Education and Research, all rights reserved.)

C-arm in a straight lateral or steep oblique position to visualize the origin of the visceral vessel. A 6 Fr sheath is placed with the tip near the origin of the vessel. After sheath placement, a 4 Fr or 5 Fr catheter is placed. A curved catheter may be useful for cannulation but may buckle when the guidewire enters the lesion, indicating that a different catheter is required to follow the wire. If the origin of the artery is patent, the catheter is used to cannulate it, whereas in flush occlusions, the catheter and sheath are used to support the wire to probe for the opening through the lesion.[40] Once the guidewire is across the lesion, the catheter can be advanced to exchange for a stiffer wire for stent placement. An 0.035 system or lower-profile system (0.014 or 0.018 inch system) may be used. A lower-profile system requires a small sheath, therefore, angiograms may be performed through the 6 Fr sheath around the treatment catheters and low-profile balloons and stents are more likely to make any sharp turns.[40] The advantage of the 0.035 systems is the stability of the system over a larger, stuff guidewire. The SMA system is typically more stable than the celiac artery due to the long segment of SMA available for wire purchase, compared to the short celiac artery with tortuous branches. Care should be taken to monitor the tip of the wire to avoid perforation or a small or collateral branch. The celiac artery is typically quite short and therefore requires accuracy in the placement of the stent, which should be placed flush with the aorta or protruding slightly into the aorta so that the entire lesion is treated.[40] Typically, stents in the celiac artery are 6 to 8 mm in diameter and 12 to 18 mm in length. The SMA may require pre-dilation prior to stent placement due to the angulation of the artery and the presence of a significant stenosis. SMA stents are typically 6 to 8 mm in diameter and tend to be longer than celiac stents, up to 3 cm not being unusual.[40] Balloon-expandable covered stents are recommended, as the high radial force, functionality at short lengths, and limited shortening with expansion make them well suited for treating orificial calcific disease.[33] Self-expanding stents may have a role in longer lesions, intraluminal dissections, and preserving significant collaterals.[33]

Hybrid treatment options

Retrograde open mesenteric stenting may be considered for patients with CMI where antegrade cannulation from femoral or upper extremity access is unsuccessful. This technique is reviewed in the AMI section.

Complications

Complication rates after open mesenteric revascularization average 20% to 40%.[41] Perioperative complications are generally related to multisystem organ dysfunction, as opposed to technical issues. Ischemia reperfusion injury results in the release of reactive oxygen species and subsequent neutrophil infiltration, systemic inflammatory syndrome, and possible multiorgan dysfunction. Pulmonary, gastrointestinal, cardiac, and renal complications are the most frequent. Prolonged ileus occurs in 8% of patients.[15] Early graft thrombosis is an uncommon (<2%) but potentially lethal complication and indicates either a technical problem due to graft kinking, intimal flap, dissection, or thrombus, poor runoff, or an underlying hypercoagulable state.[15]

Endovascular revascularization of CMI can be associated with both local and systemic complications from the intervention and underlying disease process. Perioperative complications have been demonstrated to be lower after endovascular intervention compared to open surgical repair. Access complications, contrast-induced renal insufficiency, target vessel dissection, device failure, and arterial embolization are possible endovascular complications in the treatment of CMI.

Long-Term Recommendations

After open or endovascular revascularization for CMI, patients should be maintained on antiplatelet agents and statin.[33] The optimal antiplatelet agent regimen and endovascular interventions for CMI remain unresolved. There is currently no evidence to support the use of dual antiplatelet therapy which may confer a higher bleeding risk.[33] A completion imaging study, typically a DUS, should be performed in the early postoperative period to confirm technical success and to serve as a baseline for follow-up and surveillance imaging.[33] As per SVS guidelines, patients should be followed as outpatients with mesenteric DUS at 1 month, every 6 months for 2 years, and then annually.[33] Patients should be educated on the symptoms of recurrent mesenteric ischemia and counseled to seek medical attention if they should occur. Endovascular intervention is associated with a higher rate of recurrent stenoses and symptoms.[33] CTA or a catheter based angiogram with measurement of intraluminal pressures may be used to confirm or refute ultrasound findings of recurrent stenosis.[33] Patients with recurrent CMI should undergo an endovascular first approach, reserving open revascularization for patients who are not amenable to endovascular intervention.[33]

Clinics Care Points

- The choice of treatment of patients with CMI should be a shared decision-making process between the patient and provider, considering the risks and benefits of the various options and the patient's goals of care.

- Endovascular revascularization is recommended as the initial treatment of patients with CMI and suitable lesions

- Open surgical revascularization should be reserved for patients with CMI who have lesions that are not amenable to endovascular therapy, endovascular failures, and a select group of younger, healthier patients in which the long-term benefits may offset the increased perioperative risks

- Patients require lifelong surveillance with mesenteric DUS due to the risk of restenosis and recurrence of CMI

VISCERAL ANEURYSMS
Introduction

Visceral artery aneurysms are a rare entity but clinically significant due to the risk of rupture. They account for approximately 5% of all intra-abdominal aneurysms.[42] The incidence of visceral aneurysms is demonstrated in **Table 4**, as well as the distribution with splenic artery aneurysms being the most common. Almost 25% of visceral aneurysms reported in the literature have presented with rupture, and the mortality rate is at least 10%.[43,44] Due to the increased use of abdominal imaging techniques, visceral artery aneurysms are being diagnosed with increased frequency.[42] Despite this, the natural history of visceral artery aneurysms is poorly defined and it is difficult to accurately assess the risk of rupture. The treatment goal of visceral aneurysms is to prevent aneurysm expansion and potential rupture by exclusion from arterial circulation while maintaining perfusion to the distal or collateral bed perfusion.[42]

Patient Evaluation Overview

There are many etiologies of visceral artery aneurysms, and the risk of development will depend on each specific etiology. Visceral artery aneurysms are categorized as true aneurysms or pseudoaneurysms. True aneurysms are those that expand locally

Table 4
Incidence of visceral aneurysms and anatomic distribution

Artery	Incidence	% of Splanchnic Aneurysms
Splenic	0.78%	60%
Hepatic	<0.4%	20%
SMA	0.008%	6%
Celiac	0.01%	4%
Gastric/gastroepiploic	NS	<4%
GDA/PDA	NS	2%,
IMA/jejunal/ileal/colic	NS	<2%

while maintaining components of the arterial wall, and their main cause is atherosclerosis.[45] Other possible causes of true aneurysms include medial degeneration, connective tissue diseases, and fibromuscular dysplasia.[46–48] Splenic artery aneurysms have been associated with pregnancy, multiparity, portal hypertension, liver transplantation, cirrhosis, and arteriovenous malformations. Pseudoaneurysms are attributed to a lack of arterial wall structure and may occur following trauma, infections such as tuberculosis or syphilis, vasculitis, inflammation, or due to iatrogenic causes. Chronic pancreatitis may result in splenic artery pseudoaneurysm formation, presenting as hemosuccus pancreaticus which is a rare cause of upper chronic and intermittent gastrointestinal hemorrhage. Segmental arterial mediolysis (SAM) is a rare condition identified as a nonatherosclerotic, non-vasculitic arteriopathy that typically affects late middle-age, and elderly patients. SAM is characterized by the development of a dissecting hematoma, aneurysm, occlusion, or hemorrhage after lysis of the arterial media, usually involving more than one visceral artery.[49–51]

Visceral artery aneurysms are also found in conjunction with rare diseases such as von Recklinghausen disease, Ehlers–Danlos syndrome, polyarteritis nodosa, and Behçet disease.[48] Case reports have also identified other causes such as systemic arteritis, endocarditis with septic emboli, and excessive acetaminophen use.[41]

Patients with visceral artery aneurysms are generally asymptomatic unless presenting with rupture, in which case, the most common presenting symptoms include epigastric pain, back pain, nausea, abdominal distension, hematochezia, or a palpable pulsatile mass. In up to 25% of splenic artery aneurysm cases, patients may present with the "double rupture" phenomenon, in which the patient initially ruptures into the lesser sac and subsequently stabilizes until free peritoneal rupture.[52]

One-third of patients with a splanchnic artery aneurysm will have an associated aortic, renal, iliac, lower extremity, or cerebral artery aneurysm, highlighting the importance of screening in these individuals. The SVS guidelines on visceral aneurysms outline the recommendations for screening for each visceral aneurysm, and this is summarized in **Table 5**.[42]

Surgical/Interventional Treatment Options

The natural history of many visceral artery aneurysms is not well understood, and the risk of rupture is difficult to quantify and is impacted by various factors including location, morphology, size, and patient characteristics. Given the challenge of diagnosis and high mortality, intervention at the time of diagnosis has been justified for

Table 5
SVS screening recommendations for concomitant aneurysms with visceral aneurysms and level of evidence

Artery	Screening Recommendation	Level of Evidence
Splenic	All patients for other intra-abdominal, intrathoracic, intracranial, and peripheral artery aneurysms	2B
Hepatic	One-time CTA (or MRA) of head, neck, and chest for patients with nonatherosclerotic etiology	2B
SMA	Abdominal axial imaging to screen for concomitant abdominal aneurysms in patients who did not have a CTA at the time of diagnosis	2B
Celiac	All patients for other arterial aneurysms	2B
Gastric/gastroepiploic	One-time CTA (or MRA) of the head, neck, and chest for patients with segmental arterial mediolysis	2C
GDA/PDA	No screening outside the abdomen is recommended	N/A
IMA/jejunal/ileal/colic	One-time CTA (or MRA) of the head, neck, and chest for patients with segmental arterial mediolysis	2B

aneurysms in some arterial beds and recommendations have been outlined in the SVS guidelines.[42] The SVS guidelines for surgical intervention are summarized in **Table 6**.[42]

General Treatment Principles

Treatment selection depends on various factors including the size, location, and morphology of the aneurysm etiology, patient presentation, comorbidities, and risk factors. There are no randomized controlled trials comparing open versus

Table 6
SVS guidelines on indication for surgical intervention on visceral artery aneurysms

Artery	Size Threshold for Repair
Splenic	True aneurysm >3 cm All pseudoaneurysms All women of childbearing age
Hepatic	True aneurysm >2 cm for low risk True aneurysm >5 cm for high risk All pseudoaneurysms All symptomatic aneurysms All aneurysms if a positive history of vasculitis
SMA	All aneurysms and pseudoaneurysms
Celiac	True aneurysm >2 cm All pseudoaneurysms
Gastric/gastroepiploic	All
GDA/PDA	All
IMA/jejunal/ileal/colic	IMA: decision per patient Jejunal and ileal: >2 cm Colic: all Medical management recommended for asymptomatic aneurysms associated with polyarteritis nodosa

endovascular intervention, however, literature has suggested a shorter hospital stay and lower cardiovascular complications with endovascular therapy.[45]

Endovascular

Several endovascular techniques are available for the treatment of visceral artery aneurysms. These techniques include deployment of coils and plugs, liquid embolic agents, covered stents, flow-diverting stents, and percutaneous injection of thrombin.[53] The technique selected is impacted by the anatomic shape and type of aneurysm, morphology of the aneurysm neck, tortuosity of the inflow artery, and necessity to preserve the inflow artery.[45] Endovascular treatment options for visceral artery aneurysms are outlined in **Table 7**, and the benefits and limitations of endovascular therapy are detailed in **Box 4** and **Table 8**.

Specific endovascular treatment considerations

Splenic Given the excellent collateral circulation to the spleen, coil embolization has a high success rate and low risk of ischemia. Stent graft placement may be appropriate for aneurysms in the proximal splenic artery, but placement in the distal splenic artery would be challenging due to the tortuosity of the vessel and the associated difficulty of getting adequate wire support to advance the stent through the tortuous anatomy.

Hepatic Surgical ligation or coil embolization of the common hepatic artery is feasible if the gastroduodenal artery is patent to facilitate collateral circulation to the liver. If anatomic conditions permit, including adequate diameter and sufficient proximal and distal sealing zones, stent graft placement may be considered. Most intrahepatic artery aneurysms are treated with embolization, but hepatectomy is sometimes required.

Superior mesenteric artery Coil embolization or stent graft exclusion are two endovascular options to treat SMA aneurysms. Endovascular embolization can be helpful in these cases if the aneurysm is distal to the origin of the SMA, has a small neck, and good collateral flow.

Celiac Coil embolization of the celiac artery is effective and carries a low risk of organ ischemia. However, this intervention is not applicable for aneurysms involving the origin of the celiac artery as there would be no seal zone or proximal space for coils.

Gastric/gastroepiploic Open surgery has been the most common treatment method for these aneurysms in the literature, but they are quite rare. Increasing reports of coil embolization have been reported.

Table 7
Endovascular treatment options for visceral artery aneurysms

Technique	Tips
Coil embolization	Embolization of distal artery, packing of aneurysm, embolization of proximal artery
Liquid embolic agents	Effective for complex visceral aneurysms, but technically challenging due to the risk of distal embolization
Covered self-expanding stent	Preserve perfusion of blood to distal target organ, but often limited by arterial anatomy as the large, rigid delivery devices can be difficult to navigate to the target artery
Flow-diverting stents	Adapted from the treatment of intracranial aneurysms, designed to reduce flow in the aneurysm while maintaining flow in the main artery

---

Box 4
Benefits and limitations of endovascular therapy of visceral artery aneurysms

Benefits
- Can be performed under local anesthesia
- Shorter hospital stay
- Lower perioperative complications
- Lower cost
- Avoid intra-abdominal reoperation

Limitations
- Require specific resources and facility
- Risk of access-related injury
- End-organ embolization
- Contrast toxicity
- Need for surveillance imaging

Pancreaticoduodenal artery/Gastroduodenal artery Coil embolization or stent graft placement are the preferred approach over open surgery, given the challenge of open surgery in these cases. Endovascular intervention is associated with fewer complications and improved outcomes.[45]

Interior mesenteric artery/jejunal/ileal/colic These aneurysms are very rare, both open and endovascular treatment methods have been reported in the literature with technical success.

Tips and tricks for endovascular treatment of visceral artery aneurysms[54]

Table 8
SVS surveillance recommendations for visceral aneurysms and level of evidence

Artery	Surveillance Recommendation	Level of Evidence
Splenic	Annual observation with CT or US to assess for growth in size Periodic surveillance after endovascular intervention to assess for endoleak or ongoing aneurysm perfusion	2B
Hepatic	Annual observation with CT or US to assess for growth in size	2B
SMA	Annual CTA to observe postsurgical changes	2B
Celiac	Annual observation with CT or US to assess for growth in size Periodic surveillance after endovascular intervention to assess for endoleak or ongoing aneurysm perfusion	2B
Gastric/gastroepiploic	Axial imaging every 12–24 mo in patients with segmental arterial mediolysis Postembolization surveillance every 1–2 y	2C
GDA/PDA	Follow-up imaging recommended after endovascular treatment to rule out persistent flow through the aneurysm sac	1B
IMA/jejunal/ileal/colic	Axial imaging every 12–24 mo in patients with segmental arterial mediolysis Postembolization surveillance every 1–2 y	2B

1. Plan in advance and ensure all required equipment is available
2. Select access to minimize tortuosity, consider axillary or brachial access if required
3. When using balloon-assisted coiling, choose the appropriate size balloon to avoid vessel dissection or spasm
4. When using stent grafts, ensure there is adequate landing zone on either side of the aneurysm to ensure successful exclusion and avoid early recanalization and stent migration
5. If landing zone is limited, consider embolization of small collaterals to create or increase the landing zone

Open

Open repair of visceral artery aneurysms is known to be a safe and durable treatment option, with the benefits of assessing the condition of the end-organ and concomitant pathology depending on the etiology of the aneurysm. In emergency conditions, arterial ligation without reconstruction has been applied as a strategy, and in certain elective cases, with adequate collateral circulation. Knowledge of mesenteric arterial anatomy and collateral beds is essential. Ligation of the main trunk of the splenic artery does not cause major complications due to collateral blood supply from the short gastric arteries and left gastroepiploic artery. The spleen also receives collaterals from the SMA, pancreatic arteries, and left inferior phrenic artery. If the splenic artery aneurysm is in the distal third of the artery or close to the hilum, a splenectomy may be performed. The celiac artery and common hepatic artery can be ligated if there is sufficient collateralization from the gastroduodenal and pancreaticoduodenal arteries.

Specific open treatment considerations

Splenic Options for open repair of a splenic artery aneurysm include resection with splenectomy, proximal and distal ligation of the aneurysm, or ligation with arterial reconstruction.[41] Aneurysm neck ligation and aneurysmectomy with reconstruction have been performed for splenic artery aneurysms in the main trunk of the artery. However, given the abundant collateral supply, reconstruction is unnecessary. Splenectomy is preferred for aneurysms near the hilum or intraparenchymal aneurysms. It is important to remember to administer post-splenectomy vaccinations to reduce the risk of post-splenectomy infection, the necessary vaccines and suggested schedule are outlined in **Box 5**.

Hepatic The common hepatic artery may be ligated if there is a patent GDA to provide collateral blood supply to the liver. Aneurysms of the hepatic artery proper, right or left hepatic artery require reconstruction using autologous vein or prosthetic conduit. Vein is preferred for size matching and infection resistance, however, careful

---

Box 5
Recommended splenectomy vaccinations and timing of administration

Recommended splenectomy vaccinations:
1. Hemophilus b conjugate (Hib) vaccine
2. Pneumococcal conjugate 13-valent vaccine
3. Meningococcal conjugate vaccine
4. Meningococcal serogroup B vaccine

Timing of vaccination relative to splenectomy:
  Elective—at least 14 days prior to splenectomy if possible
  Emergent—at least 14 days after surgery or prior to discharge, whichever is earliest

---

Box 6
Complications of open and endovascular repair of visceral aneurysms long-term recommendations

General
  Bleeding
  Infection (wound infection, abscess)
  End-organ infarction (splenic, hepatic, mesenteric)
  Systemic complications (respiratory, cardiac, neurologic)

Open repair
  Wound infection
  Hernia

Endovascular repair
  Access site complications (bleeding, thrombosis, pseudoaneurysm)
  Aneurysm sac reperfusion (growth, rupture)
  Arterial thrombosis/coil embolization (end-organ infarction)

---

attention must be paid to prevent compression, bending, or twisting of the graft. Inflow source options include the aorta, iliac artery, splenic artery, and renal artery.

Superior mesenteric artery Open surgical treatment options for SMA aneurysm include aneurysmectomy, aneurysmorrhaphy, and ligation with or without revascularization. The need for revascularization depends on the degree of collateral circulation from the pancreaticoduodenal and middle colic arteries. The viability of the bowel should be interrogated prior to completion of the case, with the option of performing a second-look laparotomy.

Celiac Options for open surgical repair of a celiac artery aneurysm depend on the presence of adequate collateral blood flow from the GDA or from the short gastric arteries. In the setting of collateral blood flow, it is possible to resect and ligate the celiac artery. When reconstruction is required, bypass from the aorta using prosthetic or autologous vein graft may be performed.

Gastric/gastroepiploic Open surgery has been the most common treatment method for these aneurysms in the literature, but they are quite rare. Increasing reports of coil embolization have been reported.

PDA/GDA In most cases, open surgical repair of these aneurysms would be difficult and an endovascular approach is preferred. Open surgery may be indicated in an emergency setting or if endovascular intervention has failed. Treatment of celiac artery occlusive disease or release of the median arcuate ligament may be considered to prevent recurrence or further aneurysm formation when an association between collateral flow and aneurysm formation is identified.

IMA/jejunal/ileal/colic These aneurysms are very rare, both open and endovascular treatment methods have been reported in the literature with technical success.

Complications

The mortality rates of a ruptured visceral artery aneurysm have been reported in the literature to range from 25% to 70%.[45] Ruptured splenic artery aneurysms in pregnancy have a maternal mortality rate of 70% and fetal mortality rate of 95%. Therefore, identification and treatment of these aneurysms prior to rupture can significantly reduce the morbidity and mortality.

Despite the limited evidence from previous retrospective studies, it is known that periprocedural complications are more likely after open repair. These complications include those related to laparotomy, wound infection, length of stay, and respiratory and cardiac complications.[55] A systematic review and meta-analysis by Barrionuevo and colleagues suggested that endovascular intervention is associated with shorter hospital stay and lower rates of cardiovascular complications.[55] The benefit of endovascular intervention seems to be greater in the setting of rupture, as open repair is more complex and has higher morbidity.[55] General complications of visceral artery aneurysm repair and those specific to open and endovascular repair are summarized in **Box 6.**

CLINICS CARE POINTS

- Given the rarity of this entity, the natural history of many visceral aneurysms is unclear. It is prudent to treat these aneurysms according to the SVS guidelines to prevent rupture given the high rates of mortality

- The anatomy and collateralization should be carefully assessed on preoperative imaging to determine the treatment strategy and need for revascularization

- Many visceral aneurysms are degenerative or atherosclerotic in nature, but other etiologies include fibromsucular dysplasia, connective tissue disorders, and inflammatory or infectious conditions. Therefore these patients require thorough history, physical examination and investigations to guide management and prognosis.

- Ruptured splenic artery aneurysms may present with the "double rupture" phenomenon, in which the patient ruptures into the lesser sac and may stablize hemodynamically until free intraperitoneal rupture.

DISCLOSURE

The authors have nothing to disclose.

REFERENCES

1. Stoney RJ, Cunningham CG. Acute mesenteric ischemia. Surgery 1993;114(3): 489–90.
2. Acosta S, Björck M. Acute thrombo-embolic occlusion of the superior mesenteric artery: A prospective study in a well defined population. Eur J Vasc Endovasc 2003;26(2):179–83. https://doi.org/10.1053/ejvs.2002.1893.
3. Duran M, Pohl E, Grabitz K, et al. The importance of open emergency surgery in the treatment of acute mesenteric ischemia. World J Emerg Surg 2015;10(1):45. https://doi.org/10.1186/s13017-015-0041-6.
4. Park WM, Gloviczki P, Cherry KJ, et al. Contemporary management of acute mesenteric ischemia: Factors associated with survival. J Vasc Surg 2002. https://doi.org/10.1067/nwa.2002.120373. Published online March 1.
5. Kärkkäinen JM, Lehtimäki TT, Manninen H, et al. Acute Mesenteric Ischemia Is a More Common Cause than Expected of Acute Abdomen in the Elderly. J Gastrointest Surg 2015;19(8):1407–14. https://doi.org/10.1007/s11605-015-2830-3.
6. Bala M, Catena F, Kashuk J, et al. Acute mesenteric ischemia: updated guidelines of the World Society of Emergency Surgery. World J Emerg Surg 2022; 17(1):54. https://doi.org/10.1186/s13017-022-00443-x.

7. Acosta S. Mesenteric ischemia. Curr Opin Crit Care 2015;21(2):171–8. https://doi.org/10.1097/mcc.0000000000000189.
8. Acosta-Mérida MA, Marchena-Gómez J, Saavedra-Santana P, et al. Surgical Outcomes in Acute Mesenteric Ischemia: Has Anything Changed Over the Years? World J Surg 2020;44(1):100–7. https://doi.org/10.1007/s00268-019-05183-9.
9. Campion EW, Clair DG, Beach JM. Mesenteric Ischemia. New Engl J Medicine 2016;374(10):959–68. https://doi.org/10.1056/nejmra1503884.
10. Acosta S, Ogren M, Sternby NH, et al. Clinical implications for the management of acute thromboembolic occlusion of the superior mesenteric artery: autopsy findings in 213 patients. Ann Surg 2005;241(3):516–22. https://doi.org/10.1097/01.sla.0000154269.52294.57.
11. Kärkkäinen JM, Acosta S. Acute mesenteric ischemia (part I) – Incidence, etiologies, and how to improve early diagnosis. Best Pract Res Clin Gastroenterology 2017;31(1):15–25. https://doi.org/10.1016/j.bpg.2016.10.018.
12. Mastoraki A, Mastoraki S, Tziava E, et al. Mesenteric ischemia: Pathogenesis and challenging diagnostic and therapeutic modalities. World J Gastrointest Pathophysiol 2016;7(1):125. https://doi.org/10.4291/wjgp.v7.i1.125.
13. Cudnik MT, Darbha S, Jones J, et al. The Diagnosis of Acute Mesenteric Ischemia: A Systematic Review and Meta -analysis. Acad Emerg Med 2013; 20(11):1087–100. https://doi.org/10.1111/acem.12254.
14. Evennett NJ, Petrov MS, Mittal A, et al. Systematic Review and Pooled Estimates for the Diagnostic Accuracy of Serological Markers for Intestinal Ischemia. World J Surg 2009;33(7):1374–83. https://doi.org/10.1007/s00268-009-0074-7.
15. Powell A, Armstrong P. Plasma biomarkers for early diagnosis of acute intestinal ischemia. Semin Vasc Surg 2014;27(3–4):170–5. https://doi.org/10.1053/j.semvascsurg.2015.01.008.
16. Furukawa A, Kanasaki S, Kono N, et al. CT Diagnosis of Acute Mesenteric Ischemia from Various Causes. Am J Roentgenol 2009;192(2):408–16. https://doi.org/10.2214/ajr.08.1138.
17. Kirkpatrick IDC, Kroeker MA, Greenberg HM. Biphasic CT with Mesenteric CT Angiography in the Evaluation of Acute Mesenteric Ischemia: Initial Experience1. Radiology 2003;229(1):91–8. https://doi.org/10.1148/radiol.2291020991.
18. Oldenburg WA, Lau LL, Rodenberg TJ, et al. Acute Mesenteric Ischemia: A Clinical Review. Arch Intern Med 2004;164(10):1054–62. https://doi.org/10.1001/archinte.164.10.1054.
19. Boley SJ, Sprayregan S, Siegelman SS, et al. Initial results from an aggressive roentgenological and surgical approach to acute mesenteric ischemia. Surgery 1977;82(6):848–55.
20. Mitsuyoshi A, Obama K, Shinkura N, et al. Survival in nonocclusive mesenteric ischemia: early diagnosis by multidetector row computed tomography and early treatment with continuous intravenous high-dose prostaglandin E(1). Ann Surg 2007;246(2):229–35. https://doi.org/10.1097/01.sla.0000263157.59422.76.
21. Smith SF, Gollop ND, Klimach SG, et al. Is open surgery or endovascular therapy best to treat acute mesenteric occlusive disease? Int J Surg 2013;11(10):1043–7. https://doi.org/10.1016/j.ijsu.2013.10.003.
22. Salsano G, Salsano A, Sportelli E, et al. What is the Best Revascularization Strategy for Acute Occlusive Arterial Mesenteric Ischemia: Systematic Review and Meta-analysis. Cardiovasc Intervent Radiol 2018;41(1):27–36. https://doi.org/10.1007/s00270-017-1749-3.
23. Swerdlow NJ, Varkevisser RRB, Soden PA, et al. Thirty-Day Outcomes After Open Revascularization for Acute Mesenteric Ischemia From the American College of

Surgeons National Surgical Quality Improvement Program. Ann Vasc Surg 2019; 61:148–55. https://doi.org/10.1016/j.avsg.2019.05.024.

24. Resch TA, Acosta S, Sonesson B. Endovascular Techniques in Acute Arterial Mesenteric Ischemia. Semin Vasc Surg 2010;23(1):29–35. https://doi.org/10.1053/j.semvascsurg.2009.12.004.

25. Oderich GS, Macedo R, Stone DH, et al. Multicenter study of retrograde open mesenteric artery stenting through laparotomy for treatment of acute and chronic mesenteric ischemia. J Vasc Surg 2018;68(2):470–80.e1. https://doi.org/10.1016/j.jvs.2017.11.086.

26. Scali ST, Ayo D, Giles KA, et al. Outcomes of antegrade and retrograde open mesenteric bypass for acute mesenteric ischemia. J Vasc Surg 2019;69(1): 129–40. https://doi.org/10.1016/j.jvs.2018.04.063.

27. Ballard JL, Stone WM, Hallett JW, et al. A critical analysis of adjuvant techniques used to assess bowel viability in acute mesenteric ischemia. Am Surg 1993;59(5): 309–11.

28. Cuzzocrea S, Chatterjee PK, Mazzon E, et al. Role of Induced Nitric Oxide in the Initiation of the Inflammatory Response After Postischemic Injury. Shock 2002; 18(2):169–76. https://doi.org/10.1097/00024382-200208000-00014.

29. Kougias P, Lau D, Sayed HFE, et al. Determinants of mortality and treatment outcome following surgical interventions for acute mesenteric ischemia. J Vasc Surg 2007;46(3):467–74. https://doi.org/10.1016/j.jvs.2007.04.045.

30. Ryer EJ, Kalra M, Oderich GS, et al. Revascularization for acute mesenteric ischemia. J Vasc Surg 2012;55(6):1682–9. https://doi.org/10.1016/j.jvs.2011.12.017.

31. Zierler RE, Jordan WD, Lal BK, et al. The Society for Vascular Surgery practice guidelines on follow-up after vascular surgery arterial procedures. J Vasc Surg 2018;68(1):256–84. https://doi.org/10.1016/j.jvs.2018.04.018.

32. Kolkman JJ, Bargeman M, Huisman AB, et al. Diagnosis and management of splanchnic ischemia. World J Gastroentero 2008;14(48):7309–20. https://doi.org/10.3748/wjg.14.7309.

33. Huber TS, Bjorck M, Chandra A, et al. Chronic Mesenteric Ischemia Clinical Practice Guideline from the Society for Vascular Surgery. J Vasc Surg 2020;73(1): 87S–115S. https://doi.org/10.1016/j.jvs.2020.10.029.

34. Wilson DB, Mostafavi K, Craven TE, et al. Clinical Course of Mesenteric Artery Stenosis in Elderly Americans. Arch Intern Med 2006;166(19):2095–100. https://doi.org/10.1001/archinte.166.19.2095.

35. Terlouw LG, Verbeten M, Noord D, et al. The Incidence of Chronic Mesenteric Ischemia in the Well-Defined Region of a Dutch Mesenteric Ischemia Expert Center. Clin Transl Gastroen 2020;11(8):e00200. https://doi.org/10.14309/ctg.0000000000000200.

36. Oderich GS, Bower TC, Sullivan TM, et al. Open versus endovascular revascularization for chronic mesenteric ischemia: Risk-stratified outcomes. J Vasc Surg 2009;49(6):1472–9.e3. https://doi.org/10.1016/j.jvs.2009.02.006.

37. Steiger K, Sandhu SJS, Veire AM, et al. Collateralization in a patient with occluded celiac and superior mesenteric arteries without symptoms. J Vasc Surg 2022; 76(6):1733. https://doi.org/10.1016/j.jvs.2022.06.017.

38. Mann MR, Kawzowicz M, Komosa AJ, et al. The marginal artery of Drummond revisited: A systematic review. Transl Res Anat 2021;24:100118. https://doi.org/10.1016/j.tria.2021.100118.

39. Mikkelsen WP. Intestinal angina Its surgical significance. Am J Surg 1957;94(2): 262–9. https://doi.org/10.1016/0002-9610(57)90654-2.

40. Schneider PA. Endovascular Skills. Guidewire and Catheter Skills for Endovascular Surgery; 2019. https://doi.org/10.1201/9780429156304. Published online.
41. Sidawy AN, Perler BA, editors. Rutherford's vascular surgery and endovascular therapy ©2018. . Elsevier; 2018. https://doi.org/10.1016/j.jvs.2018.08.001.
42. Chaer RA, Abularrage CJ, Coleman DM, et al. The Society for Vascular Surgery clinical practice guidelines on the management of visceral aneurysms. J Vasc Surg 2020;72(1):3S–39S. https://doi.org/10.1016/j.jvs.2020.01.039.
43. Cochennec F, Riga CV, Allaire E, et al. Contemporary Management of Splanchnic and Renal Artery Aneurysms: Results of Endovascular Compared with Open Surgery from Two European Vascular Centers. Eur J Vasc Endovasc 2011;42(3): 340–6. https://doi.org/10.1016/j.ejvs.2011.04.033.
44. Wagner WH, Allins AD, Treiman RL, et al. Ruptured Visceral Artery Aneurysms. Ann Vasc Surg 1997;11(4):342–7. https://doi.org/10.1007/s100169900058.
45. Obara H, Kentaro M, Inoue M, et al. Current management strategies for visceral artery aneurysms: an overview. Surg Today 2020;50(1):38–49. https://doi.org/10.1007/s00595-019-01898-3.
46. Carroccio A, Jacobs TS, Faries P, et al. Endovascular Treatment of Visceral Artery Aneurysms. Vasc Endovasc Surg 2007;41(5):373–82. https://doi.org/10.1177/1538574407308552.
47. Watada S, Obara H, Shimoda M, et al. Multiple Aneurysms of the Splenic Artery Caused by Fibromuscular Dysplasia. Ann Vasc Surg 2009;23(3):411.e7. https://doi.org/10.1016/j.avsg.2008.04.015.
48. Gehlen JMLG, Heeren PAM, Verhagen PF, et al. Visceral Artery Aneurysms. Vasc Endovasc Surg 2011;45(8):681–7. https://doi.org/10.1177/1538574411418129.
49. Beerle C, Soll C, Breitenstein S, et al. Spontaneous rupture of an intrahepatic aneurysm of the right hepatic artery caused by segmental arterial mediolysis. BMJ Case Rep 2016;2016. https://doi.org/10.1136/bcr-2015-214109. bcr2015214109.
50. Obara H, Matsubara K, Inoue M, et al. Successful endovascular treatment of hemosuccus pancreaticus due to splenic artery aneurysm associated with segmental arterial mediolysis. J Vasc Surg 2011;54(5):1488–91. https://doi.org/10.1016/j.jvs.2011.04.053.
51. Obara H, Matsumoto K, Narimatsu Y, et al. Reconstructive surgery for segmental arterial mediolysis involving both the internal carotid artery and visceral arteries. J Vasc Surg 2006;43(3):623–6. https://doi.org/10.1016/j.jvs.2005.11.033.
52. Zubaidi A. Rupture of Multiple Splenic Artery Aneurysms: A Common Presentation of a Rare Disease with a Review of Literature. Saudi J Gastroenterology 2009;15(1):55–8. https://doi.org/10.4103/1319-3767.45061.
53. Hemp JH, Sabri SS. Endovascular Management of Visceral Arterial Aneurysms. Techniques Vasc Interventional Radiology 2015;18(1):14–23. https://doi.org/10.1053/j.tvir.2014.12.003.
54. Elika Kashef, MBBS. "Endovascular Management of Visceral Artery Aneurysms." Endovascular Today, Bryn Mawr Communications, 24 Apr. 2020, Available at: https://evtoday.com/articles/2020-apr/endovascular-management-of-visceral-artery-aneurysms.
55. Barrionuevo P, Malas MB, Nejim B, et al. A systematic review and meta-analysis of the management of visceral artery aneurysms. J Vasc Surg 2019;70(5):1694–9. https://doi.org/10.1016/j.jvs.2019.02.024.

Nonatherosclerotic Renovascular Hypertension

Jessie Dalman[a], Dawn M. Coleman, MD[b],*

KEYWORDS

- Pediatric renovascular hypertension (pRVH) • Midoaortic syndrome (MAS)
- Renovascular hypertension (RVH) • Renal artery stenosis
- Fibromuscular dysplasia (FMD)

KEY POINTS

- Renovascular hypertension is a secondary form of high blood pressure resulting from impaired blood flow ot the kidneys, typically from aortorenal stenoses, that activate the renin-angiotensin-aldosterone system.
- A common cause of hypertension in adults, RVH results from atherosclerotic renal artery stenosis in the majority of cases, although differential diagnosis should consider fibromuscular dysplasia and other inflammatory arteritides.
- RVH is the third most common cause of high blood pressure in children, and midaortic syndrome should be considered as a severe phenotype.
- Medical management remains the mainstay of treatment for adult and pediatric RVH, with clinical guidlelines supporting the use of ACEi, ARBs, calcium channel blockers and beta-blockers with class I indication. ACEi/ARB treatment is often most effective, but requires close surveillance given risk of acute renal injury.
- While percutaneous transluminal renal angioplasty is the standard of care for adults with renal artery stenosis, open surgical revascularization offers significant blood pressure improvement and durability to children with developmental aortorenal stenoses.
- Phenotype should drive individualized surgical decision making and treatment plans for patients with RVH, and multidiscipinary care may benefit pediatric patients in particular.

BACKGROUND

Renovascular hypertension (RVH) is a secondary form of high blood pressure resulting from impaired blood flow to the kidneys with subsequent activation of the renin-angiotensin-aldosterone system. Often, this occurs due to abnormally small, narrowed, or blocked blood vessels supplying one or both kidneys (ie: renal artery occlusive disease) and is correctable. Juxtaglomerular cells release renin in response to

[a] University of Michigan, 1500 E Medical Center Drive, Ann Arbor, MI, USA; [b] Duke University, DUMC 3538, Durham, NC 27710, USA
* Corresponding author.
E-mail address: Dawn.coleman@duke.edu

Surg Clin N Am 103 (2023) 733–743
https://doi.org/10.1016/j.suc.2023.05.007
0039-6109/23/© 2023 Elsevier Inc. All rights reserved.

surgical.theclinics.com

decreased pressure, which in turn catalyzes the cleavage of circulating angiotensinogen synthesized by the liver to the decapeptide angiotensin I. Angiotensin-converting enzyme then cleaves angiotensin I to form the octapeptide angiotensin II, a potent vasopressor and the primary effector of renin-induced hypertension. The effects of angiotensin II are mediated by signaling downstream of its receptors. Angiotensin receptor type 1 is a G-protein-coupled receptor that activates vasoconstrictor and mitogenic signaling pathways resulting in peripheral arteriolar vasoconstriction and increased renal tubular reabsorption of sodium and water which promotes intravascular volume expansion. Angiotensin II stimulates the adrenal cortical release of aldosterone, which promotes renal tubular sodium reabsorption, resulting in volume expansion. Angiotensin II acts on glial cells and regions of the brain responsible for blood pressure regulation increasing renal sympathetic activation. Angiotensin II simulates the release of vasopressin from the pituitary which stimulates thirst and water reabsorption from the kidney to expand the intravascular volume and cause peripheral vasoconstriction (increased sympathetic tone). All of these mechanisms coalesce to increase arterial pressure by way of arteriolar constriction, enhanced cardiac output, and the retention of sodium and water.

A common cause of hypertension (HTN) in adults, it is estimated to affect only 8% to 10% of children with HTN.[1] Renal artery occlusive disease is the third most common cause of pediatric HTN, second only to the coarctation of the thoracic aorta and intrinsic kidney disease.[2] Though the overall incidence of pediatric RVH is low, this disease accounts for a much higher proportion of high blood pressure in children than in adults. RVH is often medically refractory and should be considered in the differential diagnosis of severe HTN in childhood, young women (<45 years), acute progression of chronic HTN, initial diastolic blood pressure (BP) > 115 mm Hg, and acute renal injury following anti-hypertensive therapy initiation (in particular with the initiation of angiotensin receptor enzyme inhibitors [ACEi] and/or angiotensin receptor antagonists [ARBs]).

In adults, RVH often results from atherosclerotic renal artery stenosis, while fibromuscular dysplasia (FMD) may affect 5% to 10% of cases. FMD is a nonatherosclerotic, noninflammatory disease of abnormal vascular remodeling, resulting in stenosis, dissection, or aneurysm in mainly the renal, carotid, and vertebral arteries of young women.[3] In medial fibroplasia, the most common form of FMD, there are alternating

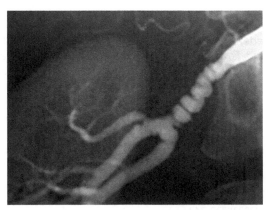

Fig. 1. Angiogram demonstrating multifocal 'string-of-beads' fibromuscular dysplasia of the main right renal artery.

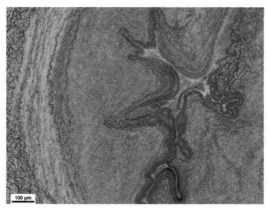

Fig. 2. Trichrome stain of a stenosed renal artery revealing intimal proliferation, fragmentation of the elastic lamina, medial thinning and excessive peri-adventitial elastin.

areas of thinned media and thickened fibromuscular ridges for which the arterial muscle is replaced by fibroplasia with loose collagen resulting in the classic "string of beads" appearance (**Fig. 1**).

Pediatric HTN is defined as an average systolic or diastolic BP (SBP or DBP) ≥95th percentile for sex, age, and height on 3 separate occasions. Pediatric RVH may result from inflammatory or infectious arteritides (ie: Takayasu's Arteritis), trauma, and malignancy. Up to 40% of pediatric patients with RVH may have a genetic etiology

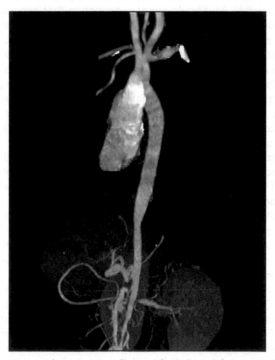

Fig. 3. CT-angiogram revealing supra-celiac mid-aortic syndrome with stenosis of the abdominal aorta, bilateral renal and SMA ostia.

such as neurofibromatosis type 1, Williams syndrome, Alagille syndrome, and tuberous sclerosis.[4–9] Most often the diagnosis remains undefined and attributed to a "developmental" arterial stenosis. The vast majority of developmental renal artery narrowings are ostial in location, representing true arterial hypoplasia. These pediatric arteries are extremely small and often exhibit intimal fibroplasia, internal elastic lamina disruptions, diminutive and discontinuous media, and excessive adventitial elastin.[10] (Fig. 2)

Midabdominal aortic syndrome (MAS) often contributes to pediatric RVH (Fig. 3). It is best classified by the most cephalad extent of the aortic narrowing as it relates to the renal arteries.[11] MAS is thought to arise from embryonic over-fusion of the paired dorsal aortas during the 4th week of development. In cases of MAS, renal arteries are most often narrowed and splanchnic involvement is common affecting 62% of patients. Additionally, multiple renal arteries and aberrant lumbar arterial anatomy are common.[11]

Patient Evaluation

Patients are frequently asymptomatic, although HTN may result in headache, epistaxis, and visual disturbance. Failure to thrive and agitation have been observed in infants with severe HTN. A careful history and physical should elicit constitutional symptoms suggesting vasculitis or endocrine dysfunction, flank pain, and hematuria. Alternate symptoms of FMD should be queried such as headache and tinnitus.[12] In children, symptoms of lower extremity exertional fatigue and/or postprandial abdominal pain are infrequent, but when present should prompt further consideration of MAS.[6]

Clinical exam should assess for the abdominal bruit, pulse abnormalities, neurologic deficits, and a complete cardiopulmonary examination that considers left ventricular hypertrophy. Additional musculoskeletal, skin and ocular abnormalities may suggest genetic etiology, especially in pediatric patients. Complete serologic evaluation should include inflammatory markers, electrolytes and renal function. Elevated plasma renin activity supports a diagnosis of RVH, while aldosterone, thyroid, and catecholamine levels will consider alternative endocrine dysfunction. Urinalysis for protein and baseline echocardiogram for structural anomalies and LVH should be performed. Additional screening for intra-cranial, cervical, and peripheral arteriopathy may be indicated for patients with underlying genetic disorders, MAS or FMD.[9,12,13]

Renal duplex ultrasonography remains the first-line diagnostic imaging modality when RVH is suspected and will offer up to 90% sensitivity in adult and pediatric patients.[14–16] Ultrasound will include renal length and yield evidence of asymmetry, identify aneurysms of the main renal artery and consider pathology of adjacent structures. Duplex ultrasonography can assess parenchymal disease based on resistive index measurements. Peak systolic velocities >180 to 200 cm/s or an elevated renal aortic ratio >3.5 are suggestive of renal artery occlusive disease.

Cross-sectional imaging with computed tomography angiography (CTA) and magnetic resonance angiography (MRA) are increasingly being employed first line and/or to confirm a diagnosis of RVH following duplex ultrasonography.[17] While both modalities carry class I indication (evidence level B) as tests to confirm the diagnosis of renal artery stenosis, CTA carries a risk of contrast-induced nephropathy and radiation exposure and both may lack the spatial resolution necessary to detect subtle and/ or distal lesions (ie: FMD webs, 2nd and 3rd order dysplastic lesions).[18]

Catheter-based angiography remains the gold standard for diagnosing renal occlusive disease offering superior spatial resolution to detect branch vessel and parenchymal lesions, adjunct opportunities for intra-vascular ultrasound and manometry, and a platform for therapeutic interventions (ie: angioplasty).[19,20] It remains a critical element of the pre-operative work-up for surgical planning.[6]

Medical Management

Medical management remains the mainstay of treatment for RVH. Clinical guidelines support the use of ACEi, ARBs, calcium channel blockers, and beta-blockers with class I indication.[18] ACEi and ARBs are potent and often effective for treating RVH. As modulators of the renin-angiotensin system, these medications risk acute renal injury, particularly in cases of solitary functioning kidneys, severe bilateral renal artery stenosis, and advanced chronic kidney disease.[21,22] As such, patients require close surveillance of renal function.

For many patients, optimum BP control will require the use of more than one agent. In patients experiencing hypertensive crises, antihypertensive medications, including calcium channel blockers, sympathetic blockers, and vasodilators, should be administered intravenously. Diuretic therapy should be used as combination therapy, as isolated use may increase renin release and worsen HTN.[23] Blood pressure, serum creatinine, and serum potassium should be regularly monitored in patients receiving these medications. Surveillance during medical management should also consider regular assessments of kidney size with renal ultrasonography.

Revascularization

Scenarios for which adult clinical guidelines support renal artery revascularization include: accelerated, resistant or malignant HTN; HTN with unexplained unilateral renal atrophy; HTN with medication intolerance; progressive kidney disease with bilateral renal artery stenosis or renal artery stenosis to a solitary functioning kidney; chronic renal insufficiency with unilateral renal artery stenosis; and recurrent unexplained congestive heart failure or sudden, unexplained pulmonary edema.[18] Additionally, cases of renal arterial dissection, aneurysm, and HTN of short duration with a curative goal may prompt revascularization in patients with FMD.[12] Medical management is favored for the very young, with a realization that definitive surgery would likely be more successful in an older and larger child. Indications for pediatric revascularization are similar, and consider hypertensive encephalopathy, failure to thrive, and in rare cases, severe lower extremity exertional fatigue with growth disturbances and mesenteric angina to justify operative therapy.

Endovascular Treatment

Percutaneous transluminal renal angioplasty is the standard of care for adults with renal artery stenosis secondary to FMD offering technical success rates that approach 100% and HTN improvement in nearly 90% of patients, and cure rates that approach 50%.[12] In these cases, risk of reintervention approximates 20% to 30%, and there is low-risk for major complications. Intravascular manometry with a trans-lesion pressure gradient should quantify the hemodynamic significant of a radiographic lesion and treatment success be determine by gradient resolution. Additionally, intravascular ultrasound may be helpful in documenting minor angiographic irregularities and intraluminal webs. Stents should be used only selectively in patients with FMD given high rates of in-stent stenosis (ie: for dissection complicating angioplasty). Liberal use of vasodilators, to include pretreatment with calcium channel blockers and catheter-directed infusion of nitroglycerin, will limit the predictable vasoreactivity and spasm that affects young arteries. Repeat balloon angioplasty is effective in treating neointimal hyperplasia that threatens primary patency and causes recurrent HTN.

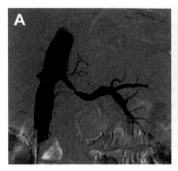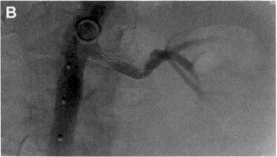

Fig. 4. Angiogram revealeing (A) occlusion of the right renal artery and stenosis of the proximal left renal artery; (B) completion angiogram following stenting of the left renal artery with persistent stenosis from incomplete stent expansion.

There is a role for endovascular therapy in select cases of pediatric RVH, being now utilized with increasing frequency for the treatment of pediatric renal artery stenosis in young patients with FMD. A meta-analysis published in 2020 supported a technical success rate of angioplasty at greater than 90%, while BP improved in nearly 70% of patients.[24] One of the larger experiences with such reported HTN cure, improved and failure rates of 23%, 40% and 37% respectively.[25] Early and late complications may result from significant recoil of lesions that are often in hypoplastic arteries and the unyielding highly fibrotic lesion, especially those in the ostial position. Importantly, a single-institution retrospective series of remedial surgery for endovascular treatment failures reports failure frequently results early (within 2 years), and remedial surgery has been reported to be made more complicated by the failed endovascular therapy,[26] Additionally, the risk of nephrectomy following angioplasty and stenting may be increased (31% compared to 15% w/angioplasty alone) and failures in endovascular therapy in patients aged <10 years resulted in a nephrectomy rate of 44%.

Open Surgical Treatment

Open surgical revascularization for recurrent and recalcitrant cases of adult renal artery stenosis should be considered for appropriate risk patients (**Fig. 4**). Open surgical revascularization offers significant BP and renal function improvement in 85% and 50% of patients respectively across high-volume centers with mortality rates of 2% to 5%. Surgical exposure through a vertical midline incision or extended subcostal incision facilitates exposure of the renal artery posterior to the venous anatomy. Venous branches often will require ligation and division to facilitate this exposure (ie: lumbar, gonadal, adrenal). Medial visceral rotation will facilitate exposure of the distal main renal artery and segmental branches as necessary for more complex reconstructions. Autogenous saphenous vein should be considered for adult renal reconstructions, although thin-walled ePTFE or hypogastric artery may serve as alternates with prosthetic conduit requiring a target vessel diameter of >4 mm.[27] Ex-vivo renal revascularization may be appropriate for cases of distal renal and segmental disease (aneurysmal or occlusive).

Surgical options for renal revascularization in pediatric renal artery stenosis are designed to minimize warm renal ischemic time, restore sustainable and regular renal perfusion, and consider the very small and significantly vasoactive arteries. We favor a supra-umbilical transverse abdominal incision with medial visceral reflection to facilitate wide exposure of the renal vasculature. Patients are routinely anticoagulated

Renal 'Kidney Artery' Revascularization

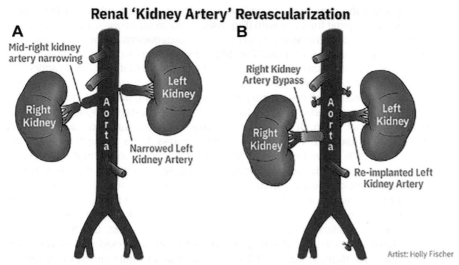

Fig. 5. Schematic of (A) mid-right renal artery stenosis and ostial left renal artery stenosis treated with (B) right aorto-renal bypass and left renal aortic reimplantation. *(From* CS Mott Children's Hospital. Surgical Treatment of Pediatric Renovascular Hypertension Conditions. Available at https://www.mottchildren.org/conditions-treatments/ped-rvh/surgical-treatment-pediatric-renovascular-hypertension; with permission*)*

intra-operatively and often not actively reversed at the case conclusion. In situ reconstructions are preferred to prevent the disruption of important pre-existing collaterals, although on occasion the kidney requires full mobilization to facilitate reimplantation without tension. Renal aortic reimplantation is favored with 180° spatulation of the

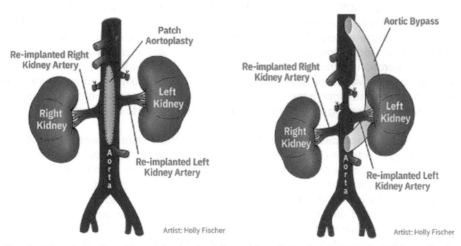

Fig. 6. Schematic of reconstructive options for midaortic syndrome including (A) patch aortoplasty with bilateral renal reimplantation onto the patched aorta and (B) supra-celiac to infra-renal aorto-aortic bypass with bilateral renal reimplantation onto the native aorta. *(Adapted from* CS Mott Children's Hospital. Surgical Treatment of Pediatric Renovascular Hypertension Conditions. Available at https://www.mottchildren.org/conditions-treatments/ped-rvh/surgical-treatment-pediatric-renovascular-hypertension; with permission)

renal artery and suture lines are created with single interrupted sutures of fine mono-filament suture to permit future growth (**Fig. 5A**). Aorto-renal bypass, when necessary, are created with hypogastric artery so as to avoid late degeneration and aneurysm that complicates intra-cavitary vein grafts (**Fig. 5B**). Ex vivo reconstructions and renal auto-transplant may be necessary for advanced and complex distal disease affecting.[6,28]

Abdominal aortic coarctation may be treated with patch aortoplasty or aorto-aortic bypass (often originating off the descending thoracic for long segment stenoses), with ePTFE favored over woven grafts due to durability and late-term degeneration asso-ciated with the latter.[6] (**Fig. 6**) Renal and mesenteric revascularization are performed concurrently as indicated. Patch aortoplasty requires large enough native aortic caliber (at least 50% diameter) to facilitate suture line creation without overlap. The patch is sized so as not to be constrictive with future growth, yet not so generous as to risk the development of unstable laminar thrombus. Aorto-aortic bypass is favored for those patients whose coarctation precludes patch aortoplasty secondary to diminutive caliber, positioned in a retro-renal position and tunneled posterior to the left diaphragmatic leaflets when originating off the thoracic aorta. Conduit should be over-sized to 60% to 70% the size of an adult aorta and fashioned with some redun-dancy in length for those children <10 years anticipating future growth and general guidelines include. This translates to 8- to 12-mm grafts in young childhood; 12- to 16-mm grafts in early adolescence; and 14- to 20-mm grafts in late adolescence.

The largest surgical experience (N = 169) with pediatric RVH comes from the Uni-versity of Michigan, of which approximately 20% of patients had NF-1, 45% had MAS and 30% underwent remedial surgery to salvage failure of a prior interventions.[6] Sec-ondary interventions to preserve primary patency were required following index oper-ation in 22 children (13%), with a median time to secondary intervention being 14 months (Range 2–159 mo, SD ± 38.43). The relative incidence of reoperation is increased in patients with MAS (N = 19, 24%) and NF-1 (N = 9, 29%). HTN was cured in 44%, improved in 46%, and unchanged in 10% with therapeutic failures defined as diastolic pressures were higher than the normal levels and not 15% lower than preop-erative levels or if ACE inhibitors were required for blood pressure control. These data are in line with other large institutional series.[29,30] Logistic regression modeling iden-tified younger age at operation and abdominal aortic coarctation to be independent predictors of reoperation, and more specifically, as age increased by 1 year, the rate of reoperation decreased by about 10%. NF-1 was identified by univariate anal-ysis to be negatively associated with HTN benefit and multiple ordinal regression modeling identified prior intervention as the single independent factor predicting that children undergoing remedial operations were less likely to be cured (33%) of their HTN.

Novel surgical approaches toward MAS include the Tissue Expander-Stimulated Lengthening of Arteries (TESLA) procedure, which involves the placement of a retro-aortic tissue expander to induce longitudinal growth of the normal distal aorta.[31] The expander is sequentially inflated through a subcutaneous port over the course of many months following which, the coarctation may be excised and the elongated aorta anastomosed directly to the normal aorta above the narrowed segment. The Mesenteric Artery Growth Improves Circulation (MAGIC) procedure involves using the mesenteric meandering artery, rather than prosthetic graft material as conduit for aortic bypass.[32,33] The value of these novel therapies await expanded experience and longer follow up.

Regardless of the revascularization approach, ongoing surveillance is essential and requires the review of home and office BP logs, urinalysis (for protein), renal function (eGFR), and regular duplex ultrasonography for renal size/mass and arterial waveforms/velocities. Serial cross-sectional imaging should be considered with some cadence every 2 to 3 years, especially during periods of robust growth. Recurrent HTN and other surveillance abnormalities should prompt catheter-based angiography for recurrent stenosis.

SUMMARY

Renovascular HTN is an important and surgically correctable form of adult and pediatric HTN. The optimal medical and surgical management of pediatric RVH remains ill-defined, in part because low-frequency limits existing data. The expansion of novel surgical and endovascular techniques has changed the landscape of patient care and patients and families are often challenged to balance different sets of recommendations. Phenotype, and possibly genotype, should drive individualized surgical decision making and treatment plan and multidisciplinary care is beneficial. Further prospective, multicenter investigation of this rare but debilitating condition is urgently required to improve the outcomes and quality of life for affected children.

DISCLOSURE

The authors have no financial disclosures, although Dr D.M. Coleman serves as the Project Lead for a PCORI-funded Engagement Award for a Pediatric Renovascular Hypertension Collaborative.

CLINICAL CARE POINTS

- Renovascular HTN is an important and surgically correctable form of adult and pediatric HTN.
- Midaortic syndrome reflects a severe phenotype of pediatric renovascular HTN.
- Medical management is the maintstay of treatment for renovascular HTN, with ACE-inhibitors and ARBs often most effective.
- Percutaneous transluminal renal angioplasty with selective stenting has become the standard of care for adults with renal artery stenosis.
- Aortorenal revascularization for pediatric renovascular HTN can be complicated, and techniques designed to limit warm renal ischemia and restore sustainable, regular renal perfusion.

REFERENCES

1. Bayazit AK, Yalcinkaya F, Cakar N, et al. Reno-vascular hypertension in childhood: a nationwide survey. Pediatr Nephrol 2007;22(9):1327–33.
2. Silverstein DM, Champoux E, Aviles DH, et al. Treatment of primary and secondary hypertension in children. Pediatr Nephrol 2006;21(6):820–7.
3. Olin JW, Froehlich J, Gu X, et al. The United States Registry for Fibromuscular Dysplasia: results in the first 447 patients. Circulation 2012;125(25):3182–90.
4. Kaas B, Huisman TA, Tekes A, et al. Spectrum and prevalence of vasculopathy in pediatric neurofibromatosis type 1. J Child Neurol 2013;28(5):561–9.
5. Salem JE, Bruguiere E, Iserin L, et al. Hypertension and aortorenal disease in Alagille syndrome. J Hypertens 2012;30(7):1300–6.
6. Coleman DM, Eliason JL, Beaulieu R, et al. Surgical management of pediatric renin-mediated hypertension secondary to renal artery occlusive disease and abdominal aortic coarctation. J Vasc Surg 2020;72(6):2035–20346 e1.

7. Warejko JK, Schueler M, Vivante A, et al. Whole Exome Sequencing Reveals a Monogenic Cause of Disease in approximately 43% of 35 Families With Midaortic Syndrome. Hypertension 2018;71(4):691–9.

8. Viering D, Chan MMY, Hoogenboom L, et al. Genetics of renovascular hypertension in children. J Hypertens 2020;38(10):1964–70.

9. Coleman DM, Wang Y, Yang ML, et al. Molecular genetic evaluation of pediatric renovascular hypertension due to renal artery stenosis and abdominal aortic coarctation in neurofibromatosis type 1. Hum Mol Genet 2022;31(3):334–46.

10. Coleman DM, Heider A, Gordon D, et al. Histologic and morphologic character of pediatric renal artery occlusive disease. J Vasc Surg 2021;73(1):161–71.

11. Stanley JC, Criado E, Eliason JL, et al. Abdominal aortic coarctation: surgical treatment of 53 patients with a thoracoabdominal bypass, patch aortoplasty, or interposition aortoaortic graft. J Vasc Surg 2008;48(5):1073–82.

12. Olin JW, Gornik HL, Bacharach JM, et al. Fibromuscular dysplasia: state of the science and critical unanswered questions: a scientific statement from the American Heart Association. Circulation 2014;129(9):1048–78.

13. Porras D, Stein DR, Ferguson MA, et al. Midaortic syndrome: 30 years of experience with medical, endovascular and surgical management. Pediatr Nephrol 2013;28(10):2023–33.

14. Taylor DC, Kettler MD, Moneta GL, et al. Duplex ultrasound scanning in the diagnosis of renal artery stenosis: a prospective evaluation. J Vasc Surg 1988;7(2): 363–9.

15. Castelli PK, Dillman JR, Kershaw DB, et al. Renal sonography with Doppler for detecting suspected pediatric renin-mediated hypertension - is it adequate? Pediatr Radiol 2014;44(1):42–9.

16. Srinivasan A, Krishnamurthy G, Fontalvo-Herazo L, et al. Spectrum of renal findings in pediatric fibromuscular dysplasia and neurofibromatosis type 1. Pediatr Radiol 2011;41(3):308–16.

17. Castelli PK, Dillman JR, Smith EA, et al. Imaging of renin-mediated hypertension in children. AJR Am J Roentgenol 2013;200(6):W661–72.

18. Hirsch AT, Haskal ZJ, Hertzer NR, et al. ACC/AHA 2005 Practice Guidelines for the management of patients with peripheral arterial disease (lower extremity, renal, mesenteric, and abdominal aortic): a collaborative report from the American Association for Vascular Surgery/Society for Vascular Surgery, Society for Cardiovascular Angiography and Interventions, Society for Vascular Medicine and Biology, Society of Interventional Radiology, and the ACC/AHA Task Force on Practice Guidelines (Writing Committee to Develop Guidelines for the Management of Patients With Peripheral Arterial Disease): endorsed by the American Association of Cardiovascular and Pulmonary Rehabilitation; National Heart, Lung, and Blood Institute; Society for Vascular Nursing; TransAtlantic Inter-Society Consensus; and Vascular Disease Foundation. Circulation 2006; 113(11):e463–654.

19. Gowda MS, Loeb AL, Crouse LJ, et al. Complementary roles of color-flow duplex imaging and intravascular ultrasound in the diagnosis of renal artery fibromuscular dysplasia: should renal arteriography serve as the "gold standard"? J Am Coll Cardiol 2003;41(8):1305–11.

20. Louis R, Levy-Erez D, Cahill AM, et al. Imaging studies in pediatric fibromuscular dysplasia (FMD): a single-center experience. Pediatr Nephrol 2018;33(9): 1593–9.

21. Wynckel A, Ebikili B, Melin JP, et al. Long-term follow-up of acute renal failure caused by angiotensin converting enzyme inhibitors. Am J Hypertens 1998; 11(9):1080–6.
22. Johansen TL, Kjaer A. Reversible renal impairment induced by treatment with the angiotensin II receptor antagonist candesartan in a patient with bilateral renal artery stenosis. BMC Nephrol 2001;2:1.
23. Meyers KE, Cahill AM, Sethna C. Interventions for pediatric renovascular hypertension. Curr Hypertens Rep 2014;16(4):422.
24. de Oliveira Campos JL, Bitencourt L, Pedrosa AL, et al. Renovascular hypertension in pediatric patients: update on diagnosis and management. Pediatr Nephrol 2021;36(12):3853–68.
25. Kari JA, Roebuck DJ, McLaren CA, et al. Angioplasty for renovascular hypertension in 78 children. Arch Dis Child 2015;100(5):474–8.
26. Eliason JL, Coleman DM, Criado E, et al. Remedial operations for failed endovascular therapy of 32 renal artery stenoses in 24 children. Pediatr Nephrol 2016; 31(5):809–17.
27. Ham SW, Kumar SR, Wang BR, et al. Late outcomes of endovascular and open revascularization for nonatherosclerotic renal artery disease. Arch Surg 2010; 145(9):832–9.
28. Stanley JC, Criado E, Upchurch GR Jr. Brophy PD, Cho KJ, Rectenwald JE, et al. Pediatric renovascular hypertension: 132 primary and 30 secondary operations in 97 children. J Vasc Surg 2006;44(6):1219–28, discussion 28-9.
29. Martinez A, Novick AC, Cunningham R, et al. Improved results of vascular reconstruction in pediatric and young adult patients with renovascular hypertension. J Urol 1990;144(3):717–20.
30. O'Neill JA Jr. Long-term outcome with surgical treatment of renovascular hypertension. J Pediatr Surg 1998;33(1):106–11.
31. Kim HB, Vakili K, Ramos-Gonzalez GJ, et al. Tissue expander-stimulated lengthening of arteries for the treatment of midaortic syndrome in children. J Vasc Surg 2018;67(6):1664–72.
32. Kim HB, Lee EJ, Vakili K, et al. Mesenteric Artery Growth Improves Circulation (MAGIC) in Midaortic Syndrome. Ann Surg 2018;267(6):e109–11.
33. Kim SS, Stein DR, Ferguson MA, et al. Surgical management of pediatric renovascular hypertension and midaortic syndrome at a single-center multidisciplinary program. J Vasc Surg 2021;74(1):79–89 e2.

Comprehensive Care of Lower-Extremity Wounds

Allison Learned, BS, NP[a], Sudie-Ann Robinson, MD[a],
Tammy T. Nguyen, MD, PhD[a,b,*]

KEYWORDS

- Chronic nonhealing wounds • Lower-extremity wounds • Diabetic foot ulcer
- Arterial ulcer • Venous ulcer • Pressure ulcer • Mixed wound • Atypical wound

KEY POINTS

- All lower-extremity wounds should be assessed for peripheral arterial disease before debridement.
- The cause for a lower-extremity chronic wound should be identified in order to guide wound treatment plan.
- Optimized wound granulation tissue should be first achieved with debridement, wound moisture balance, and infection control.
- Wound treatment plan should be reassessed every 1 to 2 weeks until 10% to 15% of wound volume reduction per week is achieved.
- Accelerated wound healing can be achieved with either collagen-based, growth factor–based, or cell-based advanced wound products.

INTRODUCTION

Chronic nonhealing lower-extremity (LE) wounds account for up to 13% of the US population, with an increasing prevalence owing to the aging population with advanced risk factors for nonhealing wounds: smoking, diabetes, hypertension, and hyperlipidemia. The management and treatment of chronic LE wounds account for an estimated annual $20 billion in health care spending in the United States. The 4 most common causes for chronic nonhealing LE wounds are arterial, venous, diabetic, pressure, and mixed etiology. These chronic LE wound types often share similar features of increased levels of proinflammatory cytokines, persistent infection, drug-resistant biofilms, and senescent cells that are not responsive to stimuli in the repair process.[1,2] This review focuses on the evaluation and treatment methodologies for chronic LE wound assessment, tissue debridement, infection control, moisture

[a] Department of Surgery, Division of Vascular Surgery, University of Massachusetts Chan Medical School, 55 North Lake Avenue, Worcester, MA 01655, USA; [b] University of Massachusetts Diabetes Center of Excellence
* Corresponding author.
E-mail address: tammy.nguyen@umassmemorial.org

Surg Clin N Am 103 (2023) 745–765
https://doi.org/10.1016/j.suc.2023.04.015
0039-6109/23/© 2023 Elsevier Inc. All rights reserved.

balance, promotion of granulation tissue with advanced wound care products, and recurrence prevention.

PATHOPHYSIOLOGY
Stages of Wound Healing

Normal wound healing requires a synchronization of 4 distinct stages: hemostasis, inflammation, proliferation, and remodeling (**Fig. 1**). When a wound is unable to progress to the next stage for more than 6 to 8 weeks, then that wound becomes chronic.[3]

> *Hemostasis:* The first stage in wound healing involves hemostasis, which serves to stop the bleeding after tissue injury.[3]
> *Inflammation*: Within the first 24 hours, the inflammatory stage is in full effect starting with an influx of leukocytes, including mastocytes, Langerhans cells, neutrophils, cytokines, and chemokines, which provides a localized and protective tissue response.[3]
> *Proliferation*: The proliferative phase starts approximately 3 to 10 days after injury and is characterized by granulation tissue formation, contraction, and fibroplasia to establish a viable epithelial barrier and angiogenesis.[3]
> *Remodeling:* During this phase, there is matrix deposition with the formation of mature type I collagen, and any disruption in this phase may lead to development of a chronic wound.[3]

CHRONIC NONHEALING WOUND TYPE

Chronic LE wounds have a differential diagnosis that includes the following: wounds of arterial insufficiency, wounds of chronic venous disease, diabetic foot ulcers (DFUs), pressure wounds, and mixed or atypical wounds (**Fig. 2**). Identifying the type of wound will dictate the treatment management.[4]

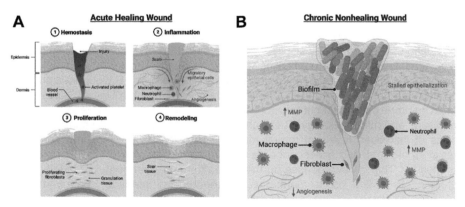

Fig. 1. Stages of wound healing in acute wounds in comparison to chronic nonhealing wounds. (*A*) Acute wound-healing model has 4 distinct stages: (1) hemostasis; (2) inflammation; (3) proliferation; and (4) remodeling. (*B*) Chronic nonhealing wounds disrupt all traditional 4 stages of wound healing. These wounds are commonly associated with a layer of biofilm that impairs epithelialization and may result in local or systemic infection. The wound bed is notable for increased inflammatory cells and metalloproteases (MMP) that can lead to local tissue destruction. The wound environment is associated with decreased fibroblast proliferation and angiogenesis, which will impair granulation tissue formation required for wound healing.

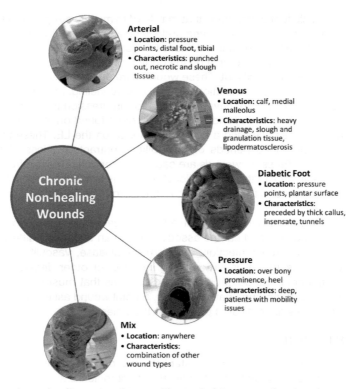

Arterial
- **Location:** pressure points, distal foot, tibial
- **Characteristics:** punched out, necrotic and slough tissue

Venous
- **Location:** calf, medial malleolus
- **Characteristics:** heavy drainage, slough and granulation tissue, lipodermatosclerosis

Diabetic Foot
- **Location:** pressure points, plantar surface
- **Characteristics:** preceded by thick callus, insensate, tunnels

Pressure
- **Location:** over bony prominence, heel
- **Characteristics:** deep, patients with mobility issues

Mix
- **Location:** anywhere
- **Characteristics:** combination of other wound types

Chronic Non-healing Wounds

Fig. 2. Chronic nonhealing wound types. The underlying cause for chronic wounds can be identified based on location on the lower extremity and distinguishing wound characteristics. This may include arterial insufficiency, venous insufficiency, diabetes, pressure, and/or mixed or atypical wounds.

Wounds of arterial insufficiency, from peripheral artery disease (PAD), represent approximately 20% of chronic LE wounds and result from a reduction of the blood flow required to maintain skin integrity, wound healing, and neuromuscular function. Arterial wounds are often seen at pressure points, distal toes, the lateral malleolus, and/or tibial areas. They are often described as punched out lesions with a deep and unhealthy wound bed, in the presence of necrotic tissue with minimal exudate unless the wound is infected. The periwound and surrounding skin may appear erythematous from dependent rubor, cool to touch (poikilothermia), hairless, thin and brittle, shiny texture, and associated with thickened dystrophic toenails.[4–6]

Venous wounds are the most common, accounting for approximately 80% to 70% of all nonhealing LE wounds. Venous wounds are most often caused by venous insufficiency and resulting venous hypertension. Signs of long-standing venous hypertension that may have preceded venous ulceration include LE edema, skin discoloration (atrophie blanche or hemosiderin), lipodermatosclerosis, stasis dermatitis, cellulitis, superficial thrombophlebitis, spontaneous bleeding, and/or ulcerations at the gaiter distribution and medial malleolus. Venous wounds are typically shallow, have flat margins with moderate to heavy exudate, and may have slough at the base with granulation tissue.[7–9]

DFUs occur in up to one-third of all diabetics and are the most common indication for nontraumatic LE amputation. These ulcers arise from underlying peripheral neuropathy, intrinsic foot denervation that may lead to muscle atrophy and foot deformities (eg, Charcot foot), anhidrosis, and underlying PAD and microvascular disease. Structural foot deformities are often the cause for a pressure point that can lead to skin breakdown and wound development on the bony prominence of the metatarsal head (mal perforans ulcer) or lateral foot. These wounds are often preceded by a callus, are associated with polymicrobial infection, exhibit deep tunneling, may demonstrate significant wound exudate, and/or have a high risk for progression to osteomyelitis.[10–12]

Pressure wounds form in dependent positions, often found on the heel of the foot, ankle, or calf and often overlying a bony prominence on the LE. These wounds are associated with prolonged periods of immobility, contractures, loss of sensation, and malnutrition.[4,13] Pressure wounds are caused by repeated trauma from constant pressure and shear force that can cause localized tissue ischemia. They may start as a bruise or shallow ulcer and then progress to skin necrosis or deep tissue erosion if not treated.

Up to 20% of chronic wounds are of mixed or atypical cause. These wounds vary in appearance and location and can be associated with an expanded differential diagnosis like systemic chronic infection, autoimmune disease, vasculitis, malignancy, pyoderma gangrenosum, calciphylaxis, drug induced, or other dermatologic disorders.[14] Given the broad range of differential diagnoses that must be considered for chronic LE wounds, a thorough patient history, careful wound assessment, and other diagnostic modalities are critical to guide best therapies.

WOUND ASSESSMENT

Initial wound care visits should aim to establish wound cause through a comprehensive patient and wound assessment.[4] Patients with chronic LE wounds benefit from a multidisciplinary approach, which includes treatment plan communication between the specialty care physician (ie, vascular surgeon for arterial and venous wounds or endocrinologist for diabetic wounds), visiting nurse, nutritionist, podiatrist, occupational and physical therapist, and social worker managed by a wound care specialist. A comprehensive multidisciplinary approach to wound healing should (1) define the arterial perfusion status of the limb, (2) identify the wound's cause, (3) wound bed preparation through debridement of devitalized tissue or biofilm, (4) treat underlying infection, (5) formulate a wound plan that will promote granulation tissue and address any underlying wound cause, and (6) offer longitudinal surveillance with serial wound checks (often weekly) until an average 10% to 15% wound area reduction per week or linear area percentage reduction over 4 weeks is achieved (**Fig. 3**).

General Principles of Wound Evaluation

The history and physical examination should consider the following: (1) symptoms of pain, (2) constitutional symptoms, (3) a careful LE pulse examination, (4) wound location, (5) the wound characteristics (color, tissue type present, drainage, odor, tunneling, exposed structures), (6) quality of the periwound tissue (macerated, dry, callused, erythematous, edema, crepitus, and so forth), (7) assessment for infection, and (8) wound dimensions (width, height, depth, and undermining/tunneling). The authors also find it useful to include a wound picture before and after debridement in the patient's medical record to track the wound-healing progress.

Assessing arterial perfusion

Assessment for PAD should be done on all LE chronic wounds with a physical pulse examination, segmental pulse volume recording (PVR), ankle-brachial index (ABI), toe pressure (TP), and/or transcutaneous pulse oximetry (TcPO2). Arterial wounds can

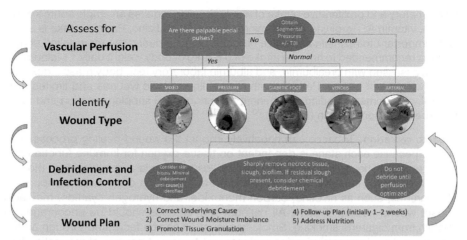

Fig. 3. Wound assessment workflow. Initial assessment decision tree for chronic nonhealing LE wounds that have been present for more than 4 weeks. First assess for vascular perfusion based on palpable pedal pulses, segmental pressures, or toe pressure (TP). Next identify the cause of the wound or wound type. Wound debridement can be tailored to the wound type and infection should be controlled in all wounds. The wound plan is formulated based on corrected the underlying cause of the wound and therapies to promote healing. The wound plan should be reassessed every 1-2 weeks after initiation in order to ensure adequate progress or need to re-evaluate the wound type.

have diminished or absent palpable pulses anywhere along the LE vascular tree. The severity of PAD can be quantified based on ABI, TP, and/or TcPO2. Chronic wounds with a systolic ankle pressure of less than 50 mm Hg or an ABI less than 0.4 or TP < 30 mm Hg for nondiabetics and TP < 40 mm Hg for diabetics are unlikely to heal without revascularization.[6,15,16] ABIs are often unreliable in diabetic patients owing to significant medial calcinosis, which stiffens the arterial vessel wall, causing a falsely elevated ABI; therefore, TP is the recommended diagnostic parameter to assess for arterial insufficiency in patients with diabetes.

Assessing venous hypertension

Assessment for venous wounds should be done on all LE chronic wounds associated with leg edema. Venous wounds are diagnosed based on a physical examination, venous reflux duplex ultrasound (DUS), venous perforator duplex ultrasound, and/or venogram to assess for venous drainage and venous valvular function. Venous wounds may be accompanied with a venous reflux study demonstrating greater than 0.5-second retrograde flow within the great saphenous vein (GSV), small saphenous vein (SSV), and/or accessory saphenous vein (ASV), greater than 1.0-second retrograde flow within the femoral or popliteal vein, or greater than 0.35- to 0.5-second retrograde flow within the perforator vein adjacent to a wound after distal manual compression under DUS. It is important to also assess for arterial insufficiency in patients with venous wounds because there is a subset of 13% to 26% of patients who will have a mixed arterial venous wound cause, which may affect the treatment plan.[17–19]

Systemic considerations

Nutrition. Malnutrition is a common factor that contributes to nonhealing wounds and often consists of either protein-energy malnutrition, mineral, or vitamin deficiency. The inflammatory and proliferative phase of wound healing requires an ample source of selenium, vitamin A, L-arginine, L-glutamine, vitamin C, and zinc. Protein intake is especially important to maintain a positive nitrogen balance during the remodeling phase, and it is recommended to have an intake of 0.8 g/kg of body weight daily.[2] Malnutrition can be assessed with prealbumin, and albumin laboratory test, body mass index, and acute weight lost history. Patients with nonhealing chronic wounds and limited oral, enteral, or parenteral feeding can benefit from nutritional supplementation and nutrition specialist consultation (**Table 1**).[20]

Tobacco cessation. Tobacco can negatively impact the wound-healing process at all stages because each stage is dependent on tissue oxygen for immune function and tissue repair. Tobacco smoking is related to tissue hypoxia and is therefore thought to be a driver for impaired wound healing. In addition, the other toxic components of cigarettes, such as nicotine, carbon monoxide, and hydrogen cyanide, may also impact wound healing directly. All patients with wounds should be encouraged to abstain from cigarette smoking. Smoking cessation can be facilitated through addiction counseling, hypnosis, nicotine replacement therapy, transcranial magnetic stimulation, or pharmacotherapy agents, such as bupropion or varenicline.[21,22]

Diabetes management. Systemic hyperglycemia is a risk factor for acute surgical and chronic nonhealing wounds. Long-term systemic hyperglycemia is a risk factor for the development of diabetes. Diabetes is diagnosed based on a fasting plasma glucose greater than 126 mg/dL, or hemoglobin $A_{1c} > 6.5\%$, or oral glucose tolerance test greater than 200 mg/dL. Patients with nonhealing LE wounds and diabetes should be comanaged with a diabetologist or endocrinologist to achieve normal glycemia. Hyperglycemia can be managed by lifestyle and diet modification and metformin, with or without the addition of sodium-glucose cotransporter 2 (SGLT-2) inhibitors or glucagon-like peptide 1 (GLP-1) or exogenous insulin to achieve normal glycemia.[23-25]

WOUND CARE AND TREATMENT

Wound management strategies should aim to promote granulation tissue promotion, which histologically is represented by proliferating fibroblasts, keratinocytes, endothelial cells, and angiogenesis (**Fig. 4**). To acheive granulation tissue, the wound bed is prepared through tissue debridement, infection or inflammation control, moisture balance, and advancement of epithelial edge (TIME framework for wound healing).[68]

Debridement

Granulation tissue may be stalled or inhibited when there is overlying necrotic, or slough tissue capped over the wound bed. Slough is devitalized, fibrous tissue that

Table 1 Nutritional supplements to enhance wound healing	
Wound Nutritional Supplements	
Zinc sulfate	200 mg daily
Vitamin C	500–1000 mg daily
Selenium	50 μg daily
Vitamin A	10,000 U daily
L-Arginine	7–10 g daily
L-Glutamine	7–10 g daily

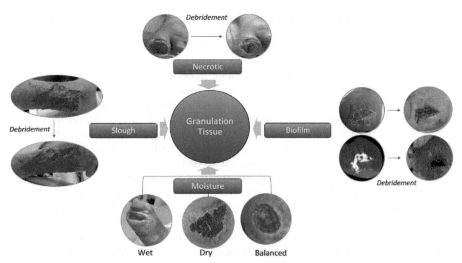

Fig. 4. General wound characteristic and management. To promote granulation tissue and wound healing, 4 major wound characteristics should be identified: necrotic tissue, slough tissue, biofilm burden, and wound moisture state. Correction of these wound characteristics will promote a wound environment suitable for granulation tissue formation. Necrotic tissue, biofilm, or slough tissue can be debrided, whereas moisture balance can be obtained with proper dressing care. Biofilm detected using fluorescent violet light is detected (*asterisk*) before debridement of a nonhealing amputated toe wound. Blue dot and white outline around the amputated toe wound were used to assess wound measurement.

may appear to be yellow or gray in color with a stringy and moist tissue consistency. Both necrotic and slough tissue should be debrided from the wound bed by sharp or chemical means to promote angiogenesis, granulation tissue formation, epidermal resurfacing, and normal extracellular matrix (ECM) formation. Furthermore, the presence of necrotic or slough tissue may harbor bacterial biofilm.[1,26,27] Bacteria biofilm represents an overgrowth of adherent layer of microbes, often polymicrobial, that can colonize the wound bed and periwound. Biofilm removal is often resistant to standard cleansing and can be sharply debrided and/or treated with Dakin solution (sodium hypochlorite), hydrogen peroxide, sodium chloride, or povidone-iodine. Dakin solution is useful for blue-green color drainage that often represents *Pseudomonas aeruginosa* biofilm.[27–29]

The goal of debridement is to establish a granulating tissue bed. Chemical debridement is a good alternative to sharp excisional or surgical debridement for wounds that have minimal to moderate slough over the wound bed or for patients who cannot tolerate a bedside sharp excisional debridement. Chemical debridement can be achieved by utilization of collagenase extracted from *Clostridium histolyticum* (Santyl or Novuxol) or *Vibrio alginolyticus*, papain, and urea (Accuzyme), or fibrinolysin and desoxyribonuclease. Alternatively, autolytic wound debridement, enhancement of the body's own endogenous enzyme to breakdown devitalized tissue, can be stimulated through the use of hydrogels, hydrocolloids, and alginates.[27,30,31]

Wound Moisture Balance

Maintaining a balanced wound moisture environment is necessary for cellular proliferation, ECM deposition, granulation tissue, and epithelialization.[1,26,32] A wet wound environment can stall a wound in the inflammatory phase and lead to periwound maceration, causing further wound breakdown. High-draining wounds can be treated with hydroconductive dressing, absorbent pads, layered compression wraps, or negative pressure wound therapy (NPWT).[1,8,33–35] The authors often use Drawtex, Hydrofera Blue, Unna boots, and/or Profore boots to manage high-draining wounds (**Fig. 5**). Unna and Profore boots are multilayered compression dressings that provide a gradient compression to treat LE edema. Multilayered compressive dressings should be changed every 2 to 3 days for high-drainage wounds. However, there are some patient circumstances when it is not technically feasible to reapply a multilayer compressive dressing every 2 to 3 days by a certified wound care nurse; then, more frequent compression dressing changes can be done with a Kerlix and ACE or Coban bandage wraps in addition to other adjuncts to help manage drainage. It is critical to ensure that the frequency of dressing changes matches the wound drainage output in order to prevent periwound maceration. The macerated periwound can be protected with a hydrocolloid adhesive dressing (such as Duoderm), barrier cream (such as zinc oxide), or tincture of benzoin to dry out the periwound. Alternatively, a dry wound environment can lead to wound desiccation, necrosis, and eschar formation and results in poorer wound-healing rates. Low drainage output pressure wounds can be treated with hydrogel, medical-grade honey, or a humectant like hyaluronic acid to regain moisture balance (see **Fig. 5**).[1,26,32]

Advanced Wound Products

With healthy granulation tissue present, accelerated wound healing can be achieved with the application of advanced wound products, such as collagen, growth factors, or cell-based products (**Fig. 6**). There is no standardized algorithm for the usage of advanced wound products, and these products are often marketed to be multipurpose. However, given the different characteristics of each chronic wound type, an individualized treatment plan is required for most chronic wounds, as reflected in

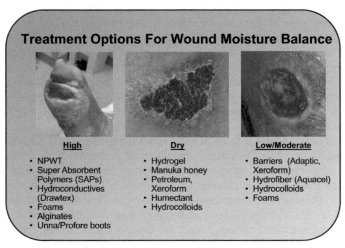

Fig. 5. Wound products to achieve moisture balance. Wound dressing for high-output drainage can either be utilization of NPWT, superabsorbent polymers, hydroconductives (ie, Drawtex or Optilock), foams, alginates, or Unna/Profore multilayer compression boot. Low output drainage or dry wounds can be treated with hydrogel, medical-grade Manuka honey, petroleum, xeroform, humectant, or hydrocolloids. Low to moderate wound drainage wounds can be treated with a barrier dressing to maintain moisture balance, such as adaptic or xeroform, hydrofiber (ie, Aquacel), hydrocolloids, or foam.

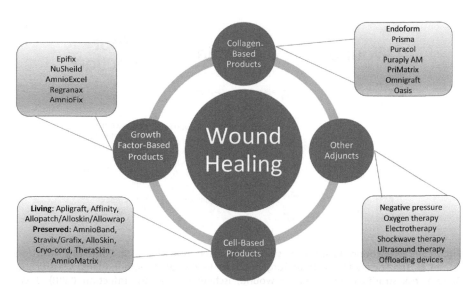

Fig. 6. Current wound product designed to promote healing. Products designed to promote wound healing are primarily focused on locally delivering (1) collagen, (2) growth factors, or (3) cells to enhance granulation tissue formation and epithelization in a chronic nonhealing wound environment.

the 50% average healing success rate for most advanced wound products on the market.[36] Advanced wound products mimic the functional and structural characteristics of autologous skin. They range from (1) collagen-based products derived from human, porcine, or bovine ECM, to (2) growth factor–based products derived from dehydrated human placental, amnion, chorion tissue, or recombinant growth factors (Regranex), to (3) cell-based products derived from living or preserved human dermis or placental tissue.[36,37] There are also several additional wound adjuncts that have varying efficacy for healing chronic wounds. The most well-studied adjunct is the use of NPWT and offloading devices for DFU and pressure wounds.[33,34]

Deeper wounds (>2 mm in depth) may respond better to collagen-based products that encourage filling at the wound depths. Once the wound is shallower (ie, < 2 mm in depth), the application of either growth factor or cell-based products should enhance periwound contraction.

CLINICAL CARE SUMMARY (BY PATHOLOGY)
Arterial Nonhealing Wounds

Approach and guidelines
Approach and guidelines the Society for Vascular Surgery (SVS) Wound, Ischemia, and foot Infection (WIfI) scoring for ischemia should be referenced to qualify the severity of wound ischemia (**Fig. 7**). The WIfI scoring system is based on a 0 to 3 scoring system and estimates that wounds with an ischemia score of ≥2 are associated with a high risk for wound-related amputation.[6,15,38] PAD should be further assessed with appropriate diagnostics to determine level of disease and opportunities for revascularization. Revascularization should be considered to facilitate healing of chronic LE wounds of arterial insufficiency. Revascularization options should be individualized to the patient, and considerations are beyond the scope of this article. However, guidelines do support open surgery LE bypass for wounds that have an ischemic

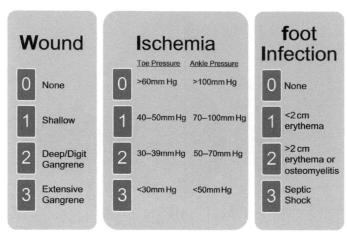

Fig. 7. SVS WIfI scoring classification system. (*Adapted from* Mills JL Sr, Conte MS, Armstrong DG, et al. The Society for Vascular Surgery Lower Extremity Threatened Limb Classification System: risk stratification based on wound, ischemia, and foot infection (WIfI). J Vasc Surg. 2014;59(1):220-34.e342; with permission.)

and wound WIfI score ≥2. Shallow wounds with a WIfI score ≤2 may likely require less robust perfusion to heal.[6,15,38] Notably, open surgical bypass for patients with GSV conduit has been shown to reduce major adverse limb events and death for patients with arterial ulcers with PAD.[39]

Treatment
Wound care. Minimal wound debridement should be performed before revascularization at the risk of additional tissue injury that could result in irreversible damage. It is prudent to favor desiccating the wound until a revascularization plan is executed to prevent bacterial infection. Wound desiccation can be achieved by using betadine paint, alcohol swabs, gauze wedged in between the toes, and/or foam dressing to wick any moisture from the wound. Any signs of tissue infection should be treated because arterial wounds have a high risk for progressing to wet gangrene or osteomyelitis.

Modifiable risk factors. Additional modifiable risk factors warrant consideration and other treatments that decrease the cardiovascular mortality, morbidity, and recurrence of arterial wounds associated with PAD. Patients that undergo revascularization benefit from a daily aspirin and 2.5 mg twice daily rivaroxaban to decrease the composite risk of acute limb ischemia, major amputation from vascular causes, myocardial infarction, ischemic stroke, or death from cardiovascular causes.[40,41] The increase in cardiovascular risk associated with PAD should also be managed with blood pressure and hyperlipidemia control with lifestyle modification, antihypertensive (angiotensin-converting enzyme inhibitor or angiotensinogen-receptor blockers), and antilipid (HMG-CoA reductase inhibitor, cholesterol gut absorption inhibitor [ezetimibe], or PCSK9 inhibitor) pharmacotherapy. The blood pressure goal for patients with PAD is systolic 120 to 140 mm Hg and diastolic greater than 70 mm Hg to reduce PAD and cardiovascular events.[42–44] The lipid goal for patients with PAD is low-density lipoprotien less than 70 mg/dL or a 50% reduction from baseline.[45] In addition, counseling and treatment for tobacco cessation, either through hypnosis, nicotine replacement therapy, transcranial magnetic stimulation, pharmacotherapy agents such as bupropion or varenicline, should be provided in patients with PAD and active tobacco use.[21,22,42]

Venous Nonhealing Wounds

Approach and guidelines

Approximately 88% of all venous wounds have venous insufficiency.[46] Venous insufficiency includes superficial venous valvular dysfunction, perforator venous valvular dysfunction, or deep venous reflux. Superficial and perforator venous valvular dysfunction can be assessed by a venous reflux DUS after distal manual compression. Superficial venous insufficiency is diagnosed when there is greater than 0.5 second of retrograde flow within the GSV, SSV, and/or ASV.[8] Perforator venous insufficiency is diagnosed when there is greater than 0.35 to 0.5 seconds of retrograde flow within a perforator vein and a diameter greater than 3.5 mm. Alternatively, deep venous reflux of the femoral or popliteal vein is defined by greater than 1.0 seconds of retrograde flow on venous reflux duplex ultrasound with Valsalva maneuver. Obstructive deep venous disease may also drive venous hypertension.[1,7,8,46,47] The SVS and American Venous Forum (AVF) Joint Clinical Practice Guidelines recommend that all wounds suspicious for a venous cause be first evaluated with an LE venous reflux study. If superficial venous reflux is identified, treatment should focus on superficial venous disease before treating deep venous reflux or obstructive disease. If only deep venous reflux or obstructive disease is identified, then a pelvic venogram, computed tomography venography, or magnetic resonance venography can be used to evaluate for venous stenosis or compressive disorders, such as scarring from deep vein thrombosis or May-Thurner disease. It is advisable to only treat superficial venous disease if there is a patent deep venous system to ensure that there will be adequate venous drainage of the LE, especially when evaluating patients with congenital venous abnormalities (Klippel-Trenaunay or Parkes Weber syndrome). If no venous insufficiency is identified in the superficial or deep venous systems, then a perforator venous reflux DUS can be useful to identify localized venous insufficiency near the venous wound.[8]

Treatment

Wound Care. Compression therapy is the first-line treatment for venous ulceration. Compression therapy goal is to provide a gradient 30 to 40 mm Hg compression from the metatarsal to below the knee or above the knee. Venous wounds often have high exudative drainage owing to stagnant venous hypertension buildup in the LE causing increased interstitial fluid shifts. Exudative drainage should be managed expeditiously to minimize further periwound maceration and breakdown, infection, and patient discomfort.[2,6,7,25,32,34,35] A multilayer gradient compression boot, either an Unna boot or a Profore boot, is often effective at treating venous ulcers because they can provide long-term gradient compression, wound hydration, or exudative drainage management through the use of orthopedic wool, crepe bandage, elastic bandage, and elastic cohesive outer bandage applied by a trained professional. Unna boot dressings may be appropriate for those venous wounds with less drainage, as zinc oxide provides more hydration. Profore boots have more absorbent layers that will wick moisture away from wounds with higher drainage. It is important that high-draining wound dressings be changed regularly to prevent further wound and periwound breakdown, and in general, the frequency of dressing changes should be tailored to the patient's drainage output. Of note, a multilayer compression boot should not be used on patients with underlying arterial insufficiency with an ABI less than 0.5 or absolute ankle pressure less than 60 mm Hg to avoid reducing arterial perfusion to the wound.[8,46]

The SVS/AVF guidelines recommend the use of advanced wound products if a venous ulcer fails to demonstrate improvement (≥10% reduction in wound size per week) after a minimum of 4 to 6 weeks on standard multilayer compression therapy.

The wound bed is first prepared by cleaning the wound with a nonirritant solution follow by debridement of necrotic or nonviable slough. Once the wound bed is prepared for enhancement of granulation tissue, advanced wound products may be applied. Advanced wound products may include growth factor–based or cell-based products; however, these should be used with caution on venous ulcers because these advanced biologics can stimulate an increase in wound drainage and lead to periwound breakdown and biofilm overgrowth if not managed expeditiously.[8,46]

Other alternative wound care adjuncts, such as negative pressure therapy, electrical stimulation, and ultrasound therapy, are not recommended by the SVS/AVF guidelines. The SVS/AVF guidelines do recommend supplemental use of pneumatic compression pumps if adequate wound healing is not observed with a multilayer compression boot alone or in replacement of and at the discretion of patient's tolerance for additional compression.[8,46]

Venous procedures. Surgical removal or ablation of the refluxing superficial/perforator vein will decrease venous hypertension, which has been shown to (1) prevent future wound development and (2) promote wound healing.[48–51] Superficial venous ablation can be accomplished by (1) thermal ablation techniques, (2) cyanoacrylate glue ablation, or (3) sclerotherapy. Early endovenous ablation (EVRA trial) has been shown to accelerate venous wound healing, and superficial venous ablation in combination with compression therapy lowers the rate of venous ulcer recurrence (ESCHAR trial).[48–50] Based on these studies and others, the SVS/AVF guidelines recommend that venous ulcer with associated incompetent superficial veins that have axial reflux directed to the bed of the ulcer be treated with venous ablation in addition to compression wound care therapy. In addition, the SVS/AVF guidelines recommend venous ablation of perforator veins if an incompetent perforator vein is located beneath or associated with the venous wound bed. Ablation of the incompetent perforator vein may be done simultaneously or upon reevaluation of the wound after the superficial venous ablation procedure.[8,46]

Venous wounds can be associated with significant iliac or caval venous reflux or obstruction. Suprainguinal deep venous insufficiency can be treated with percutaneous balloon angioplasty with stenting. The SVS/AVF guidelines recommend first-line endovascular treatment for suprainguinal deep venous insufficiency over deep venous valvular reconstructions or open operative bypass procedures owing to decreased patient procedural risk.[8,46]

Modifiable risk factors. In addition to compression therapy and venous interventions, regular low-impact aerobic exercise and leg elevation will optimize venous return. There are inconclusive data on the utility of prophylactic antiplatelet therapy for venous wounds.[8,46,52] Leukocyte activation drugs, intravenous micronized purified flavonoid fraction or oral pentoxifylline, have shown promising results in wound healing when combined with routine compression therapy.[9,53,54]

Diabetic Foot Ulcer

Approach and guidelines
More than 25% of patients with diabetes have macrovasculature and microvasculature PAD leading to noncompressible arteries, resulting in falsely elevated ABI (>1.2), and therefore, TP or TcPO2 with PVRs may be more useful noninvasive studies.[5,10] Early engagement of a multidisciplinary care approach to managing the patient's diabetes, podiatric needs, and PAD is critical for limb salvage.[11,12] Recent studies demonstrate that strict glycemic control decreases the risk of long-term

DFU and in turn LE amputation.[11,55–57] Given the importance of preventing hyperglycemia in DFU prevention and long-term outcomes, patients who present with a suspected DFU should be screened for prediabetes and diabetes (**Table 2**).

Treatment

Wound care. DFU characteristics can vary significantly, and therefore, their treatment and management may be variable. The wound should be thoroughly washed with soap or chlorhexidine scrub. Then, sharp or chemical debridement of all devitalized, callus, fibrinous, or necrotic tissue should be done. Daily collagenase is a good alternative for chemical debridement if the wound does not have too much drainage.[27,34,56] High-drainage output DFU can be managed with NPWT or frequent daily dressing changes with antibacterial-coated foam (such as Hydrofera Blue, Drawtex, or Mesalt) and compression dressing. The authors' experience with NPWT has been mixed, and results highly depend on consistent home wound care that is able to accommodate 2 to 3 times per week dressing changes with adequate seal.[34] The macerated periwound should also be managed as described above. High-drainage output DFU can also be a sign of local infection and can be expected to decrease drainage once the infection is treated and the wound begins to heal. Alternatively, there are low-drainage output DFUs that are often accompanied by thick periwould callus Thick callus can be treated with 40% urea cream to soften and allow dead skin buildup to be exfoliated. Once a wound moisture balance is acheived in a DFU, tissue granulation can be promoted using advanced wound products. It is important that any DFU wound plan be supplemented with physical offloading to prevent further external pressure. Offloading of DFU can be achieved with a total contact cast, podiatric forefront offloading shoe, or donut foam dressing.[1,11,12]

Infection control. Common bacterial organisms seen in a DFU are *Staphylococcus aureus*, Streptococcus, and *P aeruginosa*. DFU can be plagued with wound biofilm, cellulitis, and progress to osteomyelitis.[6,12,15,29,56] The authors prefer oral doxycycline, trimethoprim/sulfamethoxazole, or amoxicillin + clavulanate for broad coverage or intravenous vancomycin and zosyn, then narrow coverage once deep tissue cultures are obtained. It is critically important to evaluate DFUs for surgical source control

Table 2
Criteria for the screening and diagnosis of prediabetes and diabetes

	Prediabetes	Diabetes
A$_{1c}$	5.7%–6.4% (39–47 mmol/mol)[a]	≥6.5% (48 mmol/mol)[b]
Fasting plasma glucose	100–125 mg/dL (5.6–6.9 mmol/L)[a]	≥126 mg/dL (7.0 mmol/L)[b]
2-h plasma glucose during 75-g OGTT	140–199 mg/dL (7.8–11.0 mmol/L)[a]	≥200 mg/dL (11.1 mmol/L)[b]
Random plasma glucose	—	≥200 mg/dL (11.1 mmol/L)[c]

Abbreviation: OGGT, oral glucose test tolerance.
[a] For all 3 tests, risk is continuous, extending below the lower limit of the range and becoming disproportionately greater at the higher end of the range.
[b] In the absence of unequivocal hyperglycemia, diagnosis requires 2 abnormal test results from the same sample or in 2 separate samples.
[c] Only diagnostic in a patient with classic symptoms of hyperglycemia or hyperglycemic crisis.
Adapted from Good to Know: ADA's Standards of Medical Care in Diabetes. Clin Diabetes. 2022;40(1):108; with permission.

if there is a deep tissue infection concerning for necrotizing soft tissue infection or osteomyelitis.

Glycemic control. The American Diabetes Association recommends a goal hemoglobin A_{1c} for nonpregnant adults less than 7% or less than 8% for patients with limited life expectancy. Capillary plasma glucose preprandial goal is 80 to 130 g/dL and postprandial is less than 180 mg/dL (**Table 3**).[58] First-line hyperglycemia therapy will depend on specific patient comorbidities. Initiation of metformin and lifestyle modification are generally recommended for all patients with diabetes. Patients with type 2 diabetes in combination with cardiovascular disease and/or renal disease may benefit from SGLT-2 inhibitors or GLP-1 to achieve glycemic goals.[23–25]

Modifiable risk factors. DFU is preventable. SVS recommends that patients with prediabetes or diabetes should have annual foot examinations with monofilament testing (Semmes-Weinstein test) and identify any pedal callus. Patients with peripheral neuropathy and a preulcer callus should be referred to Podiatry for prescription accommodative orthotic shoe inserts or custom diabetic footwear.[10,11,58] Even if a DFU has healed, there is a 40% recurrence rate so the preventative measures outlined above should continue as part of the patient's routine care.[55]

Pressure Wounds

Approach and guidelines
Identifying the external cause or causes of the pressure wound is a critical component to developing an effective wound care plan and to prevent future pressure wounds because pressure wound recurrence rates are approximately 5% to 20% depending on the wound location.[59,60] Offloading modality should be tailored to the patient's anatomic needs, such as egg crate foam pads, donut dressing or cushion, assisted extremity turns or repositioning every 2 hours, waffle air cushion boots, or lamb/sheep wool padding. Pressure wounds are staged based on depth of the pressure injury (stage 1 [shallow] through 4 [full thickness]), and treatment plans will depend on the individualized wound characteristics.[1,13]

Treatment
Wound care. Pressure wound location, size, depth, and staging can vary significantly between patients because their nuanced cause highly depends on the patient. Wound care plan should use debridement, moisture balance, and granulation tissue promotion as outlined above based on the TIME framework.[68] Any wound care treatment plan implemented must be supplemented with physical offloading techniques described above.

Table 3 Summary of glycemic recommendations for many nonpregnant adults with diabetes	
A_{1c}	<7.0% (53 mmol/mol)[a,#]
Preprandial capillary plasma glucose	80–130 mg/dL[a] (4.4–7.2 mmol/L)
Peak postprandial capillary plasma glucose[b]	<180 mg/dL[a] (10.0 mmol/L)

[a] More or less stringent glycemic goals may be appropriate for individual patients.
[b] Postprandial glucose may be targeted if A_{1c} goals are not met despite reaching preprandial glucose goals. Postprandial glucose measurements should be made 1 to 2 h after the beginning of the meal, generally peak levels in patients with diabetes.
Adapted from Good to Know: ADA's Standards of Medical Care in Diabetes. Clin Diabetes. 2022;40(1):108; with permission.

Infection control. Pressure wounds may commonly be infected by *S aureus*, Strepto-coccus, and *P aeruginosa*. These wounds can progress to necrotizing soft tissue infection or osteomyelitis and should be carefully evaluated for periwound crepitus, tracking erythema, cellulitis, or fluctuance. The wound biofilm can be sharply or chemically debrided as described above. In the authors' practice, they often initiate broad-spectrum oral or intravenous antibiotics and then narrow coverage once deep tissue cultures are obtained.[13]

Surgical skin graft and flaps. Most pressure wounds should be able to heal with a consistent offloading and wound treatment plan; however, some clean wounds remain slow to progress. These wounds may benefit from a split-thickness, regional/pedicle flap, or microvascular flaps for coverage. For pressure wounds that are superficial and without exposure of vital tissues, such as bone, vessels, nerves, or tendons, a split-thickness skin graft may be appropriate. In contrast, larger wound defects owing to their size or location may be more appropriate for regional/pedicle flaps.[61] Microvascular free flaps are usually reserved for pressure wounds that require healing for proper weight-bearing, such as the heel of the foot or amputation stumps.[13,62]

Mixed Cause/Atypical Nonhealing Wounds

Approach and guidelines

Mixed or atypical wound cause is the most difficult chronic nonhealing LE wounds to treat because there can be multiple underlying causes or no clear cause identified. Differential diagnosis is broad and should include the following: malignant or fungating wounds that are friable with heavy biofilm and drainage,[63] vasculitis and other inflammatory associated wounds, such as rheumatoid arthritis, systemic lupus erythematous, scleroderma, thromboangiitis obliterans, antineutrophil cytoplasmic antibody vasculitis, granulomatosis with polyangiitis, microscopic polyangiitis, or Churg-Strauss syndrome. The appearance of these wounds can vary depending on the extent of arterial involvement and range from palpable purpura, livedo reticularis, pain, skin lesions with or without nodules, to tissue necrosis.[64] Pyoderma gangrenosum wounds have rapid onset and progression that often develop as a pustule or bulla with subsequent ulceration with purulent drainage.[64] Calciphylaxis wounds are associated with patients with renal failure that have calcific uremic deposits in the arterial wall that can cause acutely painful, indurated plaques that develop necrosis and ulceration.[64] Effective treatment requires an understanding of the cause, and patients benefit from multidisciplinary care. Full-thickness skin biopsies at multiple wound locations (periwound, wound border, and center of wound) can provide meaningful information about the histology, immunohistochemistry, and bacterial pathologic condition of a wound that can be useful for diagnosis and to guide treatment. Skin biopsies can be either incisional or punched.[14] The authors prefer to use a 4- to 6-mm punch biopsy in clinic with local anesthetic. This method allows for a clean uniform sampling that maintains the full-thickness skin integrity.

Treatment

Wound care. Mixed cause or atypical wounds are often plagued with heavy biofilm, and initial wound care should be initiated with a thorough cleanse with soap or chlorhexidine scrub. The wound characteristic should be carefully evaluated and only minimally debrided until PAD and malignancy have been ruled out. High-drainage output wounds are often associated with superficial or deep bacterial infection. The authors have avoided using NPWT on these wounds primarily because they either lack wound depth or present with a high-bacterial burden that requires more frequent dressing changes. Once the wound is carefully debrided and infection is controlled, the authors follow the standard treatment algorithm outlined above to promote wound moisture balance and granulation tissue.

Infection control. Some mixed wounds may be nonhealing because of on-going biofilm or soft tissue infection that has not been fully eradicated. Wound swab cultures may be unrevealing because they are often contaminated with surface skin flora. Wounds with clear signs of cellulitis should be treated with oral or intravenous antibiotics depending on the severity. Chronically infected wounds can be very painful, and adequate biofilm debridement may only be achieved in the operating room. The wound biofilm that cannot be sharply debrided can be treated with Dakin solution (sodium hypochlorite), hydrogen peroxide, sodium chloride, or povidone-iodine.[28,65] Patients may have intolerance to these treatments owing to burning or painful sensation. In these circumstances, the authors have found it useful to prescribe washes instead of leaving these solutions on the skin for prolong period of time or diluting the strength (one-half or one-quarter) for patient tolerance.

SUMMARY

Chronic lower-extremity wounds are *a major clinical and public health problem that disproportionately impacts vulnerable populations.* The medical cost, utilization of emergency care, and medical disability owing to chronic LE wounds impact societal productivity and is a growing medical problem.[66] Treatment of chronic LE wounds should focus on multidisciplinary care owing to the multifactorial components required for adequate wound healing. The cause of chronic LE wounds may include arterial insufficiency, venous insufficiency, diabetes, pressure, and/or mixed or atypical wounds (see **Fig. 2**). Treating the underlying cause or causes of chronic LE wounds will require the wound specialist to coordinate care with medical specialists who can assist in managing the systemic causes of LE wounds. In addition, wound healing should also include a multidisciplinary care team of visiting nurse, nutritionist, podiatrist, occupational and physical therapist, and social worker who are vital for the initiation, implementation, and maintenance of the wound care plan set by the wound specialist.[1,4,67] A chronic LE wound should be systematically assessed and reassessed for the underlying wound cause. Chronic LE wound treatment should be focused on building healthy granulation tissue using the TIME framework through wound debridement, infection control, moisture balance, and advanced wound care products to promote wound epithelializatin and edge healing.

CLINICS CARE POINTS

Wound care assessment and treatment should be tailored to the chronic nonhealing wound type based on the identified artieral, venous, diabetes, pressure or mixed/atypical cause. Arterial wound management:

- The SVS recommends that wounds with a WIfI ischemia score of ≥2 are associated with a high risk for wound-related amputation and open surgery LE bypass with GSV conduit is the gold standard to acheive revascularization for wound healing.

- Patients that undergo revascularization benefit from a daily aspirin and 2.5 mg twice daily rivaroxaban to decrease the composite risk of acute limb ischemia, major amputation from vascular causes, myocardial infarction, ischemic stroke, or death from cardiovascular causes.

Venous wound management:
- The SVS and AVF Joint Clinical Practice Guidelines recommend that all wounds suspicious for a venous cause be first evaluated with an LE venous reflux study and treatment

---

should focus on superficial venous disease before treating deep venous reflux or obstructive disease.
- Gradient compression therapy (30-40 mm Hg) Is the gold standard treatment for venous ulcers.

Diabetic foot ulcer management:
- Approximately 40% of DFU recur and therefore patients with DFU should be managed by a multidiciplinary team made of podiatry, endocrinology, vascular surgery, infectious disease, physcial therapy, and nutritionist.

- The American Diabetes Association recommends a goal hemoglobin A1c for nonpregnant adults less than 7% or less than 8% for patients with limited life expectancy with diabetes.

Pressure wound management:
- Offloading modality should be tailored to the patient's anatomic needs, such as egg crate foam pads, donut dressing or cushion, assisted extremity turns or repositioning every 2 hours, waffle air cushion boots, or lamb/sheep wool padding.

Mixed cause/atypical wound management:
- Identifying the cause of the wound is imperative to formulating a successful wound care plan. The differential diagnosis is broad and skin biopsy may assist in diagnosis.

DISCLOSURE

None.

REFERENCES

1. Bowers S, Franco E. Chronic Wounds: Evaluation and Management. Am Fam Physician 2020;101(3):159–66.
2. Frykberg RG, Banks J. Challenges in the Treatment of Chronic Wounds. Adv Wound Care 2015;4(9):560–82 [published Online First: Epub Date]|.
3. Eming SA, Martin P, Tomic-Canic M. Wound repair and regeneration: mechanisms, signaling, and translation. Sci Transl Med 2014;6(265):265sr6 [published Online First: Epub Date]|.
4. Kirsner RS, Vivas AC. Lower-extremity ulcers: diagnosis and management. Br J Dermatol 2015;173(2):379–90 [published Online First: Epub Date]|.
5. Aday AW, Matsushita K. Epidemiology of Peripheral Artery Disease and Polyvascular Disease. Circ Res 2021;128(12):1818–32 [published Online First: Epub Date]|.
6. Mills JL, Conte MS, Armstrong DG, et al. The Society for Vascular Surgery Lower Extremity Threatened Limb Classification System: risk stratification based on wound, ischemia, and foot infection (WIfI). J Vasc Surg 2014;59(1):220, 234 e1-2.
7. Eberhardt RT, Raffetto JD. Chronic venous insufficiency. Circulation 2014;130(4): 333–46 [published Online First: Epub Date]|.
8. O'Donnell TF Jr, Passman MA. Clinical practice guidelines of the Society for Vascular Surgery (SVS) and the American Venous Forum (AVF)–Management of venous leg ulcers. Introduction. J Vasc Surg 2014;60(2 Suppl):1S–2S [published Online First: Epub Date]|.
9. Tassiopoulos AK, Golts E, Oh DS, et al. Current concepts in chronic venous ulceration. Eur J Vasc Endovasc Surg 2000;20(3):227–32.
10. Armstrong DG, Lavery LA. Diabetic foot ulcers: prevention, diagnosis and classification. Am Fam Physician 1998;57(6):1325–32, 37-1332.
11. Hingorani A, LaMuraglia GM, Henke P, et al. The management of diabetic foot: A clinical practice guideline by the Society for Vascular Surgery in collaboration

with the American Podiatric Medical Association and the Society for Vascular Medicine. J Vasc Surg 2016;63(2 Suppl):3S–21S [published Online First: Epub Date]|.

12. Schaper NC, van Netten JJ, Apelqvist J, et al. Practical Guidelines on the prevention and management of diabetic foot disease (IWGDF 2019 update). Diabetes Metab Res Rev 2020;36(Suppl 1):e3266 [published Online First: Epub Date]|.

13. Boyko TV, Longaker MT, Yang GP. Review of the Current Management of Pressure Ulcers. Adv Wound Care 2018;7(2):57–67 [published Online First: Epub Date]|.

14. Janowska A, Dini V, Oranges T, et al. Atypical Ulcers: Diagnosis and Management. Clin Interv Aging 2019;14:2137–43 [published Online First: Epub Date]|.

15. Robinson WP, Loretz L, Hanesian C, et al. Society for Vascular Surgery Wound, Ischemia, foot Infection (WIfI) score correlates with the intensity of multimodal limb treatment and patient-centered outcomes in patients with threatened limbs managed in a limb preservation center. J Vasc Surg 2017;66(2):488–498 e2 [published Online First: Epub Date]|.

16. Vallabhaneni R, Kalbaugh CA, Kouri A, et al. Current accepted hemodynamic criteria for critical limb ischemia do not accurately stratify patients at high risk for limb loss. J Vasc Surg 2016;63(1):105–12 [published Online First: Epub Date]|.

17. Grey JE, Harding KG, Enoch S. Venous and arterial leg ulcers. BMJ 2006; 332(7537):347–50 [published Online First: Epub Date]|.

18. Hedayati N, Carson JG, Chi YW, et al. Management of mixed arterial venous lower extremity ulceration: A review. Vasc Med 2015;20(5):479–86 [published Online First: Epub Date]|.

19. Humphreys ML, Stewart AH, Gohel MS, et al. Management of mixed arterial and venous leg ulcers. Br J Surg 2007;94(9):1104–7 [published Online First: Epub Date]|.

20. Herberger K, Muller K, Protz K, et al. Nutritional status and quality of nutrition in chronic wound patients. Int Wound J 2020;17(5):1246–54 [published Online First: Epub Date]|.

21. McDaniel JC, Browning KK. Smoking, chronic wound healing, and implications for evidence-based practice. J Wound, Ostomy Cont Nurs 2014;41(5):415–23 [quiz: E1-2].

22. Silverstein P. Smoking and wound healing. Am J Med 1992;93(1A):22S–4S [published Online First: Epub Date]|.

23. American Diabetes A. Standards of Medical Care in Diabetes-2022 Abridged for Primary Care Providers. Clin Diabetes 2022;40(1):10–38 [published Online First: Epub Date]|.

24. Clegg LE, Penland RC, Bachina S, et al. Effects of exenatide and open-label SGLT2 inhibitor treatment, given in parallel or sequentially, on mortality and cardiovascular and renal outcomes in type 2 diabetes: insights from the EXSCEL trial. Cardiovasc Diabetol 2019;18(1):138 [published Online First: Epub Date]|.

25. Gerstein HC, Sattar N, Rosenstock J, et al. Cardiovascular and Renal Outcomes with Efpeglenatide in Type 2 Diabetes. N Engl J Med 2021;385(10):896–907 [published Online First: Epub Date]|.

26. Dowsett C, Ayello E. TIME principles of chronic wound bed preparation and treatment. Br J Nurs 2004;13(15):S16–23.

27. Manna B, Nahirniak P, Morrison CA. Wound debridement. Treasure Island (FL): StatPearls; 2022.

28. Alves PJ, Barreto RT, Barrois BM, et al. Update on the role of antiseptics in the management of chronic wounds with critical colonisation and/or biofilm. Int Wound J 2021;18(3):342–58 [published Online First: Epub Date]|.

29. Percival SL, McCarty SM, Lipsky B. Biofilms and Wounds: An Overview of the Evidence. Adv Wound Care 2015;4(7):373–81 [published Online First: Epub Date]|.

30. Falabella AF, Carson P, Eaglstein WH, et al. The safety and efficacy of a proteolytic ointment in the treatment of chronic ulcers of the lower extremity. J Am Acad Dermatol 1998;39(5 Pt 1):737–40 [published Online First: Epub Date]|.

31. Patry J, Blanchette V. Enzymatic debridement with collagenase in wounds and ulcers: a systematic review and meta-analysis. Int Wound J 2017;14(6): 1055–65 [published Online First: Epub Date]|.

32. Okan D, Woo K, Ayello EA, et al. The role of moisture balance in wound healing. Adv Skin Wound Care 2007;20(1):39–53 [quiz: 53-5].

33. Dumville JC, Webster J, Evans D, et al. Negative pressure wound therapy for treating pressure ulcers. Cochrane Database Syst Rev 2015;(5):CD011334. https://doi.org/10.1002/14651858.CD011334.pub2 [published Online First: Epub Date]|.

34. Liu Z, Dumville JC, Hinchliffe RJ, et al. Negative pressure wound therapy for treating foot wounds in people with diabetes mellitus. Cochrane Database Syst Rev 2018;10(10):CD010318 [published Online First: Epub Date]|.

35. Polignano R, Bonadeo P, Gasbarro S, et al. A randomised controlled study of four-layer compression versus Unna's Boot for venous ulcers. J Wound Care 2004; 13(1):21–4 [published Online First: Epub Date]|.

36. Snyder D, Sullivan N, Margolis D, et al. Skin substitutes for treating chronic wounds. Rockville (MD), 2020.

37. Dussoyer M, Michopoulou A, Rousselle P. Decellularized Scaffolds for Skin Repair and Regeneration. Appl Sci 2020;10(10):3435.

38. Mills JL, Sr. The impact of organized multidisciplinary care on limb salvage in patients with mild to moderate WIfl ischemia grades. J Vasc Surg 2020;71(6): 2081–2 [published Online First: Epub Date]|.

39. Farber A, Menard MT, Conte MS, et al. Surgery or Endovascular Therapy for Chronic Limb-Threatening Ischemia. N Engl J Med 2022. https://doi.org/10. 1056/NEJMoa2207899 [published Online First: Epub Date]|.

40. Bonaca MP, Bauersachs RM, Anand SS, et al. Rivaroxaban in Peripheral Artery Disease after Revascularization. N Engl J Med 2020;382(21):1994–2004 [published Online First: Epub Date]|.

41. Hiatt WR, Bonaca MP, Patel MR, et al. Rivaroxaban and Aspirin in Peripheral Artery Disease Lower Extremity Revascularization: Impact of Concomitant Clopidogrel on Efficacy and Safety. Circulation 2020;142(23):2219–30 [published Online First: Epub Date]|.

42. Bevan GH, White Solaru KT. Evidence-Based Medical Management of Peripheral Artery Disease. Arterioscler Thromb Vasc Biol 2020;40(3):541–53 [published Online First: Epub Date]|.

43. Diehm C, Schuster A, Allenberg JR, et al. High prevalence of peripheral arterial disease and co-morbidity in 6880 primary care patients: cross-sectional study. Atherosclerosis 2004;172(1):95–105 [published Online First: Epub Date]|.

44. Fudim M, Jones WS. New Curveball for Hypertension Guidelines? Circulation 2018;138(17):1815–8 [published Online First: Epub Date]|.

45. Belch JJF, Brodmann M, Baumgartner I, et al. Lipid-lowering and anti-thrombotic therapy in patients with peripheral arterial disease: European Atherosclerosis

Society/European Society of Vascular Medicine Joint Statement. Atherosclerosis 2021;338:55–63 [published Online First: Epub Date]|.

46. O'Donnell TF Jr, Passman MA, Marston WA, et al. Management of venous leg ulcers: clinical practice guidelines of the Society for Vascular Surgery (R) and the American Venous Forum. J Vasc Surg 2014;60(2 Suppl):3S–59S [published Online First: Epub Date]|.

47. Bergan JJ, Schmid-Schonbein GW, Smith PD, et al. Chronic venous disease. N Engl J Med 2006;355(5):488–98 [published Online First: Epub Date]|.

48. Barwell JR, Davies CE, Deacon J, et al. Comparison of surgery and compression with compression alone in chronic venous ulceration (ESCHAR study): randomised controlled trial. Lancet 2004;363(9424):1854–9 [published Online First: Epub Date]|.

49. Gohel MS, Barwell JR, Taylor M, et al. Long term results of compression therapy alone versus compression plus surgery in chronic venous ulceration (ESCHAR): randomised controlled trial. BMJ 2007;335(7610):83. BE[published Online First: Epub Date]|.

50. Gohel MS, Heatley F, Liu X, et al. A Randomized Trial of Early Endovenous Ablation in Venous Ulceration. N Engl J Med 2018;378(22):2105–14 [published Online First: Epub Date]|.

51. Lawrence PF, Hager ES, Harlander-Locke MP, et al. Treatment of superficial and perforator reflux and deep venous stenosis improves healing of chronic venous leg ulcers. J Vasc Surg Venous Lymphat Disord 2020;8(4):601–9 [published Online First: Epub Date]|.

52. de Oliveira Carvalho PE, Magolbo NG, De Aquino RF, et al. Oral aspirin for treating venous leg ulcers. Cochrane Database Syst Rev 2016;2(2):CD009432 [published Online First: Epub Date]|.

53. Coleridge-Smith P, Lok C, Ramelet AA. Venous leg ulcer: a meta-analysis of adjunctive therapy with micronized purified flavonoid fraction. Eur J Vasc Endovasc Surg 2005;30(2):198–208 [published Online First: Epub Date]|.

54. Jull AB, Arroll B, Parag V, et al. Pentoxifylline for treating venous leg ulcers. Cochrane Database Syst Rev 2012;12(12):CD001733 [published Online First: Epub Date]|.

55. Armstrong DG, Boulton AJM, Bus SA. Diabetic Foot Ulcers and Their Recurrence. N Engl J Med 2017;376(24):2367–75 [published Online First: Epub Date]|.

56. Boulton AJM, Armstrong DG, Kirsner RS, et al. Diagnosis and Management of Diabetic Foot Complications. Arlington (VA): American Diabetes Association; 2018.

57. Lane KL, Abusamaan MS, Voss BF, et al. Glycemic control and diabetic foot ulcer outcomes: A systematic review and meta-analysis of observational studies. J Diabetes Complications 2020;34(10):107638 [published Online First: Epub Date]|.

58. Good to Know: ADA's Standards of Medical Care in Diabetes. Clin Diabetes 2022;40(1):108. https://doi.org/10.2337/cd22-pe01 [published Online First: Epub Date]|.

59. Morgan JE. Recurrence of pressure ulcers. A study of five cases. JAMA 1976;236(21):2430–1.

60. Paker N, Bugdayci D, Goksenoglu G, et al. Recurrence rate after pressure ulcer reconstruction in patients with spinal cord injury in patients under control by a plastic surgery and physical medicine and rehabilitation team. Turk J Phys Med Rehabil 2018;64(4):322–7 [published Online First: Epub Date]|.

61. Wong JK, Amin K, Dumville JC. Reconstructive surgery for treating pressure ulcers. Cochrane Database Syst Rev 2016;12(12):CD012032 [published Online First: Epub Date]].

62. Bhattacharya S, Mishra RK. Pressure ulcers: Current understanding and newer modalities of treatment. Indian J Plast Surg 2015;48(1):4–16 [published Online First: Epub Date]].

63. Vardhan M, Flaminio Z, Sapru S, et al. The Microbiome, Malignant Fungating Wounds, and Palliative Care. Front Cell Infect Microbiol 2019;9:373 [published Online First: Epub Date]].

64. Shanmugam VK, Angra D, Rahimi H, et al. Vasculitic and autoimmune wounds. J Vasc Surg Venous Lymphat Disord 2017;5(2):280–92 [published Online First: Epub Date]].

65. Leaper DJ, Durani P. Topical antimicrobial therapy of chronic wounds healing by secondary intention using iodine products. Int Wound J 2008;5(2):361–8 [published Online First: Epub Date]].

66. Sen CK. Human Wounds and Its Burden: An Updated Compendium of Estimates. Adv Wound Care 2019;8(2):39–48 [published Online First: Epub Date]].

67. Kim PJ, Evans KK, Steinberg JS, et al. Critical elements to building an effective wound care center. J Vasc Surg 2013;57(6):1703–9 [published Online First: Epub Date]].

68. Harries RL, Bosanquet DC, Harding KG. Wound bed preparation: TIME for an update. Int Wound J 2016;13(Suppl 3):8–14.

Lower Extremity Bypass

Ajibola George Akingba, MD, PhD[a], Warren Bryan Chow, MD, MS[b],
Vincent Lopez Rowe, MD[b],*

KEYWORDS

- Lower extremity bypass • Great saphenous vein • Graft
- Chronic limb threatening ischemia

KEY POINTS

- Single-segment great saphenous vein outperforms endovascular therapy for chronic limb-threatening ischemia patients.
- Single-segment great saphenous vein is the best conduit for lower extremity bypass.
- Additional adjuncts should be used to assure the most effective bypass construction.
- There is no significant difference in outcome based on the configuration of the bypass graft tunnel.

 Video content accompanies this article at http://www.www.surgical.theclinics.com.

HISTORY

Vascular interventions for the salvage of lower extremity function compromised by progressive atherosclerotic occlusive disease dates back over 75 years with the first bypass reported in 1949 by Dr Jean Kunlin.[1] In his report, Dr Kunlin documents consulting on a patient with toe gangrene and rest pain. The patient had undergone a prior toe amputation which did not heal and now was facing limb loss. The angiogram showed an occluded superficial femoral artery with reconstitution of the below knee popliteal artery and single-vessel runoff via the posterior tibial artery. Dr Kunlin moved forward with a femoral artery to below-knee popliteal artery bypass with ipsilateral reversed greater saphenous vein (GSV). The bypass was successful in providing sufficient perfusion to heal the toe amputation site. One important surgical detail of this lower extremity bypass (LEB) technique was an end-to-side configuration for the proximal and distal anastomoses that maintained blood flow through preexisting collateral vessels. The same patient required a contralateral bypass months later which was also

[a] DC VAMC, Uniformed Services University of Health Sciences, 50 Irving Street, Washington, DC 20422, USA; [b] Division of Vascular Surgery and Endovascular Therapy, David Geffen School of Medicine at UCLA, 200 Peter Morton Medical Building, Suite 526, Los Angeles, CA 90095, USA
* Corresponding author.
E-mail address: vrowe@mednet.ucla.edu

Surg Clin N Am 103 (2023) 767–778
https://doi.org/10.1016/j.suc.2023.04.014
0039-6109/23/© 2023 Elsevier Inc. All rights reserved.

successful. Unfortunately, 1 year after the second bypass, the patient succumbed to a major adverse cardiovascular event. In the years following that initial report by Kunlin, numerous authors documented bypasses to more distal targets in the tibial region of the calf and ankle.[2–4] Reports of LEB for limb salvage sparked a significant paradigm shift from the conventional techniques of that period which relied on homograft-based conduits and endarterectomy. Thanks to this pioneering group of surgeons, the LEB with GSV had affirmed itself as the procedure of choice in limb salvage.

INDICATIONS

The indications for LEB are based on a well-described collection of symptoms, including gangrenous changes to the foot and toes, ischemic rest pain, and nonhealing ulcers. Although there is no consensus for the duration of an ulcer to be considered nonhealing, anecdotally, 4 to 6 weeks allows clinicians a suitable timetable for healing attempts without revascularization. However, the subjective time frame should be adjusted based on additional clinical variables, such as location of the ulcer, exposure of bone or tendon, pain and disability of the patient, and presence of infection related to the ulcer. Any adverse factors should spark consideration for expedient revascularization.

In very select clinical situations, disabling claudication can be considered an indication for LEB. A careful evaluation of the anatomic disease distribution, patient symptoms, tobacco use, and success of prior medical therapy weigh heavily into the clinical decision for intervention. Adherence to the recent Society of Vascular Surgery guidelines for management of patients with intermittent claudication is recommended.[5]

Last, in the case of extensive necrosis and tissue loss, the authors endorse the use of LEB over an endovascular approach. In such cases, maximizing expedient perfusion to the foot is imperative for successful healing of subsequent partial foot amputations and possible tissue transfer procedures.

PREOPERATIVE EVALUATION

The preoperative evaluation of the chronic limb-threatening ischemia (CLTI) patient is complex. The care team is faced with patients harboring numerous comorbidities, often including diabetes mellitus, cardiac disease, hypertension, hyperlipidemia, and kidney disease, at various levels of control or progression; accompanied by a component of deconditioning and limited mobility. The nuances in preoperative and perioperative care can challenge the most proficient limb preservation teams. In addition to standard preoperative metrics and laboratory studies, the assessment of patient functional status is helpful.[6] An Understanding of the limitations of the patient function and mobility significantly impacts the outcome following bypass and may provide insight into the role of primary amputation. Other indices such as frailty and preoperative anesthetic metrics are helpful; however, in a patient facing limb loss, the ultimate decision outcome measure is an attempt at limb salvage versus amputation. In such dire consequences, limb salvage attempts frequently supersede primary amputation.

Enhanced recovery after surgery (ERAS) protocols help prepare the patient for the physiologic insult of upcoming surgery. The protocol follows the premise that control of comorbidities in the perioperative period will lead to better recovery. First reported in 1997 with early application in general and orthopedic surgery, the protocol used a multimodal approach to decrease postoperative morbidity.[7] Specifically in vascular surgery, a systematic review of ERAS in 2019 documented moderate benefits in application of ERAS open aortic surgery, but limited adoption of ERAS for LEB.[8] The investigators cited an overall decrease in length of stay and hospital costs as significant benefits of ERAS in LEB but agree that barriers in early mobilization, one of the tenets of ERAS, are challenging in the postoperative LEB patient. Similar to the earlier systematic review, recently published ERAS guidelines provide insight for patients with aortic surgery.[9] With the visible momentum and success by ERAS adhering centers, the expectation that limb salvage centers will solidify pathways to allow seamless implementation in the CLTI subset and improve perioperative outcomes is hopeful.

Cardiovascular events are the most devastating perioperative complication facing the CLTI patient. A thorough evaluation of the cardiovascular reserve is critical before undergoing an LEB. Many clinicians have suggested preemptive coronary revascularization procedures to lower the risk surrounding the time of the LEB; however, the outcomes of Preoperative Coronary Revascularization Prior to Major Vascular Reconstruction trial challenged the notion.[10] In the 2004 study, 5859 Veterans Administration patients were randomized to preoperative coronary revascularization or no coronary revascularization before major vascular reconstructions. Surprisingly, no benefit was identified at the 30-day or 2-year follow-up between the revascularized and non-revascularized groups. Follow-up reports including subset analyses reinforced the initial findings, limiting the recommendation for preoperative cardiac revascularization to a small subset of patients with a history of congestive heart failure, chest pain, and recent myocardial infarctions.[11]

Despite the profound comorbidities challenging limb salvage teams with improved preoperative strategy for patients including preoperative conditioning protocols, medical therapy, and anesthetic regimens, the outcomes for open revascularization will continue to improve even for the most frail and debilitated patient.

TECHNIQUE

Since the initial work of Dr Kunlin, key tenets in the technique of LEB have remained.[1] An end-to-side anastomosis meticulously constructed to the unabated inflow vessel, optimal outflow target, and use of GSV still form the foundation of technical success in open lower extremity revascularizations. With the foundations firmly in place, the remainder of this section addresses specific areas of technical considerations.

Inflow and Outflow Vessels

The inflow to any vascular bypass must be free of significant perianastomotic occlusive disease. To combat local disease, a local endarterectomy at or proximal to the anastomotic site and may be performed at the time of anastomotic construction. For an endarterectomy of up to 3 cm in length, the use of the proximal anastomosis as a patch is preferred. However, for longer endarterectomy sites, separate autologous patch closure (vein or occluded superficial femoral artery) with origination of the proximal anastomosis off the distal end of the patch is preferred by the authors. If the common femoral artery is selected as the inflow vessel for an LEB, any hemodynamically significant proximal disease should also be addressed, either by open surgery (eg, aorto-femoral bypass) or endovascular technique (iliac artery angioplasty with or without stenting). If the occlusive lesions are isolated to the tibial region, inflow from the superficial femoral artery or even below knee popliteal artery as durable as the common femoral artery.[12,13]

Similarly, for the outflow vessel choice, an artery with unabated flow to the foot is ideal. However, if the conduit length is compromised, selection of the least diseased outflow target followed by postoperative endovascular therapy to treat residual distal disease is feasible. Owing to the cumbersome nature of gaining a stable access to a tibial vessel at the time of the LEB, our recommendation for this scenario would be for early postoperative treatment. In the tibial vessels, where calcification and limitation in exposure add to the challenge of anastomosis construction, the authors' preference is to avoid local endarterectomy in the smaller fragile tibial vessels.

Global Limb Anatomic Staging System

To provide a balanced mechanistic approach to limb revascularization, the investigators have proposed an anatomic grading and staging criteria to define the optimal target arterial pathway to the foot. The Global Limb Anatomic Staging System (GLASS)[14] is the product from intense analysis of data evaluated by the Global Vascular Guidelines authors.[15,16] GLASS stages the femoral popliteal and infrapopliteal vessels in conjunction with patient comorbidity assessment to find the optimal revascularization strategy. As more literature delineates the application of GLASS, adoption into the evaluation and treatment planning for CLTI patients will become more pervasive.

Conduit

Overwhelmingly, the quality and type of conduit heavily impact the outcome and longevity of LEB. Since the first recorded bypass, single-segment GSV has proven to be the highest quality conduit of choice.[1] The results of the Best Endovascular versus Best Surgical Therapy in Patient with Critical Limb Ischemia (BEST-CLI) trial, our largest randomized trial comparing endovascular and open bypass for treatment of CLTI patients, documented the superiority of single-segment GSV over endovascular therapy and disadvantaged conduits.[17] Based on this revelatory finding, the outcome of preoperative vein mapping became a more crucial decision point in the algorithm of treatment in patients with CLTI.

When suitable GSV is not available, numerous alternatives exist, including arm veins, spliced veins, short saphenous vein, prosthetic conduits, and cryopreserved artery or vein. These are termed "disadvantaged" conduits based on well-documented inferior outcomes when compared with GSV.[17] A detailed account of the historical outcomes is beyond the scope of this article. With highly variable and poor predictability in outcomes, the selection of a disadvantaged conduit lies in the experience of the clinician or institution. The authors have surgically evaluated each option and have yet to establish a strong preference. Attempts to interplay autologous and prosthetic conduits in a composite format should be avoided. The benefit of the segment of autologous conduit will be completely eradicated by the deleterious effects of the prosthetic portion. If a mix of conduits is required, configuration in a sequential manner with each conduit and anastomosed to the native artery only and not to each other is recommended.

Vein Harvest

The only existing controversy regarding GSV use in LEB is the harvest method. Traditional harvest techniques with continuous incisions remain a viable and effective option. Endoscopic vein harvest was popularized first in the cardiac surgery literature, but translation to LEB incorporation has shown mixed results when compared with traditional methods (**Table 1**). The largest series analyzed harvest techniques using the Vascular Quality Initiative (VQI) data.[18] The authors reported no statistically significant difference in wound complications and slightly worse patency of the bypass grafts at 1 year with endovascular harvest. Conflicting studies followed with proponents alluding to overcoming the operative learning curve and patient selection as key determinants to successful outcomes. Other variables for consideration include

Table 1
Comparison of recent studies evaluating the endoscopic vein harvest technique

Author/Year	Patients	Wound Comp	Patency
Gazoni et al,[35] 2006	144	↑	↑
Wartman et al,[36] 2013	76	NS	NS
Santo et al,[37] 2014	251	↑	↓
Eid et al,[38] 2014	88	↑	↓
Jauhari et al,[39] 2014	2343 Meta-analysis	NS	↓
Teixeria et al,[40] 2015	5066 VQI	NS	↓
Khan et al,[41] 2016	153	↑	NS 60 mo
Mirza et al,[42] 2018	505	↑	↓
Kronick et al,[43] 2019	113	↑	↑

From Teixeira PG, Woo K, Weaver FA, Rowe VL. Vein harvesting technique for infrainguinal arterial bypass with great saphenous vein and its association with surgical site infection and graft patency. J Vasc Surg. 2015;61(5):1264-71.e2; with permission.

the body mass index (BMI) of the patient and length of conduit required. For the use of only the thigh segment of GSV, the use of an endoscopic harvest approach can alleviate the need for a continuous thigh incision. In summation, the conflicting opinions and recommendations only support the notion that the presence of high-quality GSV is still the dominant variable and not the method of harvest.

Vascular Control

The construction of the distal anastomosis often presents the greatest challenge to the surgeon. With more CLTI patients presenting with renal dysfunction and accompanied vessel wall calcification, establishing safe vascular control can be problematic. Even the gentlest application of a non-crushing vascular clamp may create enough vessel wall disruption with the plaque interface to form isolated dissections. The use of pneumatic tourniquet for proximal control avoids the aforementioned problems. Placement technique involves application of the pneumatic tourniquet at thigh or proximal calf level, exsanguination of the leg with Esmarch circumferential wrapping, followed by inflation of the pneumatic tourniquet to 250 to 300 mg of mercury[19] (Video 1). The subsequent bloodless operative field allows precise anastomotic construction and optimal visualization for trainee instruction. Tourniquet use for all tibial level bypasses is highly recommended. In extreme arterial calcified vessels, arterial inflow may persist after the target vessel arteriotomy even with inflation pressures to 300 mg of mercury. Adjunct clamping of the inflow vessels at the proximal anastomosis assists in diminishing bleeding.

Bypass Graft Tunnel

Although the tunneling of the LEB graft seems intuitive, it may present certain challenges. With revision of the bypass graft stenosis shifting predominantly to an endovascular approach, the choice of tunnel configuration is mainly surgeon preference and dictated by other clinical variables such as size of the leg, possibility of skin necrosis in the thigh, and available conduit length. In a review of the tunneling configuration in patients undergoing LEB, no difference in patency was identified at 1-year follow-up period.[20] The author's preference is for a sub-sartorial tunnel through the thigh and then subcutaneous routing through the perigeniculate area into the target outflow vessel (Video 2). If crossing the interosseous membrane is required to reach the anterior tibial target, initiation of the tunnel creation from the lateral side is recommended. With caudal retraction of the anterior tibial neurovascular bundle, clear visualization of the interosseous membrane is obtained. A generous cruciate incision of the membrane and blunt passage of a surgical clamp under the tibia through the musculature completes the maneuver.

Completion Imaging

Despite the known consequences faced with the success or failure of the LEB, the investigative initiative to perform any completion study is only moderate. A review of vascular registry data showed only 48% of LEBs with single-segment GSV had any form of completion imaging which included angiogram or duplex.[21,22] The rate of completion imaging and complexity of the bypass construction correlated positively and reached a peak of 58% for LEB using spliced vein grafts (**Fig. 1**). Interestingly, the 1-year patency rate was not statistically different for LEB grafts that had a completion image compared with those that did not. The preference of the authors is for intraoperative completion duplex. The duplex modality has the added benefit of providing a real-time hemodynamic feedback to the surgeon regarding the bypass graph configuration and the evaluation for areas of stenosis.

OUTCOMES

The patency outcome of LEB is a highly critical variable in limb salvage, confirming the need for optimal patency of each graft. Historically, individual surgeon or institutional series of LEBs provided performance benchmarks for patency of bypass grafts. More recently, surgical outcome benchmarks has shifted to reliance on larger clinical trials and extrapolation of outcome characteristics from national data sets.

The Prevent III trial evaluated the efficacy of the competitive smooth muscle cell proliferation inhibitor edifoligide (E2F decoy) to reduce intimal hyperplasia in lower extremity vein bypass grafts.[13] The study randomized 1404 patients in a double-blinded

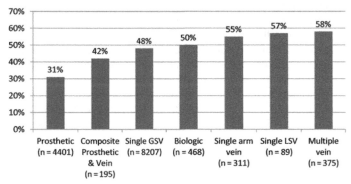

Fig. 1. Percentages of patients undergoing completion imaging determined by the type of bypass configuration. GSV, great saphenous vein; LSV, lessor saphenous vein. (*From* Woo K, Palmer OP, Weaver FA, Rowe VL; Society for Vascular Surgery Vascular Quality Initiative. Outcomes of completion imaging for lower extremity bypass in the Vascular Quality Initiative. J Vasc Surg. 2015;62(2):412-416; with permission.)

fashion and included 83 centers in the United States and Canada. Despite the nonstatistically significant difference in the two groups for the overall trial outcome, patency and limb salvage benchmarks were established from this cohort. In comparison of the treatment group and nontreatment group, primary patency was 61.5% compared with 59.3% and limb salvage rates of 87.7% compared with 89.2% at 18 months follow-up, respectively. Additional analyses of the study cohort confirmed shorter bypass lengths and GSV greater than or equal to 3.5 mm positively predicted improved outcomes in patients.

The Bypass versus Angioplasty in Severe Ischemia of the Leg (BASIL) multicenter randomized trial was one of the first comparative trials evaluating success of LEB compared with endovascular therapy. Four hundred and fifty-two patients with infrainguinal disease were randomized, 228 for surgery-first and 224 to angioplasty-first. The primary endpoint was amputation (of trial leg)-free survival. Although early results showed no significant difference in amputation-free survival, after 2 years, the LEB group showed a survival advantage that leads to the investigators recommending LEB in patients with suitable life expectancy.[23,24]

The Circulase investigators trial is similar in construction to the PREVENT III. The randomized controlled double-blinded trial evaluated the effect of lipo-ecraprost, a lipid-encapsulated prostaglandin E_1 prodrug.[25] The treatment group received the study drug intravenously in small aliquots starting within 72 hours postrevascularization followed by 5 days a week for 8 weeks. The study randomized 322 patients, 213 patients underwent surgical bypass, and 71 underwent endovascular revascularization before receiving study medication. At 180 days follow-up, there was no significant difference in primary-assisted patency or amputation-free survival between treatment and placebo cohorts. Despite the negative study, another benchmark of outcomes from an unequivocally accepted scientific structured format was established.

A close evaluation of the three trial results formed the foundation for investigators to provide the Global Vascular Guidelines. The guidelines were created to provide standards in the comprehensive care to the CLTI patient. The investigators created the objective performance goals (OPGs) for LEB, recommending benchmarks for limb preservation centers. Unfortunately, the OPGs are less generalizable for patient with increased complexity and comorbidities. Renal failure patient, patients over the age of 80, and those requiring disadvantaged conduits were considered outliers of the suggested benchmarks. Subsequent analyses which included these outlier subsets predictably demonstrated worse outcome for limb preservation, emphasizing the limitations of OPGs for broad application.

During the search for the benchmarks with the recommendations of OPGs, endovascular interventions become a majority component of limb salvage. Comparisons on the modalities were inevitable. To allow similar study endpoints, recommendation for transition to assimilate outcome nomenclature that would align consistently with endovascular studies was proposed. Endpoints such as primary patency, secondary patency, and other named outcome variables had new replacement definitions instituted with seamless adoption into vascular surgery literature (**Fig. 2**).

Similar to the comparative trial of BASIL, the BEST-CLI results were released with much anticipation this past year.[17] With over 1800 patients randomized, outcome data evaluating treatment modalities for patients with CLTI showed that a single segment of GSV provided the optimal outcome for revascularization of the lower extremity. In patients with a disadvantaged conduit, the outcomes were similar between endovascular and open bypass, reinforcing the long-standing premise that exceptional conduit was the most critical component in limb salvage.

Outcome	Definition
MALE	Major Adverse Limb Event: Above ankle amputation of the index limb or major reintervention (new bypass graft, jump/interposition graft revision, or thrombectomy/thrombolysis).
MALE+POD	Perioperative death (30 days), or any MALE
MACE	Major Adverse Cardiovascular Event: MI, stroke or death (any cause).
AMPUTATION	Above ankle amputation of the index limb.
AFS	Amputation-Free Survival: Above ankle amputation of the index limb or death (any cause).
RAO	Any reintervention or above ankle amputation of the index limb.
RAS	Any reintervention, above ankle amputation of the index limb, or stenosis
DEATH	Death (any cause).

Fig. 2. New replacement definitions instituted with seamless adoption into vascular surgery literature. (*From* Conte MS, Geraghty PJ, Bradbury AW, et al. Suggested objective performance goals and clinical trial design for evaluating catheter-based treatment of critical limb ischemia. J Vasc Surg. 2009;50(6):1462-73.e733; with permission.)

Racial Disparity Outcomes

For the past two decades, the disparity in the outcomes of LEB and limb salvage based on race has been richly documented in the literature.[26–30] Unfortunately, despite the in-depth discussion of the problems, plausible solutions have eluded the vascular community. A depth of analysis of patient demographics is now reaching to alternative variables to explain the disparity in the surgical outcomes. The inclusion of social determinants of health allows adjustment of the patient demographics and outcome data based on socioeconomic factors, access to care, educational levels, and environmental factors.[31,32] Simultaneously, the conversation is shifting from continued reporting of the difference in outcomes to institution of programs and multi-specialty teams leading on the pathway of sustainable solutions. The challenge of the solution in limb salvage is intensified due to the in depth of interplay between science, culture, and the newly evaluated social factors. A continued study is required.

Surveillance

LEB graft patency can be critical for continue limb salvage, and abnormalities can often be expeditiously treated with less invasive endovascular methods more easily than rescuing a thrombosed graft. For these reasons, the authors strongly recommend life-long surveillance of these bypass grafts in concordance with the Society of Vascular Surgery Practice Guidelines.[33] This includes early postoperative clinical examination including ankle brachial index (ABIs) and duplex ultrasound at 3-, 6-, and 12-month postoperatively and annually thereafter. More frequent duplex studies can be performed if there are any concerning clinical signs or symptoms or abnormalities seen on prior ultrasounds. Duplex ultrasound is the ideal modality because it is noninvasive and relatively inexpensive; however, it is subject to the skills of the ultrasonographer and the interpreting physician.

SPECIAL CIRCUMSTANCE

Patients presenting with tissue necrosis and gangrene pose a more formidable challenge in limb preservation. The first decision is defining which process, infectious, or ischemic, is dominant in the presentation. If the infection is dominant, adequate therapy for source control before LEB is mandatory. In severe cases of infection, partial or complete foot guillotine amputations are recommended for source control. Once the infection has cleared, LEB may proceed. If the LEB is to tibial targets, care should be taken to maximize the distance between the distal anastomosis and the necrotic tissue.

In situations with predominant dry gangrene, revascularization should proceed as planned, followed by subsequent partial foot amputation. The timing of the toe or partial foot amputation remains debatable with little literature to support either treatment preference.[34] The authors generally prefer amputation at or soon after the time of LEB to decrease the risk of secondary infections. In cases of extensive gangrene interspersed throughout the foot, a period of observation to examine the response to revascularization may be required before the definitive partial foot amputation.

SUMMARY

From the original description of LEB to current analysis comparing newer modalities, the LEB continues to provide the surgeon with the most reliable method of limb revascularization. Care should be taken to use all adjuncts including judicious target vessel control, completion imaging, and vein harvesting techniques to assure optimal outcomes, because a functioning LEB remains the key to successful limb salvage with preserved function.

DISCLOSURE

The authors have nothing to disclose.

SUPPLEMENTARY DATA

Supplementary data related to this article can be found online at https://doi.org/10.1016/j.suc.2023.04.014.

REFERENCES

1. Kunlin J. Le traitement de l'arterite obliterante par la greffe veineuse. Arch Mal Coeur 1949;42:371–2.
2. Linton RR, Darling RC. Surgery. 1962;51:62–65.
3. McCaughan JJ. Successful arterial grafts to the anterior tibial, posterior tibial (below the peroneal), and peroneal arteries. Angiology 1961;12:91–4.
4. McCaughan JJ Jr. Bypass graft to the posterior tibial artery at the ankle. Case reports. Am Surg 1966;32(2):126–30.
5. Woo K, Siracuse JJ, Klingbeil K, et al. Society for Vascular Surgery appropriate use criteria for management of intermittent claudication. J Vasc Surg 2022; 76(1):3–22.
6. Plotkin A, Khan T, Shin L, et al. Functional Ambulatory Status as a Potential Adjunctive Decision-Making Tool Following WIfI Assessment. J Vasc Surg 2020; 72(2):738–46.
7. Kehlet H. Multimodal approach to control postoperative pathophysiology and rehabilitation. Br J Anaesth 1997;78:606–17.
8. McGinigle KL, Eldrup-Jorgensen J, McCall R, et al. A systematic review of enhanced recovery after surgery for vascular operations. J Vasc Surg 2019; 79(2):629–40.

9. McGinigle KL, Spangler EL, Pichel AC, et al. Perioperative care in open aortic vascular surgery: A consensus statement by the Enhanced Recovery After Surgery (ERAS) Society and Society for Vascular Surgery. J Vasc Surg 2022;75(6): 1796–820.

10. McFalls EL, Ward HB, Moritz TE, et al. Coronary-Artery Revascularization before Elective Major Vascular Surgery. N Engl J Med 2004;351:2975–3804.

11. Raghunathan A, Rapp JH, Littooy F, et al. Postoperative Outcomes for Patients Undergoing Elective Revascularization for Critical Limb Ischemia and Intermittent Claudication: A Subanalysis of the Coronary Artery Revascularization Prophylaxis (CARP) Trial. J Vasc Surg 2006;43(6):1175–82.

12. Tran K, Ho VT, Itoga NK, et al. Comparison of mid-term graft patency in common femoral versus superficial femoral artery inflow for infra-geniculate bypass in the vascular quality initiative. Vascular 2020;28(6):722–30.

13. Conte MS, Bandyk DF, Clowes AW. PREVENT III Investigators. Results of PREVENT III: a multicenter, randomized trial of edifoligide for the prevention of vein graft failure in lower extremity bypass surgery. J Vasc Surg 2006;43(4):742–51.

14. Wijnand JGJ, Zarkowsky D, Wu B, van Haelst STW, Vonken EPA, Sorrentino TA, Pallister Z, Chung J, Mills JL, Teraa M, Verhaar MC, de Borst GJ, Conte MS. The Global Limb Anatomic Staging System (GLASS) for CLTI: Improving Inter-Observer Agreement. J Clin Med 2021;10(16):3454.

15. Conte MS, Bradbury AW, Kolh P, et al. GVG Writing Group for the Joint Guidelines of the Society for Vascular Surgery (SVS), European Society for Vascular Surgery (ESVS), and World Federation of Vascular Societies (WFVS). Global Vascular Guidelines on the Management of Chronic Limb-Threatening Ischemia. Eur J Vasc Endovasc Surg 2019;58(1S):S1–109.e33.

16. Conte MS, Bradbury AW, Kolh P, et al, GVG Writing Group. Global vascular guidelines on the management of chronic limb-threatening ischemia. J Vasc Surg 2019;69(6S):3S–125S.e40. Erratum in: J Vasc Surg. 2019;70(2):662.

17. Farber A, Menard MT, Conte MS, et al, the BEST-CLI Investigators. Bypass or endovascular therapy for treatment of chronic limb threatening ischemia. N Engl J Med 2022;387:2305–16.

18. Teixeira PGR, Woo K, Weaver FA, et al. Vein harvesting technique for infra-inguinal arterial bypass with greater saphenous vein and its association with surgical site infection and graft patency. J Vasc Surg 2015;61:1264–71.

19. Bernhard VM, Boren CH, Towne JB. Pneumatic tourniquet as a substitute for vascular clamps in distal bypass surgery. Surgery 1980;87(6):709–13.

20. Saldana-Ruiz N, Dominguez J, Ham SW, et al. Impact of Infrainguinal Bypass Tunneling Technique on Patency, Amputation, and Survival in Patients with Chronic Limb-threatening Ischemia. J Vasc Surg 2021;74(4):1242–50.

21. Woo K, Palmer O, Weaver FA, et al. Use of Completion Imaging During Infra-Inguinal Bypass in the Vascular Quality Initiative. J Vasc Surg 2015;61:1258–63.

22. Woo K, Palmer O, Weaver FA, et al. Outcomes of Completion Imaging for Lower Extremity Bypass in the Vascular Quality Initiative. J Vasc Surg 2015;62:412–6.

23. Adam DJ, Beard JD, Cleveland T. BASIL trial participants. Bypass versus angioplasty in severe ischaemia of the leg (BASIL): multicentre, randomised controlled trial. Lancet 2005;366(9501):1925–34.

24. Bradbury AW, Adam DJ, Bell J, et al. BASIL trial Participants. Bypass versus Angioplasty in Severe Ischaemia of the Leg (BASIL) trial: An intention-to-treat analysis of amputation-free and overall survival in patients randomized to a bypass surgery-first or a balloon angioplasty-first revascularization strategy. J Vasc Surg 2010;51(5 Suppl):5S–17S.

25. Nehler MR, Brass EP, Anthony R, et al. Circulase Investigators. Adjunctive parenteral therapy with lipo-ecraprost, a prostaglandin E1 analog, in patients with critical limb ischemia undergoing distal revascularization does not improve 6-month outcomes. J Vasc Surg 2007;45(discussion 960–1):953–60.

26. Rowe VL, Kumar SR, Glass H, et al. Race Independently Impacts Outcome of Infra-Popliteal Bypass for Symptomatic Arterial Insufficiency. Vasc and Endovas Surg 2007;41:397–401.

27. O'Donnell TFX, Powell C, Deery SE, et al. Regional variation in racial disparities among patients with peripheral artery disease. J Vasc Surg 2018;68(2):519–26.

28. Rivero M, Nader ND, Blochle R, et al. Poorer limb salvage in African American men with chronic limb ischemia is due to advanced clinical stage and higher anatomic complexity at presentation. J Vasc Surg 2016;63(5):1318–24.

29. Holman KH, Henke PK, Dimick JB, et al. Racial disparities in the use of revascularization before leg amputation in Medicare patients. J Vasc Surg 2011;54(2):420–6.

30. Rowe VL, Weaver FA, Lane JS, et al. Racial/Ethnic Differences in Patterns of Treatment Acute PAD in the United States, 1998-2006. J Vasc Surg 2010;51:21S–6S.

31. Hawkins RB, Charles EJ, Mehaffey JH, et al, Virginias Vascular Group. Socioeconomic Distressed Communities Index associated with worse limb-related outcomes after infrainguinal bypass. J Vasc Surg 2019;70(3):786–94.

32. Arya S, Binney Z, Khakharia A, et al. Race and Socioeconomic Status Independently Affect Risk of Major Amputation in Peripheral Artery Disease. J Am Heart Assoc 2018;7(2):e007425.

33. Zierler RE, Jordan WD, Lal BK, et al. The Society for Vascular Surgery practice guidelines on follow-up after vascular surgery arterial procedures. J Vasc Surg 2018;68(1):256–84.

34. Setacci C, Sirignano P, Mazzitelli G, Setacci F, Messina G, Galzerano G, de Donato1 G. Diabetic Foot: Surgical Approach in Emergency International Journal of Vascular Medicine. Int J Vasc Med 2013;2013:296169.

35. Gazoni LM, Carty R, Skinner J, et al. Endoscopic versus open saphenous vein harvest for femoral to below the knee arterial bypass using saphenous vein graft. J Vasc Surg 2006;44(2):282–7.

36. Wartman SM, Woo K, Herscu G, et al. Endoscopic vein harvest for infrainguinal arterial bypass. J Vasc Surg 2013;57(6):1489–94.

37. Santo VJ, Dargon PT, Azarbal AF, et al. Open versus endoscopic great saphenous vein harvest for lower extremity revascularization of critical limb ischemia. J Vasc Surg 2014;59(2):427–34.

38. Eid RE, Wang L, Kuzman M, et al. Endoscopic versus open saphenous vein graft harvest for lower extremity bypass in critical limb ischemia. J Vasc Surg 2014;59(1):136–44.

39. Jauhari YA, Hughes CO, Black SA, et al. Endoscopic vein harvesting in lower extremity arterial bypass: a systematic review. Eur J Vasc Endovasc Surg 2014;47(6):621–39.

40. Teixeira PG, Woo K, Weaver FA, Rowe VL. Vein harvesting technique for infrainguinal arterial bypass with great saphenous vein and its association with surgical site infection and graft patency. J Vasc Surg 2015;61(5):1264–71.

41. Khan SZ, Rivero M, McCraith B, et al. Endoscopic vein harvest does not negatively affect patency of great saphenous vein lower extremity bypass. J Vasc Surg 2016;63(6):1546–54.

42. Mirza AK, Stauffer K, Fleming MD, et al. Endoscopic versus open great saphenous vein harvesting for femoral to popliteal artery bypass. J Vasc Surg 2018; 67(4):1199–206.
43. Kronick M, Liem TK, Jung E, et al. Experienced operators achieve superior patency and wound complication rates with endoscopic great saphenous vein harvest compared with open harvest in lower extremity bypasses. J Vasc Surg 2019;70(5):1534–42.

Advanced Endovascular Techniques for Limb Salvage

Arash Fereydooni, MD, MS, MHS[a], Venita Chandra, MD[a,b],*

KEYWORDS

- Drug-coated balloon • Drug-eluting stent • Intravascular lithotripsy • Atherectomy
- Serrated balloon • Deep venous arterialization • Retrograde pedal access
- Pedal angioplasty

KEY POINTS

- Coupled with drug-coated devices, intravascular lithotripsy, and atherectomy can be useful in the management of long-segment, highly calcified femoropopliteal lesions, and more studies are necessary in determining their utility.
- An array of 0.014-inch platform devices including serrated balloons, intravascular lithotripsy, and dissection stents have been developed specifically for the tibial segment.
- Deep and superficial vein arterialization can be performed through percutaneous, open surgical, or hybrid approaches in no-option chronic limb-threatening ischemia patients with encouraging results for limb salvage.

INTRODUCTION

In recent years, endovascular therapy for the treatment of peripheral artery disease (PAD) has substantially increased in the United States and is performed more commonly than open surgery.[1–3] In the management of chronic limb-threatening ischemia (CLTI), most recent guidelines suggest vein bypass may be preferred for average-risk patients with advanced limb threat and high complexity disease, while those with less complex anatomy, intermediate severity limb threat, or high patient risk may be favored for endovascular intervention.[4,5] With advances in endovascular technology, most PAD lesions are amenable to various endovascular treatment modalities. There are a variety of devices for the treatment of lesions refractory to percutaneous transluminal angioplasty (PTA) in patients who are poor candidates for open bypass. These include devices such as drug-coated balloons and stents, atherectomy, lithotripsy, and so forth as well as advanced techniques involving deep vein arterialization, pedal artery interventions, and retrograde access. This review

^a Division of Vascular and Endovascular Surgery, Department of Surgery, Stanford University, Stanford, CA, USA; ^b Stanford School of Medicine, 780 Welch Road, Palo Alto, CA 94304, USA
* Corresponding author. Stanford School of Medicine, 780 Welch Road, Palo Alto, CA 94304.
E-mail address: vchandra@stanford.edu

Surg Clin N Am 103 (2023) 779–799
https://doi.org/10.1016/j.suc.2023.05.002
0039-6109/23/© 2023 Elsevier Inc. All rights reserved.

surgical.theclinics.com

summarizes current endovascular techniques for de novo and recurrent lower extremity arterial occlusive disease as well as the novel devices and strategies for limb salvage.

DRUG-COATED DEVICES

Most drug-coated devices for the treatment of PAD in the United States are coated with paclitaxel which inhibits neointimal hyperplasia.[6] These are used in aortoiliac and femoropopliteal occlusive disease, which are at high risk for restenosis or reinterventions. Several randomized clinical trials (RCTs) have substantiated the better primary patency and higher rate of freedom from target lesion recurrence (TLR) with drug-coated balloons (DCB) compared to plain balloon angioplasty in the femoropopliteal segment across a wide breadth of lesions and including long term follow-up, up to 5 years.[7–13] This benefit, however, to date has not been demonstrated in the below-the-knee vasculature.[12,14,15]

Similar patency benefits have been seen with DES. The RCT comparing Zilver PTX (Cook Medical, Bloomington, Ind)drug-eluding stent (DES) with PTA in the treatment of femoropopliteal lesions showed that there was a significant increase in 5-year primary patency with drug-eluting stent (DES) and freedom from TLR.[16,17] Covered stents avoid in-growth of neointimal tissue, a drawback of bare metal stents (BMS). A prospective, randomized trial compared heparin-bonded stent grafts with BMS in 141 patients with TASC B, C, or D femoropopliteal disease and demonstrated in lesions greater than 200 mm, heparin-bonded covered stents were associated with statistically greater 12-month primary patency rates and Ankle Brachial Indices (ABIs).[18] Paclitaxel-coated devices came under scrutiny after a meta-analysis of RCTs demonstrated a significant increase in 2-year and 5-year all-cause mortality[19] while another meta-analysis showed increased risk of major amputation for DCBs.[20] However, these findings were not reproducible in multiple studies and after individual analysis of each trial.[21]

Despite promising evidence, tibial revascularization with DES remains a rarely-used technique in the United States due, in part, to lack of a Food and Drug Administration–approved indication. While BMS has shown no advantage over PTA in tibials,[22,23] several studies have shown the superiority of balloon-expanding DES in the tibial segment compared with BMS. Although their use for complex tibial lesions remains off-label in the United States, DES are associated with 23% to 35% increases in 1-year patency and 42% to 50% reductions in odds of amputation when compared to PTA and BMS.[24–31] In patients with complex infrapopliteal lesions, the data remains unclear. A few randomized studies focused on longer lesions have shown minimal to no clinical benefit with DES compared to balloon angioplasty, despite improved angiographic outcomes.[32,33] The multicenter randomized SAVAL study evaluated 1-year primary vessel patency and safety following the use of the Saval DES, which is designed specifically for infrapopliteal interventions.[34] The primary effectiveness endpoint of superior 12-month primary patency was not met – 68% in the DES group and 71% in the PTA group – nor was the major adverse limb-free event – 91.6% and 95.3% respectively for the DES and PTA groups.[34] Therefore, stent placement in the tibial segment should be reserved for situations when balloon angioplasty has not resolved a traumatic or iatrogenic perforation or dissection. Self-expanding stents are preferable in tibial lesions distal to the vessel origin whereas balloon-expandable in areas close to the origin of a tibial vessel for precise deployment.[35] There should be minimal oversizing in the tibial arteries, with sizes typically less than 4 mm.[35] Improved below the knee scaffolds are an unmet clinical need, and we hope to see new technologies designed specifically for complex infrapopliteal disease soon.

ATHERECTOMY

Instead of displacing atheromatous tissue into the vessel wall as in PTA and stenting, atherectomy removes plaque from arteries by vaporizing, shaving, or cutting to acquire luminal gain.[36-39] Atherectomy has been considered a tool to prepare the vessel for definitive treatment. There is a wide number of publications with varied definitions of success and outcomes, but very few comparative studies. Laser ablation atherectomy utilizes a pulsed high-energy ultraviolet beam to vaporize the lesion without damaging the surrounding tissue.[40-42] Several laser atherectomy devices have been approved by the Food and Drug Administration (FDA) for peripheral artery intervention, including Auryon (Angiodynamics), Turbo-Elite, Turbo-Power, Turbo-Tandem, and Turbo-Booster (Spectranetics).[43] Orbital or rotational atherectomy devices have an eccentrically or concentrically-mounted, diamond-coated crown that rotates at high speeds to ablate calcified lesions with each pass of the device.[40] Orbital atherectomy is performed with the Diamondback 360° Orbital Atherectomy System (OAS) (Cardiovascular Systems), Rotablator system (Boston Scientific), Pathway Jetstream PV system (Boston Scientific), and Phoenix atherectomy catheter (Volcano Corporation).[39,44,45] Excisional or directional atherectomy debulks the plaque as the device is advanced across the lesion through rotations of a carbide cutter disc that packs the excised plaque into a nosecone.[36,40] Four excisional systems have been FDA-approved in PAD including the TurboHawk (Medtronic), SilverHawk (Medtronic), HawkOne (Medtronic, **Fig. 1**), and Pantheris Optical Coherence Tomography Imaging Atherectomy System (Avinger).[39] The annual increase in atherectomy utilization in the Vascular Quality Initiative (VQI) registry has been shown to be driven primarily by the use of orbital atherectomy.[46] Despite significant variation in peri-operative outcomes, there is no difference in 1-year primary patency and major ipsilateral amputation rates among the different atherectomy modalities for isolated femoropopliteal revascularization.[46]

In the treatment of infrapopliteal disease, excisional atherectomy is associated with improved 1-year primary patency and major ipsilateral amputation rates compared to laser atherectomy.[46] Atherectomy, however, does come with a higher rate of complications compared to angioplasty alone. Excisional atherectomy in the DEFINITIVE LE study had a 4.2% rate of perforation and bail-out stenting rate of 3.7%.[47]

It is well known that the impact of drug-coated technologies is decreased in heavily calcified vessels.[48] The concept of using atherectomy as a vessel prep for definitive treatment was evaluated by the VIVA REALITY study which assessed the utility of directional atherectomy in 102 patients with long-segment, calcified femoropopliteal lesions followed by treatment with drug-coated balloons.[49] The 12-month primary patency was very promising in these extremely challenging patients at 76.6% and freedom from TLR 92.6% with a provisional stent rate of less than 10%.[49]

Despite the promising data on luminal gain and vessel prep benefits with atherectomy, the utilization of atherectomy has been questioned and plagued by the complexity of the disease, variability of the studies, lack of direct comparative studies as well as variability in practice patterns.[38,50-55] In a recent retrospective observational study, it was shown that in the treatment of femoropopliteal disease, atherectomy is predominantly used in the outpatient setting and is associated with higher incidence of distal embolization than PTA.[56] Atherectomy was associated with a better initial technical success and improved 1-year femoropopliteal primary patency; however,

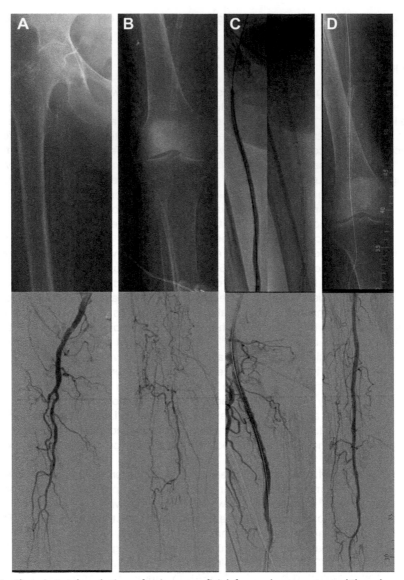

Fig. 1. Chronic total occlusion of prior superficial femoral artery stents (*A*) and proximal popliteal artery (*B*) treated with directional atherectomy of the superficial femoral artery and popliteal artery using a Medtronic Hawk-One device, followed by drug-coated balloon angioplasty of the below and behind knee popliteal artery over an 0.018-inch platform (*C*, *D*). Of note, the use of Hawk-One device for in-stent restenosis is outside of instructions for use.

these changes were not associated with any differences in major amputation or reintervention rate after at 1-year[56] As such, the recent Global Chronic Limb-threatening Ischemia Guidelines do not recommend atherectomy as the preferred endovascular technique for infrainguinal disease owing to its lack of high-quality comparative data to demonstrate its superiority to PTA.[5] The 2018 guidelines from the Society for Cardiovascular Angiography and Interventions recommend the use of atherectomy devices for "adjunctive" lesion preparation purposes in the treatment of femoropopliteal disease.[57] These recommendations are class IIa at best and are based on level C evidence.

ALTERNATE ACCESS

Another promising endovascular approach to complex peripheral lesions is retrograde access. This method allows for crossing lesion from the distal aspect, where plaque morphology may be more amenable to a wire crossing across.[35] It is hypothesized that a "hibernating" (patent) lumen may be present within the space between the proximal and distal caps, with the distal cap easier to cross.[58] The chronic total occlusion (CTO) crossing approach based on plaque cap morphology (CTOP) has been developed.[58] Type I has 2 concave caps when evaluating from the cranial to caudal flow. Type II has a concave proximal cap and a convex distal cap. Type III has a convex proximal and concave distal cap. Type IV has 2 convex caps. It has been shown CTOP type I lesions are easiest to cross in antegrade fashion and type IV the most difficult. Lesion length greater than 10 cm, severe calcification, and CTO types II, III, and IV benefited from retrograde tibio-pedal access (**Fig. 2**).[58]

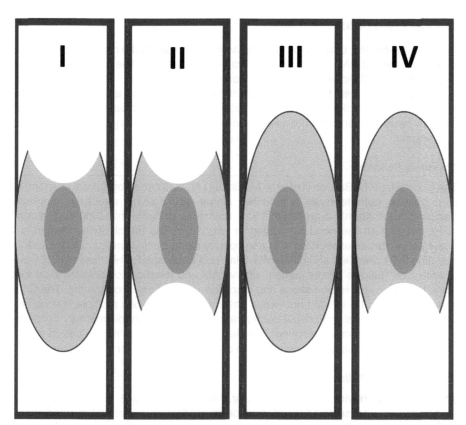

Fig. 2. The chronic total occlusion crossing approach based on plaque cap morphology (CTOP) classification. Type I: concave proximal and distal caps, Type II: concave proximal and convex distal caps, Type III: convex proximal and concave distal caps, Type IV: convex proximal and distal caps.

There have been promising outcomes with retrograde access in tibial segment and similar complication rates as transfemoral access.[59,60] Retrograde access often involves the distal PT and AT and dorsalis pedis using a shortened access needle. Intra-arterial injection of verapamil, nitroglycerin, and heparin mixture can prevent vasospasm and thrombosis. Low-profile sheaths, such as those used in radial access, have outer diameters smaller by one French size and may be used for access. Sheathless access also allows for the use of a catheter instead to facilitate wire exchange. The major concerns with retrograde access during tibial revascularization are dissection, thrombosis, and compromise of a vessel that may be a future distal bypass target.[35] Nonetheless, these complications are reported at low rates in the current literature with an overall rate of less than 2% perioperative complications.[61] Use of atraumatic 0.014-inch wires, minimizing sheath exchanges, and manual pressure to achieve hemostasis are helpful in preserving vessel integrity in retrograde access.[35] In the subintimal arterial flossing with antegrade-retrograde intervention (SAFARI) technique, a subintimal plane is accessed from an antegrade and retrograde approach, and a "flossing" wire maintained in the subintimal plane is used for intervention.[62] Simultaneous double balloon angioplasty to disrupt dividing septum between the two different planes can facilitate through-and-through wire access.[35]

SPECIALTY BALLOONS

In the United States, plain balloon angioplasty has remained the mainstay of endovascular treatment of PAD, particularly in infrapopliteal lesions. The uncontrolled expansion with the standard angioplasty balloon may lead to increased torsional, longitudinal, and radial stresses that can strain the vessel wall and lead to increased incidence of dissection, elastic recoil, and abrupt vessel closure. However, there are now newer options that provide controlled dilatation techniques to mitigate these challenges.

Chocolate Balloon

The Chocolate PTA Balloon (TriReme Medical, LLC, distributed by Cordis Corporation) is a balloon catheter with a mounted nitinol constraining structure specifically designed for uniform, controlled inflation, and rapid deflation resulting in atraumatic dilatation without the need for cutting or scoring.[63] The intent of this design is to disperse the forces associated with angioplasty along the increased contact surface, resulting in a controlled and differential dilatation approach to minimize overall vessel trauma. The "pillows" make contact with vessel and function to minimize local force while the "grooves" relieve stress and stop dissections from propagating. The Chocolate device can be inflated numerous times and used across multiple lesions, as it returns to its original, cylindrical configuration due to the shape memory properties of nitinol, providing rapid deflation. This design is thought to minimize vessel trauma, reduce the rate of dissection, and lead to a decreased need for bailout stenting.[63]

Serrated/Scoring Balloons

The Serranator device (Cagent Vascular, Wayne, PA, USA) is a balloon with 3 embedded external serrated metal strips designed to create linear interrupted scoring patterns during dilation.[64] This mechanism provides a controlled, predictable result in lumen gain while minimizing vessel injury.[64] In the PRELUDE (Prospective Study for the Treatment of Atherosclerotic Lesions in the Superficial Femoral and/or Popliteal Arteries Using the Serranator Device) of 25 patients with femoropopliteal lesions, the 1- and 6-month patency rates were 100% and 64%, respectively.[65] A Serranator balloon for the treatment of the infrapopliteal arteries is currently under investigation.

The Ultrascore Focused Force PTA balloon (BD/Bard Peripheral Vascular, Tempe, AZ, USA) is another available scoring balloon for both above- and below-knee lesions with a 0.014-inch platform and is currently under study.[64] Several reports have also provided encouraging results regarding the safety of AngioSculpt (Philips, Japan, Inc.).[66–68] This device consists of a semi-compliant balloon surrounded by helical nitinol element, the purposes of which are to expand and provide a scoring effect on advanced stenotic lesions. Recently, it has been shown that primary patency after 12 months in patients that underwent a combination of DEB and AngioSculpt was comparable to patients that underwent AngioSculpt balloon angioplasty only.[67] VascuTrak (Bard) is a 0.014-inch semi-compliant balloon that has two longitudinal wires designed to provide concentrated force against plaque at low inflation pressures. The 12-month results of the DCB-Trak registry showed the treatment of 32 femoro-popliteal lesions using VascuTrak scoring-balloon along with DCB had no clinically-driven TLRs after 12 months.[69]

Lithotripsy

Intravascular lithotripsy (IVL) applied a commonly used technology for treating renal calculi to a balloon catheter designed to address calcified vascular lesions. By delivering focused ultrasonic energy via small electrical emitters within a balloon, IVL disrupts the calcium within all the layers of the arterial wall causing microfracture in the calcium and theoretically increasing the compliance of the vessel and enabling balloon angioplasty at a low pressure.[70] IVL is rarely a stand-alone technique and it is used for vessel preparation before another planned intervention, such as PTA, DCB, or stenting. **Fig. 3** shows an example of a patient who underwent revascularization of the superficial femoral artery with IVL and DCB and posterior tibial artery with specialty balloons such as Serranator.

To this date, there is only one RCT comparing IVL to other endovascular modalities. In Disrupt III trial, a comparison of IVL + DCB versus PTA + DCB in 306 patients with femoropopliteal lesions causing claudication or CLTI, IVL proved to have a higher technical success rate (66% v 52%; $P = .02$), and have a higher primary patency at 1 year (80.5% vs 68.0%, $P = .017$).[71] The requirement for provisional stenting was significantly lower in the IVL group (4.6% vs 18.3%, $P < .0001$).[71] Freedom from clinically-driven TLR and restenosis rates were similar between the 2 groups at 1 year.[71] At 2 years, primary patency remained significantly greater in the IVL arm (70.3% vs 51.3%, $P = .003$).[71]

Sub-analysis of the infrapopliteal segment in the larger PAD Disrupt III study demonstrated a residual stenosis less than 50% in 99% of treated lesions and a mean residual stenosis of 23% overall.[72] Analysis of safety profile of IVL in the tibial segment has also shown no major adverse events at 30 days and only one dissection despite use in challenging heavily calcified lesions.[73] The efficacy of IVL in tibial arteries is currently being studied. Disrupt BTK II is a post-market, prospective, multicenter, single-arm study to enroll 250 patients across 40 sites globally that will be followed for 2 years to assess the long-term durability of IVL in this difficult-to-treat patient population.

PEDAL ARTERY INTERVENTIONS

Currently, non-RCT data and expert opinion support pedal artery interventions primarily in patients with CLTI with both tibial and pedal artery disease if optimal healing does not occur after successful tibial artery intervention and those with post-surgical

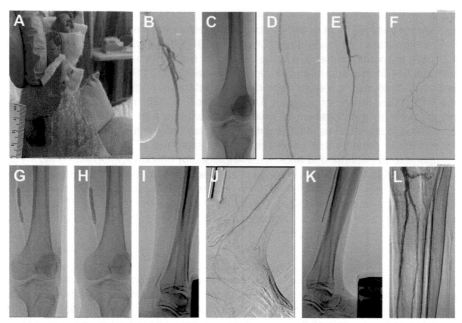

Fig. 3. This is a 78-year-old male with left lateral foot wound, tone-brachial index (TBI:0.41), toe pressure of 53 mm-Hg and monophasic DP and PT waveforms (*A*). On pre-intervention angiography patient had patent proximal superficial femoral artery (SFA), heavily calcified SFA with focal high grade distal SFA lesion (*B-D*) and single vessel peroneal runoff (*E*) with the reconstitution of lateral plantar artery (*F*). The SFA lesion was treated with 6 mm and 7 mm intravascular lithotripsy balloons, followed by 7 mm drug-coated balloon (*G, H*). An 0.014-inch platform Armada XT balloon was used to help cross the posterior tibial (PT) artery lesion (*I*). The entire length of the PT lesion was then treated with a tapered Nanocross balloon (*J*), followed by serration angioplasty 3 mm Serranator balloon (*K*). On completion angiogram patient had two vessel run-offs (PT and peroneal). On follow up patient had a TBI of 0.67, a toe pressure of 78 and triphasic DP and PT waveforms and had healed his wound. (*L*) On completion angiogram patient had two vessel run-offs (PT and peroneal). On follow up patient had a TBI of 0.67, a toe pressure of 78 and triphasic DP and PT waveforms and had healed his wound.

ischemic wounds from forefoot amputations, as surgery may separate the anterior and posterior circulations of the foot.[74–80] Furthermore, in a retrospective review of patients with CLTI, patients with one vessel runoff after revascularization and in-line flow into a patent pedal arch were compared to those with in-line flow to distal end of tibial vessel without direct flow into a patent pedal arch.[81] Patients with in-line flow into a patent pedal arch had a higher amputation-free survival (88.2% vs 65.6%, *P*<.01) as well as better limb salvage rate (98.4% vs 89.3%, *P* = .03).[81] Similarly, in RENDEZVOUS study, a retrospective analysis for the clinical impact of pedal artery revascularization versus non-revascularization strategy for patients with critical limb ischemia, patients who underwent pedal artery angioplasty showed a higher rate of wound healing (57.5% vs 37.3%, *P* = .003) and shorter time to wound healing (211 days vs 365 days; *P* = .008).[82]

Pedal artery interventions use 0.014-inch support catheters, guidewires, and low-profile angioplasty balloons. Pedal artery interventions are typically performed from antegrade access into the common femoral artery using a flexible 6Fr sheath to allow for more pushability and use of two 0.014-inch systems, if needed.[83] Moreover, placing the distal position of the sheath in the P2 or P3 segment of the popliteal artery optimizes the visualization of chronic total occlusion cap morphology, collaterals, and reconstitution points.[83] The antero-posterior fluoroscopy view of the foot should include the proximal first metatarsal interspace and forefoot in order to show the pedal-plantar loop passing from the dorsal portion to the plantar portion, along with the origins of the tarsal arteries. The lateral oblique view must project the fifth meta-tarsal bone outward from the base of the foot and include the heel and proximal fore-foot to visualize common planter artery bifurcation into the medial and lateral plantar arteries as well as dorsalis pedis artery and the pedal plantar loop.[84]

In the pedal-plantar loop access technique, the plantar arcade is accessed from a patent tibial artery to recanalize an occluded AT or PT in a retrograde fashion.[85] This technique has a technical success rate up to 85%.[85,86] Intraluminal recanalization is necessary as subintimal recanalization is associated with branch exclusion in this area. Hydrophilic 0.014-inch wires are typically used in combination with tapered small-diameter balloons inflated for prolonged duration of approximately 3 minutes.[35] Surveillance after pedal artery intervention is of utmost importance. In addition to the conventional noninvasive testing (eg, ABI, duplex ultrasound, and transcutaneous ox-ygen pressure), pedal acceleration time studies can also be used. This technique uses duplex ultrasound to directly visualize the pedal arch, delineate the pedal artery anat-omy, and determine pedal flow hemodynamics. This method has been shown to correlate with ABI and toe-brachial index (TBI) measurements and predict wound healing.[87,88]

Not all patients are candidates for pedal arch angioplasty. Several studies have shown the impact of pedal arch quality on tissue loss and time to healing in patients undergoing infrainguinal endovascular revascularization.[89] There is a strong associa-tion between medial arterial calcification (MAC) of the foot arteries and metatarsal ar-tery obstruction, suggesting that advanced MAC is associated with blood flow restriction to the forefoot.[90] Small artery disease (SAD) and MAC are considered ex-pressions of the same obstructing disease, adversely impacting the fate of CLTI pa-tients.[91] Patients with SAD and high MAC scores are more likely to have adverse limb events than those with big artery disease (BAD) of foot.[90,91] Therefore, in patients with end-stage renal disease and long-standing diabetes mellitus who tend to have significant occlusive SAD and extensive MAC, pedal angioplasty may not be success-ful and these patients may be better served with venous arterialization procedures (**Fig. 4**).

VENOUS ARTERIALIZATION

Up to 20% of patients with CLTI are considered "no-option CLTI," as they do not have an adequate bypass conduit and have occlusive disease of pedal arteries – a "desert" foot.[92] Patients with no-option CLTI often progress to amputation and have a reported lower quality of life than patients who have revascularization options.[93] Deep vein arterialization (DVA) has been reserved for select patients as last attempt to avoid ma-jor amputation. DVA delivers arterial blood flow to the healthy venous bed in the foot to facilitate wound healing. This can be done via open surgical, endovascular, or hybrid approach. Studies have demonstrated a 71% to 75% limb salvage rate at 12 months and 46% secondary patency rate at 12 months in patients undergoing DVA.[94,95] Often, the initiation of clinically apparent wound healing takes place several weeks after DVA. Reported angiographic changes include the development of a wound blush around week 2 that continues to improve for 4 to 8 weeks post-procedure.[96] There is

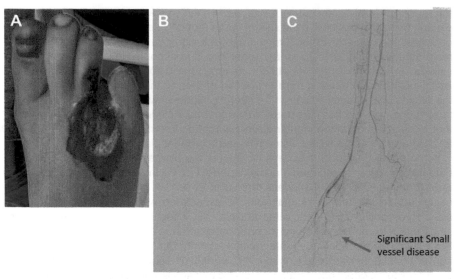

Fig. 4. (A) This is 45-year-old male with type I diabetes and end-stage renal disease status-post-successful renal transplantation who has had a non-healing forefoot ulcer. (B, C) He underwent angioplasty of anterior and posterior tibial arteries as well as angioplasty of dorsalis pedis artery and deep plantar arteries. However, given the extensive medial arterial calcification and small arterial disease, the revascularization attempt was not successful. Deep vein arterialization was offered but patient declined and elected to undergo primary below knee amputation of his right leg.

persistent improvement in wound healing that continues to occur even after thrombosis of the DVA, supporting the hypothesis that DVA may promotes wound healing through neovascularization.[92]

In preoperative evaluation, a venous duplex ultrasound of the lower extremity is necessary to assess for a patent and complete venous arch, confirm adequate vein diameter of 2.5 to 3 mm and rule out deep vein thrombosis.[92] The medial marginal vein fills the greater saphenous vein (GSV) while lateral plantar vein fills posterior tibial vein and dorsal venous arch. Due to the long period between the DVA procedure and initiation of wound healing, native arterial flow to the distal extremity should be preserved.[92] Thus, in patients with single vessel runoff, proximal recanalization of an occluded tibial vessel may be necessary to provide additional arterial inflow site for DVA, while maintaining native arterial flow.[92]

Open surgical DVA consists of a surgical arteriovenous bypass with mechanical disruption of the pedal venous valves. The common femoral artery, superficial femoral artery, popliteal artery, and proximal tibial arteries can all be used for arterial inflow. Described conduits include GSV, polytetrafluoroethylene with vein patch or cephalic vein.[97] Distal venous targets include the posterior tibial vein and dorsal venous arch. The vein conduit can be fashioned in a reversed manner or in situ with valve lysis. The valves distal to the bypass anastomosis and in the pedal arch must be disrupted by retrograde ballooning, valvulotome, dilators, direct valvulectomy, and cutting balloons. **Fig. 5** shows open DVA procedure involving a connection between the posterior tibial vein at the ankle and the below knee popliteal artery. While waiting for the arterialization of the venous system to occur, post-operative wound care involves negative pressure therapy, offloading, and topical products.[97] Approximately 5 to 7 days after the completion of open DVA, the proximal posterior tibial vein can be ligated to prevent

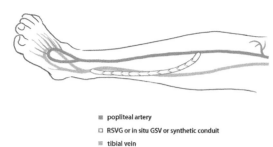

- popliteal artery
- RSVG or in situ GSV or synthetic conduit
- tibial vein

Fig. 5. Depiction of open surgical deep venous arterialization (DVA) procedure with bypass from proximal arterial inflow to distal venous target with reversed saphenous vein graft (*RSVG*), in situ great saphenous vein (*GSV*), or synthetic conduit. (*From* Ho VT, Gologorsky R, Kibrik P, et al. Open, percutaneous, and hybrid deep venous arterialization technique for no-option foot salvage. J Vasc Surg. 2020;71(6):2152-2160; with permission.)

arterial steal from the foot and cardiac overload.[97] In hybrid DVA approach, an open surgical bypass (in situ or reversed GSV) is created with the typical proximal arterial and distal venous anastomoses, but the valvulotomy or embolization of distal collateral venous branches is performed through an endovascular approach as opposed to use of valvulotome during an open surgical DVA.[97]

Endovascular DVA can be performed using off-the-shelf devices or the LimFlow system (LimFlow SA, Paris, France), which is currently in clinical trials in the United States. In endovascular DVA, tibial vessels are used as arterial inflow sites to allow maintenance of antegrade flow to the leg. The venous access site is the posterior tibial vein or peroneal vein via the lateral plantar vein. An 0.014-inch wire is advanced into the posterior tibial vein followed by the placement of 4/5Fr sheath. Ipsilateral femoral artery is also accessed using a 7Fr sheath and the inflow tibial vessel is selected. A simultaneous angiogram and venogram is performed to identify the optimal crossover point. A crossing device or LimFlow system can be used for arterial to venous crossover, often involving a needle deployed from the arterial catheter into the vein. The site of the arteriovenous fistula is balloon dilated.[97] The valves through the midfoot and pedal venous arch are disrupted.[97] Distally, a self-expanding, covered stent graft is deployed to below the medial malleolus (**Fig. 6**).[97] This typically occludes the large venous branches near the ankle and heel. If there is a concern for a steal phenomenon via retrograde arterial blood flow diversion, the early outflow veins that branch off of the posterior tibial veins in the foot can be occluded to increase resistance in the venous outflow bed.[97] The international multicenter study of the LimFlow device in 32 patients with no-option CLTI demonstrated a 97% technical success rate, limb salvage rate of 79.8%, wound healing rate of 72.7% at 24 months and 45% reintervention rate for the recanalization of occluded DVA.[98] Results from the PROMISE I trial, to evaluate safety and efficacy of the LimFlow system in the United States, showed a technical success of 100%, with all of patients experiencing greater than 50% wound healing and 40% patency at 6 months.[99] The recently published PROMISE II trial enrolled 105 with CLTI who underwent DVA with LimFlow System. These patients had 99% technical success with 66.1% amputation-free survival at 6 months, limb-salvage rate of 76%, and complete wounds healing rate of 25%.[100]

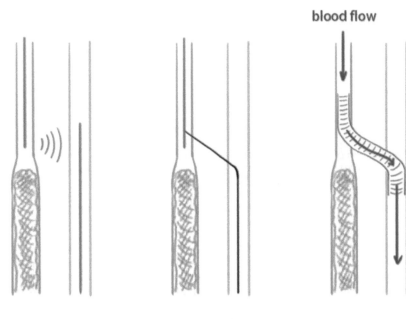

blood flow

1. Catheters are aligned with ultrasound signal

2. Crossover and insertion of guidewire

3. Predilatation and insertion of covered stent

Fig. 6. Depiction of percutaneous deep venous arterialization procedure with retrograde venous access and antegrade arterial access to place bridging stent. (*From* Ho VT, Gologorsky R, Kibrik P, et al. Open, percutaneous, and hybrid deep venous arterialization technique for no-option foot salvage. J Vasc Surg. 2020;71(6):2152-2160; with permission.)

RISING INNOVATIVE TECHNOLOGY

Intravascular ultrasound (IVUS) provides a cross-sectional view of the artery with the visualization of plaque burden and morphology, luminal diameter, and true lumen re-entry after chronic total occlusion recanalization.[101] This technology is available in 0.014- and 0.018-inch platform, extending its utility to the infrapopliteal region. Studies have shown luminal discrepancy in angiographic and IVUS images after angioplasty or stenting.[102] A recent meta-analysis comparing IVUS-guided peripheral vascular intervention and angiography-guided peripheral vascular intervention found comparable primary patency, TLR, and amputation rates, but decreased rates of periprocedural complications, such as dissection or perforation with IVUS use.[102] There was no difference in amputation or mortality.

Tack Endovascular System is another rising technology for the treatment of focal dissections. Mechanical dilatation with angioplasty results in controlled dissections in up to nearly one-third of infrapopliteal lesions.[103] Dissections are thought to lead to procedural complications and restenosis.[104,105] Treatment of post-PTA dissections in the infrapopliteal arteries typically involves prolonged secondary balloon inflations and/or placement of a coronary stent, the latter of which remains off-label in the United States and is prone to fracture.[28,29] The Tack Endovascular System is self-expanding implant designed to exert a low outward radial force to create focal tissue apposition with a reduction in metal burden relative to stents due to their short longitudinal length and open-cell design. The TOBA II BTK trial (Tack Optimized Balloon Angioplasty Study of the Tack Endovascular System in Below the Knee Arteries) reported a 24-month amputation-free survival rate of 92.2% and 24-month freedom from clinically-driven TLR of 73.6%.[106,107]

Bioabsorbable scaffolds are another drug delivery modality that forgo permanent stent placement. The Absorb Esprit Everolimus-eluting Bioresorbable Vascular Scaffold (Abbott Vascular, Santa Clara, CA, USA) is a fully biodegradable polymer that provides a controlled release of everolimus through hydrolysis.[108] In the infrapopliteal arteries, this device has demonstrated a 2-year primary patency of 90.3% and restenosis of 8%.[109] In ESPRIT I study of 35 patients with external iliac artery and superficial femoral artery disease, the technical success was 100% and at 2 years, there were no amputations, with a stenosis rate of 16.1% and TLR of 8.8%.[110] The LIFE-BTK trial is currently underway and will randomize patients to receive the Espirit everolimus bioresorbable scaffold or PTA in the infrapopliteal arteries.[64]

The Temporary Spur Stent System is a novel retrievable stent designed for the treatment of severely calcified infrapopliteal disease using a series of radially expandable spikes that create multiple channels to deliver antiproliferative drugs for increased uptake into the vessel wall.[111] This device is not FDA-approved and currently has breakthrough device designation. DEEPEROUS is a 100-patient prospective, non-randomized, and multicenter trial that will assess the safety and efficacy of the Temporary Spur Stent System compared against meta-analysis of published data for PTA in treating patients with infrapopliteal disease.

VALUE AND COST OF DRUG-ELUTING TECHNOLOGY

Despite the promising results with drug-eluting technology, questions remain regarding the value and cost of these devices owing to their higher initial cost.[112] Reinterventions, on the other hand, are quite costly and the potential for decreased reintervention rates over time with drug-eluting technology may lead to cost-savings despite the increased initial cost.[113] The value of rising endovascular technology should be assessed based on its outcomes (improved patency and TLR), appropriateness of use (safety and correct indications such as the inhibition of restenosis cascade In claudication and CLTI) and patient experience (ambulation, wound healing, amputation rate, and quality of life). A retrospective analysis of data from the Florida State Ambulatory Database, using peripheral intervention model that assumed an 8% per year transition from BMS to DES, showed cost savings of more than 1.6 million dollars over 5 years when compared with a model that assumed only BMS were used.[114] In a prospective economic analysis of DCB versus PTA for femoropopliteal lesions in patients with claudication, the decision analytical cost-effectiveness model demonstrated that DCB was economically dominant with projected 2-year cost savings of $576 and gain in quality-adjusted life-year (QALY) of 0.01 years. In a metanalysis of 7 RCTs, DCB was the most cost-effective strategy for endovascular intervention in the SFA.[115] The incremental cost-effectiveness ratio (ICER) between DCB and DES was largely driven by cost differences of device rather than patency. However, the use of more than one DCB per procedure was no longer cost-effective compared to DES.[115]

In a decision-analytic Markov model using Dutch and German reimbursement data, it was shown that compared to PTA, use of DCB for treating femoropopliteal disease in patient with CLTI is associated with improved patient outcomes and expected overall cost savings to payers in the Dutch and German healthcare systems, rendering it a cost-effective and likely dominant treatment strategy.[116] In a similar study of UK's National Health Service, a decision analytical model over 24 month period demonstrated that use of DCB or DES for femoropopliteal disease improved reintervention rate and in result improved QALY and ICER over POBA/BMS.[117]

In 2018, the Centers for Medicare and Medicaid Services (CMS) ended the transitional pass-through add-on payment for DCB, without creating a new ambulatory payment classification rate for these devices.[118] Since DCB is more expensive, but reimbursed the same as PTA devices, healthcare systems may still benefit from no readmission and reduction in costs and amputation rates. However, there may be less direct benefit in outpatient settings and this will pose a challenge to the quality of vascular care provided, as growing number of interventions are performed in office-based setting.[118] While Drug-eluting technologies appear to be cost-effective across a variety of health systems for both claudication and CLTI, the CMS decision unfortunately confers little to no financial benefit to using the most effective and advanced technology and places the financial burden of providing appropriate care on hospitals and physicians.

SUMMARY

As the number of patients with CLTI is increasing, new endovascular revascularization strategies beyond the mostly plain balloon-based technologies may provide new solutions. Coupled with drug-coated devices, IVL, and atherectomy can be useful in the management of long-segment, highly calcified femoropopliteal lesions. An array of 0.014-inch platform devices including serrated balloons, IVL, and dissection stents have been developed specifically for the tibial segment. Deep and superficial vein arterialization can be performed through a percutaneous, open surgical, or hybrid approaches in no-option CLTI patients with encouraging results for limb salvage.

DISCLOSURE

Dr V. Chandra: Cook Medical, Medtronic, Alucent Medical, Shockwave Medical, Penumbra, Gore.

REFERENCES

1. Goodney PP, Beck AW, Nagle J, et al. National trends in lower extremity bypass surgery, endovascular interventions, and major amputations. J Vasc Surg 2009; 50(1):54–60.

2. Thomas MP, Jung Park Y, Grey S, et al. Temporal trends in peripheral arterial interventions: Observations from the blue cross blue shield of Michigan cardiovascular consortium (BMC2 PVI). Catheter Cardiovasc Interv 2017;89(4): 728–34.

3. Siracuse JJ, Menard MT, Eslami MH, et al. Comparison of open and endovascular treatment of patients with critical limb ischemia in the Vascular Quality Initiative. J Vasc Surg 2016;63(4):958–65.e951.

4. Farber A, Menard MT, Conte MS, et al. Surgery or Endovascular Therapy for Chronic Limb-Threatening Ischemia. N Engl J Med 2022;387(25):2305–16.

5. Conte MS, Bradbury AW, Kolh P, et al. Global vascular guidelines on the management of chronic limb-threatening ischemia. J Vasc Surg 2019;69(6, Supplement):3S–125S.e140.

6. Mills JL, Conte MS, Murad MH. Critical review and evidence implications of paclitaxel drug-eluting balloons and stents in peripheral artery disease. J Vasc Surg 2019;70(1):3–7.

7. Iida O, Soga Y, Urasawa K, et al. Drug-coated balloon vs standard percutaneous transluminal angioplasty for the treatment of atherosclerotic lesions in the superficial femoral and proximal popliteal arteries: one-year results of the MDT-2113 SFA Japan randomized trial. J Endovasc Ther 2018;25(1):109–17.

8. Osheiba MA, Khan S. TCTAP C-024 The Use of Intravascular Lithotripsy and Intravascular Ultrasound to Aid Percutaneous Coronary Intervention to a Calcific Vein Graft. J Am Coll Cardiol 2021;77(14_Supplement):S85–7.

9. Iida O, Soga Y, Urasawa K, et al. Drug-coated balloon versus uncoated percutaneous transluminal angioplasty for the treatment of atherosclerotic lesions in the superficial femoral and proximal popliteal artery: 2-year results of the MDT-2113 SFA Japan randomized trial. Catheter Cardiovasc Interv 2019; 93(4):664–72.

10. Laird JR, Schneider PA, Tepe G, et al. Durability of treatment effect using a drug-coated balloon for femoropopliteal lesions: 24-month results of IN. PACT SFA. J Am Coll Cardiol 2015;66(21):2329–38.

11. Laird JA, Schneider PA, Jaff MR, et al. Long-term clinical effectiveness of a drug-coated balloon for the treatment of femoropopliteal lesions: five-year outcomes from the IN. PACT SFA randomized trial. Circulation: Cardiovasc Interv 2019;12(6):e007702.

12. Schneider PA, Laird JR, Tepe G, et al. Treatment effect of drug-coated balloons is durable to 3 years in the femoropopliteal arteries: long-term results of the IN. PACT SFA randomized trial. Circ Cardiovasc Interv 2018;11(1):e005891.

13. Brodmann M, Werner M, Meyer D-R, et al. Sustainable antirestenosis effect with a low-dose drug-coated balloon: the ILLUMENATE European randomized clinical trial 2-year results. JACC Cardiovasc Interv 2018;11(23):2357–64.

14. Zeller T, Beschorner U, Pilger E, et al. Paclitaxel-coated balloon in infrapopliteal arteries: 12-month results from the BIOLUX P-II randomized trial (BIOTRONIK'S-first in man study of the Passeo-18 LUX drug releasing PTA balloon catheter vs. the uncoated Passeo-18 PTA balloon catheter in subjects requiring revascularization of infrapopliteal arteries). JACC Cardiovasc Interv 2015;8(12):1614–22.

15. Zeller T, Baumgartner I, Scheinert D, et al. Drug-eluting balloon versus standard balloon angioplasty for infrapopliteal arterial revascularization in critical limb ischemia: 12-month results from the IN. PACT DEEP randomized trial. J Am Coll Cardiol 2014;64(15):1568–76.

16. Dake MD, Ansel GM, Jaff MR, et al. Durable clinical effectiveness with paclitaxel-eluting stents in the femoropopliteal artery: 5-year results of the Zilver PTX randomized trial. Circulation 2016;133(15):1472–83.

17. Müller-Hülsbeck S, Benko A, Soga Y, et al. Two-year efficacy and safety results from the IMPERIAL randomized study of the eluvia polymer-coated drug-eluting stent and the zilver PTX polymer-free drug-coated stent. Cardiovasc Intervent Radiol 2021;44(3):368–75.

18. Lammer J, Zeller T, Hausegger KA, et al. Heparin-bonded covered stents versus bare-metal stents for complex femoropopliteal artery lesions: the randomized VIASTAR trial (Viabahn endoprosthesis with PROPATEN bioactive surface [VIA] versus bare nitinol stent in the treatment of long lesions in superficial femoral artery occlusive disease). J Am Coll Cardiol 2013;62(15):1320–7.

19. Katsanos K, Spiliopoulos S, Kitrou P, et al. Risk of death following application of paclitaxel-coated balloons and stents in the femoropopliteal artery of the leg: a

systematic review and meta-analysis of randomized controlled trials. J Am Heart Assoc 2018;7(24):e011245.

20. Katsanos K, Spiliopoulos S, Teichgräber U, et al. Editor's Choice - Risk of Major Amputation Following Application of Paclitaxel Coated Balloons in the Lower Limb Arteries: A Systematic Review and Meta-Analysis of Randomised Controlled Trials. Eur J Vasc Endovasc Surg 2022;63(1):60–71.

21. Behrendt C-A, Sedrakyan A, Peters F, et al. Editor's choice–long term survival after femoropopliteal artery revascularisation with paclitaxel coated devices: a propensity score matched cohort analysis. Eur J Vasc Endovasc Surg 2020; 59(4):587–96.

22. Hsu CCT, Kwan GN, Singh D, et al. Angioplasty versus stenting for infrapopliteal arterial lesions in chronic limb-threatening ischaemia. Cochrane Database Syst Rev 2018;(12):CD009195.

23. Wu R, Yao C, Wang S, et al. Percutaneous transluminal angioplasty versus primary stenting in infrapopliteal arterial disease: a meta-analysis of randomized trials. J Vasc Surg 2014;59(6):1711–20.

24. Katsanos K, Kitrou P, Spiliopoulos S, et al. Comparative effectiveness of plain balloon angioplasty, bare metal stents, drug-coated balloons, and drug-eluting stents for the treatment of infrapopliteal artery disease: systematic review and Bayesian network meta-analysis of randomized controlled trials. J Endovasc Ther 2016;23(6):851–63.

25. Fusaro M, Cassese S, Ndrepepa G, et al. Drug-eluting stents for revascularization of infrapopliteal arteries: updated meta-analysis of randomized trials. JACC Cardiovasc Interv 2013;6(12):1284–93.

26. Almasri J, Adusumalli J, Asi N, et al. A systematic review and meta-analysis of revascularization outcomes of infrainguinal chronic limb-threatening ischemia. J Vasc Surg 2019;69(6):126S–36S.

27. Fereydooni A, Bai H, Baril D, et al. Embolic Protection Devices are Not Associated with Improved Outcomes of Atherectomy for Lower Extremity Revascularization. Ann Vasc Surg 2022;86:168–76.

28. Huntress LA, Fereydooni A, Dardik A, et al. Endovascular Revascularization Incorporating Infrapopliteal Coronary Drug-Eluting Stents Improves Clinical Outcomes in Patients with Critical Limb Ischemia and Tissue Loss. Ann Vasc Surg 2020;63:234–40.

29. Bosiers M, Scheinert D, Peeters P, et al. Randomized comparison of everolimus-eluting versus bare-metal stents in patients with critical limb ischemia and infrapopliteal arterial occlusive disease. J Vasc Surg 2012;55(2):390–8.

30. Rastan A, Brechtel K, Krankenberg H, et al. Sirolimus-eluting stents for treatment of infrapopliteal arteries reduce clinical event rate compared to bare-metal stents: long-term results from a randomized trial. J Am Coll Cardiol 2012;60(7):587–91.

31. Hicks CW, Canner JK, Lum YW, et al. Drug-eluting stents are associated with improved outcomes for the treatment of infrainguinal bypass graft stenoses. J Vasc Surg 2019;69(3):875–82.

32. Scheinert D, Katsanos K, Zeller T, et al. A prospective randomized multicenter comparison of balloon angioplasty and infrapopliteal stenting with the sirolimus-eluting stent in patients with ischemic peripheral arterial disease: 1-year results from the ACHILLES trial. J Am Coll Cardiol 2012;60(22):2290–5.

33. Siablis D, Kitrou PM, Spiliopoulos S, et al. Paclitaxel-coated balloon angioplasty versus drug-eluting stenting for the treatment of infrapopliteal long-segment

arterial occlusive disease: the IDEAS randomized controlled trial. JACC Cardiovasc Interv 2014;7(9):1048–56.

34. CIRSE. SAVAL trial finds no gains with custom drug-eluting stents in PAD below the knee. Vascular News 2022;5685.
35. Feldman ZM, Mohapatra A. Endovascular management of complex tibial lesions. Semin Vasc Surg 2022;35(2):190–9.
36. Franzone A, Ferrone M, Carotenuto G, et al. The role of atherectomy in the treatment of lower extremity peripheral artery disease. BMC Surg 2012;12(1):S13.
37. Shafique S, Nachreiner RD, Murphy MP, et al. Recanalization of Infrainguinal Vessels: Silverhawk, Laser, and the Remote Superficial Femoral Artery Endarterectomy. Semin Vasc Surg 2007;20(1):29–36.
38. Engelberger S, van den Berg JC. Atherectomy in complex infrainguinal lesions: a review. J Cardiovasc Surg 2015;56(1):43–54.
39. Bhat TM, Afari ME, Garcia LA. Atherectomy in Peripheral Artery Disease: A Review. J Invasive Cardiol 2017;29(4):135–44.
40. Akkus NI, Abdulbaki A, Jimenez E, et al. Atherectomy devices: technology update. Med Devices (Auckl) 2014;8:1–10.
41. DeBakey ME. Endovascular therapy: principles of peripheral interventions. John Wiley & Sons; 2008.
42. Taylor KD, Reiser C. From Laser Physics to Clinical Utilization: Design and Ablative Properties of Cardiovascular Laser Catheters. In: Topaz O, editor. Lasers in Cardiovascular interventions. London: Springer London; 2015. p. 1–14.
43. Giannopoulos S, Kokkinidis DG, Jawaid O, et al. Turbo-power™ laser atherectomy combined with drug-coated balloon angioplasty is associated with improved one-year outcomes for the treatment of Tosaka II and III femoropopliteal in-stent restenosis. Cardiovasc Revasc Med 2020;21(6):771–8.
44. Topfer LA, Spry C. New Technologies for the Treatment of Peripheral Artery Disease. 2018. In: CADTH Issues in Emerging Health Technologies. Ottawa (ON): Canadian Agency for Drugs and Technologies in. Health 2016;172.
45. Zeller T, Krankenberg H, Steinkamp H, et al. One-Year Outcome of Percutaneous Rotational Atherectomy with Aspiration in Infrainguinal Peripheral Arterial Occlusive Disease: The Multicenter Pathway PVD Trial. J Endovasc Ther 2009; 16(6):653–62.
46. Bai H, Fereydooni A, Zhang Y, et al. Trends In Utilization and Outcomes of Orbital, Laser, and Excisional Atherectomy for Lower Extremity Revascularization. J Endovasc Ther 2022;29(3):389–401.
47. McKinsey JF, Zeller T, Rocha-Singh KJ, et al. Lower Extremity Revascularization Using Directional Atherectomy. 12-Month Prospective Results of the DEFINITIVE LE Study. JACC Cardiovasc Interv 2014;7(8):923–33.
48. Fanelli F, Cannavale A, Gazzetti M, et al. Calcium Burden Assessment and Impact on Drug-Eluting Balloons in Peripheral Arterial Disease. Cardiovasc Intervent Radiol 2014;37(4):898–907.
49. Rocha-Singh KJ, Sachar R, DeRubertis BG, et al. Directional atherectomy before paclitaxel coated balloon angioplasty in complex femoropopliteal disease: the VIVA REALITY study. Catheter Cardiovasc Interv 2021;98(3):549–58.
50. Katsanos K, Spiliopoulos S, Reppas L, et al. Debulking Atherectomy in the Peripheral Arteries: Is There a Role and What is the Evidence? Cardiovasc Intervent Radiol 2017;40(7):964–77.
51. Panaich SS, Arora S, Patel N, et al. In-Hospital Outcomes of Atherectomy During Endovascular Lower Extremity Revascularization. Am J Cardiol 2016;117(4): 676–84.

52. Ambler GK, Radwan R, Hayes PD, et al. Atherectomy for peripheral arterial disease. Cochrane Database Syst Rev 2014;3:Cd006680.
53. Diamantopoulos A, Katsanos K. Atherectomy of the femoropopliteal artery: a systematic review and meta-analysis of randomized controlled trials. J Cardiovasc Surg 2014;55(5):655–65.
54. Todd KE Jr, Ahanchi SS, Maurer CA, et al. Atherectomy offers no benefits over balloon angioplasty in tibial interventions for critical limb ischemia. J Vasc Surg 2013;58(4):941–8.
55. Ramkumar N, Martinez-Camblor P, Columbo JA, et al. Adverse Events After Atherectomy: Analyzing Long-Term Outcomes of Endovascular Lower Extremity Revascularization Techniques. J Am Heart Assoc 2019;8(12):e012081.
56. Bai H, Fereydooni A, Zhuo H, et al. Comparison of Atherectomy to Balloon Angioplasty and Stenting for Isolated Femoropopliteal Revascularization. Ann Vasc Surg 2020;69:261–73.
57. Feldman DN, Armstrong EJ, Aronow HD, et al. SCAI consensus guidelines for device selection in femoral-popliteal arterial interventions. Catheter Cardiovasc Interv 2018;92(1):124–40.
58. Saab F, Jaff MR, Diaz-Sandoval LJ, et al. Chronic Total Occlusion Crossing Approach Based on Plaque Cap Morphology: The CTOP Classification. J Endovasc Ther 2018;25(3):284–91.
59. El-Sayed H, Bennett ME, Loh TM, et al. Retrograde pedal access and endovascular revascularization: a safe and effective technique for high-risk patients with complex tibial vessel disease. Ann Vasc Surg 2016;31:91–8.
60. Perry M, Callas PW, Alef MJ, et al. Outcomes of peripheral vascular interventions via retrograde pedal access for chronic limb-threatening ischemia in a multi-center registry. J Endovasc Ther 2020;27(2):205–10.
61. El-Sayed HF. Retrograde pedal/tibial artery access for treatment of infragenicular arterial occlusive disease. Methodist Debakey Cardiovasc J 2013;9(2):73–8.
62. Spinosa DJ, Harthun NL, Bissonette EA, et al. Subintimal arterial flossing with antegrade–retrograde intervention (SAFARI) for subintimal recanalization to treat chronic critical limb ischemia. J Vasc Interv Radiol 2005;16(1):37–44.
63. Mustapha JA, Lansky A, Shishehbor M, et al. A prospective, multi-center study of the chocolate balloon in femoropopliteal peripheral artery disease: The Chocolate BAR registry. Catheter Cardiovasc Interv 2018;91(6):1144–8.
64. Kim TI, Schneider PA. New Innovations and Devices in the Management of Chronic Limb-Threatening Ischemia. J Endovasc Ther 2020;27(4):524–39.
65. Holden A, Hill A, Walker A, et al. PRELUDE Prospective Study of the Serranator Device in the Treatment of Atherosclerotic Lesions in the Superficial Femoral and Popliteal Arteries. J Endovasc Ther 2019;26(1):18–25.
66. Sato R, Sato T, Shirasawa Y, et al. A case series of favorable vessel dilatation using a nitinol scoring element-equipped helical balloon catheter (AngioSculpt®). J Vasc Access 2019;20(1_suppl):93–6.
67. Lugenbiel I, Grebner M, Zhou Q, et al. Treatment of femoropopliteal lesions with the AngioSculpt scoring balloon - results from the Heidelberg PANTHER registry. Vasa 2018;47(1):49–55.
68. Kronlage M, Werner C, Dufner M, et al. Long-term outcome upon treatment of calcified lesions of the lower limb using scoring angioplasty balloon (AngioSculpt™). Clin Res Cardiol 2020;109(9):1177–85.
69. Baumhäkel M, Chkhetia S, Kindermann M. Treatment of femoro-popliteal lesions with scoring and drug-coated balloon angioplasty: 12-month results of the DCB-Trak registry. Diagn Interv Radiol 2018;24(3):153–7.

70. Dini CS, Tomberli B, Mattesini A, et al. Intravascular lithotripsy for calcific coronary and peripheral artery stenoses. EuroIntervention 2019;15(8):714–21.

71. Tepe G, Brodmann M, Bachinsky W, et al. Intravascular Lithotripsy for Peripheral Artery Calcification: Mid-term Outcomes From the Randomized Disrupt PAD III Trial. JACC Cardiovascu Interv 2022;1(4):100341.

72. Adams G, Soukas PA, Mehrle A, et al. Intravascular lithotripsy for treatment of calcified infrapopliteal lesions: results from the disrupt PAD III observational study. J Endovasc Ther 2022;29(1):76–83.

73. Brodmann M, Holden A, Zeller T. Safety and feasibility of intravascular lithotripsy for treatment of below-the-knee arterial stenoses. J Endovasc Ther 2018;25(4): 499–503.

74. Azuma N, Uchida H, Kokubo T, et al. Factors influencing wound healing of critical ischaemic foot after bypass surgery: is the angiosome important in selecting bypass target artery? Eur J Vasc Endovasc Surg 2012;43(3):322–8.

75. Varela C, Acín F, de Haro J, et al. The role of foot collateral vessels on ulcer healing and limb salvage after successful endovascular and surgical distal procedures according to an angiosome model. Vasc Endovasc Surg 2010;44(8): 654–60.

76. Alexandrescu V, Hubermont G. The challenging topic of diabetic foot revascularization: does the angiosome-guided angioplasty may improve outcome. J Cardiovasc Surg 2012;53(1):3–12.

77. Iida O, Nanto S, Uematsu M, et al. Importance of the angiosome concept for endovascular therapy in patients with critical limb ischemia. Catheter Cardiovasc Interv 2010;75(6):830–6.

78. Neville RF, Attinger CE, Bulan EJ, et al. Revascularization of a specific angiosome for limb salvage: does the target artery matter? Ann Vasc Surg 2009; 23(3):367–73.

79. Huizing E, Schreve MA, de Vries J-PP, et al. Below-the-ankle angioplasty in patients with critical limb ischemia: a systematic review and meta-analysis. J Vasc Interv Radiol 2019;30(9):1361–8.e2.

80. Palena LM, Manzi M. Techniques for Successful BTK Revascularization. An overview of BTK vessel anatomy, related angiosomes, and techniques for optimal outcomes. Endovascular Today 2019;18(5).

81. Higashimori A, Iida O, Yamauchi Y, et al. Outcomes of One straight-line flow with and without pedal arch in patients with critical limb ischemia. Catheter Cardiovasc Interv 2016;87(1):129–33.

82. Nakama T, Watanabe N, Haraguchi T, et al. Clinical Outcomes of Pedal Artery Angioplasty for Patients With Ischemic Wounds: Results From the Multicenter RENDEZVOUS Registry. JACC Cardiovasc Interv 2017;10(1):79–90.

83. Tummala S, Briley K. Advanced limb salvage: Pedal artery interventions. Semin Vasc Surg 2022;35(2):200–9.

84. Manzi M, Cester G, Palena LM, et al. Vascular imaging of the foot: the first step toward endovascular recanalization. Radiographics 2011;31(6):1623–36.

85. Gandini R, Del Giudice C, Simonetti G. Pedal and plantar loop angioplasty: technique and results. J Cardiovasc Surg 2014;55(5):665–70.

86. Graziani L. Crossing the Rubicon: A Closer Look at the Pedal Loop Technique. Ann Vasc Surg 2017;45:315–23.

87. Sommerset J, Karmy-Jones R, Dally M, et al. Plantar acceleration time: a novel technique to evaluate arterial flow to the foot. Ann Vasc Surg 2019;60:308–14.

88. Sommerset J, Teso D, Karmy-Jones R, et al. Pedal flow hemodynamics in patients with chronic limb-threatening ischemia. J Vasc Ultrasound 2020;44(1): 14–20.

89. Troisi N, Turini F, Chisci E, et al. Impact of Pedal Arch Patency on Tissue Loss and Time to Healing in Diabetic Patients with Foot Wounds Undergoing Infrainguinal Endovascular Revascularization. Korean J Radiol 2018;19(1):47–53.

90. Ferraresi R, Mauri G, Losurdo F, et al. BAD transmission and SAD distribution: a new scenario for critical limb ischemia. J Cardiovasc Surg 2018;59(5):655–64.

91. Ferraresi R, Ucci A, Pizzuto A, et al. A Novel Scoring System for Small Artery Disease and Medial Arterial Calcification Is Strongly Associated With Major Adverse Limb Events in Patients With Chronic Limb-Threatening Ischemia. J Endovasc Ther 2021;28(2):194–207.

92. Ilyas S, Powell RJ. Management of the no-option foot: Deep vein arterialization. Semin Vasc Surg 2022;35(2):210–8.

93. Kodama A, Takahara M, Iida O, et al. Health Related Quality of Life Over Time After Revascularisation in Patients With Chronic Limb Threatening Ischaemia. Eur J Vasc Endovasc Surg 2021;62(5):777–85.

94. Lu X, Idu M, Ubbink D, et al. Meta-analysis of the clinical effectiveness of venous arterialization for salvage of critically ischaemic limbs. Eur J Vasc Endovasc Surg 2006;31(5):493–9.

95. Schreve MA, Vos CG, Vahl AC, et al. Venous Arterialisation for Salvage of Critically Ischaemic Limbs: A Systematic Review and Meta-Analysis. Eur J Vasc Endovasc Surg 2017;53(3):387–402.

96. Nakama T, Obunai K, Kojima S, et al. Angiographic findings of the development of a reverse blood supply after percutaneous deep venous arterialization. Cardiovasc Interv 2020;13(12):1489–91.

97. Ho VT, Gologorsky R, Kibrik P, et al. Open, percutaneous, and hybrid deep venous arterialization technique for no-option foot salvage. J Vasc Surg 2020; 71(6):2152–60.

98. Schmidt A, Schreve MA, Huizing E, et al. Midterm Outcomes of Percutaneous Deep Venous Arterialization With a Dedicated System for Patients With No-Option Chronic Limb-Threatening Ischemia: The ALPS Multicenter Study. J Endovasc Ther 2020;27(4):658–65.

99. JA Mustapha M, Saab FA, Daniel Clair M, et al. Interim results of the PROMISE I trial to investigate the LimFlow system of percutaneous deep vein arterialization for the treatment of critical limb ischemia. J Invasive Cardiol 2019;31(3):57–63.

100. Shishehbor MH, Powell RJ, Montero-Baker MF, et al. Transcatheter Arterialization of Deep Veins in Chronic Limb-Threatening Ischemia. N Engl J Med 2023;388(13):1171–80.

101. Sheikh AB, Anantha-Narayanan M, Smolderen KG, et al. Utility of intravascular ultrasound in peripheral vascular interventions: systematic review and meta-analysis. Vasc Endovasc Surg 2020;54(5):413–22.

102. Hitchner E, Zayed M, Varu V, et al. A prospective evaluation of using IVUS during percutaneous superficial femoral artery interventions. Ann Vasc Surg 2015; 29(1):28–33.

103. Giannopoulos S, Varcoe RL, Lichtenberg M, et al. Balloon angioplasty of infrapopliteal arteries: a systematic review and proposed algorithm for optimal endovascular therapy. J Endovasc Ther 2020;27(4):547–64.

104. Armstrong EJ, Brodmann M, Deaton DH, et al. Dissections After Infrainguinal Percutaneous Transluminal Angioplasty: A Systematic Review and Current State of Clinical Evidence. J Endovasc Ther 2019;26(4):479–89.

105. Spiliopoulos S, Karamitros A, Reppas L, et al. Novel balloon technologies to minimize dissection of peripheral angioplasty. Expert Rev Med Devices 2019; 16(7):581–8.
106. Narins CR. Access strategies for peripheral arterial intervention. Cardiol J 2009; 16(1):88–97.
107. Geraghty PJ, Adams GL, Schmidt A, et al. Twelve-month results of Tack-optimized balloon angioplasty using the Tack Endovascular System in below-the-knee arteries (TOBA II BTK). J Endovasc Ther 2020;27(4):626–36.
108. Varcoe RL, Schouten O, Thomas SD, et al. Initial experience with the absorb bio-resorbable vascular scaffold below the knee: six-month clinical and imaging outcomes. J Endovasc Ther 2015;22(2):226–32.
109. Varcoe RL, Thomas SD, Lennox AF. Three-Year Results of the Absorb Everolimus-Eluting Bioresorbable Vascular Scaffold in Infrapopliteal Arteries. J Endovasc Ther 2018;25(6):694–701.
110. Lammer J, Bosiers M, Deloose K, et al. Bioresorbable Everolimus-Eluting Vascular Scaffold for Patients With Peripheral Artery Disease (ESPRIT I) 2-Year Clinical and Imaging Results. JACC Cardiovasc Interv 2016;9(11): 1178–87.
111. Brunacci N, Schurmann-Kaufeld S, Haase T, et al. Preclinical Evaluation of the Temporary Drug-Coated Spur Stent System in Porcine Peripheral Arteries. J Endovasc Ther 2021;28(6):938–49.
112. Bosiers M, Deloose K, Keirse K, et al. Are drug-eluting stents the future of SFA treatment? J Cardiovasc Surg 2010;51(1):115–9.
113. DeCock E, Sapoval M, Julia P, et al. A budget impact model for paclitaxel-eluting stent in femoropopliteal disease in France. Cardiovasc Intervent Radiol 2013;36(2):362–70.
114. Sridharan ND, Liang N, Robinson D, et al. Implementation of drug-eluting stents for the treatment of femoropopliteal disease provides significant cost-to-system savings in a single-state outpatient simulation. J Vasc Surg 2018;68(5):1465–72.
115. Sridharan ND, Boitet A, Smith K, et al. Cost-effectiveness analysis of drug-coated therapies in the superficial femoral artery. J Vasc Surg 2018;67(1): 343–52.
116. Pietzsch JB, Geisler BP, Iken AR, et al. Cost-Effectiveness of Urea Excipient-Based Drug-Coated Balloons for Chronic Limb-Threatening Ischemia from Fem-oropopliteal Disease in the Netherlands and Germany. Cardiovasc Intervent Radiol 2022;45(3):298–305.
117. Katsanos K, Geisler BP, Garner AM, et al. Economic analysis of endovascular drug-eluting treatments for femoropopliteal artery disease in the UK. BMJ Open 2016;6(5):e011245.
118. Shishehbor MH, Jaff MR, Beckman JA, et al. Public Health Impact of the Centers for Medicare and Medicaid Services Decision on Pass-Through Add-On Pay-ments for Drug-Coated Balloons: A Call to Action. JACC Cardiovasc Interv 2018;11(5):496–9.

Management of Vascular Injuries in Penetrating Trauma

Nicolas A. Stafforini, MD[a], Niten Singh, MD[a],*

KEYWORDS

- Penetrating vascular injuries • Management • Trauma

KEY POINTS

- The approach to penetrating trauma has been driven by historical military experience.
- The approach to penetrating vascular trauma is often with open techniques necessitating an understanding of exposures.
- Endovascular interventions continue to evolve with experience.

INTRODUCTION TO PENETRATING VASCULAR TRAUMA

Management of vascular trauma remains a challenge and traumatic injuries result in significant morbidity and mortality. Vascular trauma can be broadly classified according to the mechanism of injury (iatrogenic, blunt, penetrating, and combination injuries). In addition, this can be further classified by anatomical area (neck, thoracic, abdominal, pelvic, and extremities) or contextual circumstances (civilian and military).

Over the years, the management of vascular trauma has evolved with significant improvement in patient outcomes. Most of the advances in the management of vascular trauma have been driven by past military experiences. During World War II, the amputation rate from vascular injuries was greater than 40%.[1] With advances in surgical techniques, anesthesia, patient management, and logistics during the Korean and Vietnam conflicts, the amputation rates decreased to approximately 13%.[2,3] Despite the advances in technology, prehospital systems protocols, and vascular surgery techniques, penetrating vascular trauma management can lead to significant morbidity and mortality if not managed expeditiously and appropriately. The lessons learned in military environments are also applicable to civilian settings—in urban areas, penetrating vascular trauma has been shown to account for 50% of deaths and majority of these injuries were caused by firearms.[4] The aim of

[a] Division of Vascular Surgery, Department of Surgery, University of Washington, 325 9th Avenue, Box 359908, Seattle, WA 98104, USA
* Corresponding author.
E-mail address: singhn2@uw.edu

Surg Clin N Am 103 (2023) 801–825
https://doi.org/10.1016/j.suc.2023.04.018
surgical.theclinics.com
0039-6109/23/© 2023 Elsevier Inc. All rights reserved.

this article is to outline the approach, diagnosis, and management of penetrating vascular trauma.

APPROACH TO PENETRATING VASCULAR TRAUMA

Standard Advance Trauma Life Support protocols should be initiated with all patients.[5] The prompt diagnosis of penetrating vascular injuries requires knowledge of the mechanism and anticipation of the expected vessel that could be injured.

Vascular injuries can be classified into soft or hard signs. Hard signs suggesting a vascular injury include pulsatile bleeding, expanding hematoma, palpable thrill, audible bruit, and stroke. In addition, signs of ischemia are often evident to include pulselessness, pain, pallor, paralysis, and poikilothermia (5 Ps). Soft signs of vascular injuries include moderate hemorrhage at the scene of injury, non-expanding hematoma, and decreased but present pulse. Penetrating vascular injuries are often accompanied by hard signs.[6]

Extremity pulse exam should be confirmed with Doppler interrogation when feasible with an ankle-brachial index (ABI). An ABI less than 0.9 is considered to be abnormal and should lead to further imaging or exploration in the operating room depending on the clinical stability.[7] Patients with penetrating extremity injuries often will present with tourniquet control of hemorrhage that precludes further testing and necessitates repair.[8]

SPECIFIC INJURIES
Cervical Injuries

Penetrating trauma to the neck describes an injury that has breached the platysma muscle and represents 5% to 10% of all trauma cases.[9] If not diagnosed and treated in a timely manner, these injuries carry a high incidence of morbidity and mortality as high as 10%.[10]

Carotid artery injuries
Internal carotid artery injuries carry a high incidence of morbidity with a reported mortality of 50% in some series.[11] The neck is divided into three anatomic zones that help guide therapy (**Fig. 1**). Zone 1 extends from the sternal notch to the cricoid cartilage. Zone 2 extends from the cricoid cartilage to the angle of the mandible. Zone 3 extends from the angle of the mandible to the skull. Zone 2 injuries are most accessible to surgical exploration whereas Zones 1 and 3 often require more extensive exposure or endovascular approaches.[12] Patients who are hemodynamically stable and without hard signs of vascular injury should undergo computed tomographic angiography (CTA) which has a 90% sensitivity and 100% specificity to identify significant vascular injuries.[13] Duplex ultrasound has been used to evaluate and diagnose penetrating neck trauma.[14] However, it is operator-dependent and can be limited by bone fragments and subcutaneous air as well as immediate availability of the sonographers.

Surgical management. The patient should be placed on a radiolucent operating table for potential imaging and the neck and chest should be prepped in the operating field along with the proximal thigh for potential saphenous vein harvest. For Zone 1 injuries, proximal control should include the ability to enter the chest if needed, for Zones 2 and 3, proximal and distal control should be obtained in the neck. Carotid injuries in Zones 1 and 3 present unique challenges. For Zone 1 injuries, if proximal control cannot be obtained through a cervical incision, a median sternotomy or a clavicular resection should be performed (**Fig. 2**).

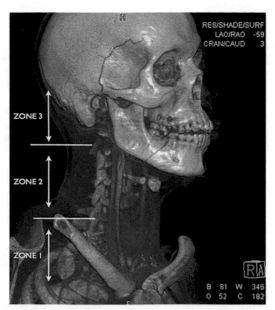

Fig. 1. Three-dimensional volume-rendering technique (3D VRT) of MDCTA performed on a young male victim of a stab wound to the neck demonstrating the anatomical trauma zones in the penetrating injury of the neck. In this young patient, the cricoid cartilage has not yet calcified and therefore is not visualized on the VRT but the thyroid gland is visible (the lower border of the cricoid cartilage will be located just above the level of the isthmus of the thyroid gland). (*From* Offiah, C., Hall, E. Imaging assessment of penetrating injury of the neck and face. Insights Imaging 3, 419–431 (2012); with permission.)

Historically, the recommendation for Zone 2 penetrating injuries was surgical exploration. However, several studies have reported that more than a half of these explorations were negative for injuries.[15,16] Exploration of Zone 2 injuries is conducted via a cervical incision anterior to the sternocleidomastoid muscle similar to a carotid endarterectomy exposure. If the injury is more distal in Zone 2 and there is a pulsatile hematoma, a proximal transverse incision above the clavicle and between the two heads of the sternocleidomastoid can be performed to obtain common carotid control prior to hematoma exploration similar to a transcervical carotid artery revascularization exposure.

For Zone 3 carotid injuries, to obtain vascular control, there are several maneuvers that can be implemented that are analogous to performing a carotid endarterectomy in a patient with a high bifurcation. These maneuvers include nasotracheal intubation, complete mobilization of the hypoglossal nerve, ligation of the posterior auricular artery, division of the posterior belly of the digastric muscle, and anterior displacement of the mandible. In the scenario where it is not possible to obtain distal control with a clamp, a Fogarty balloon can gently be placed within the field of view. In this scenario, ligation of the distal internal carotid artery (ICA) is often required due to the back bleeding from the ICA and potential for continued hemorrhage.

After obtaining vascular control, the decision to repair is made based on the extent of the injury, the stability of the patient, and the availability of appropriately sized conduit. Small partial lacerations can undergo a primary repair with or without a patch angioplasty. Repair of more extensive injuries will require an interposition graft or a bypass graft. Vein graft is the conduit of choice given the decreased rate of infection

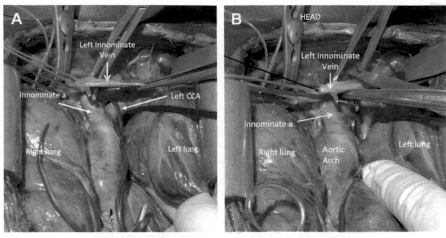

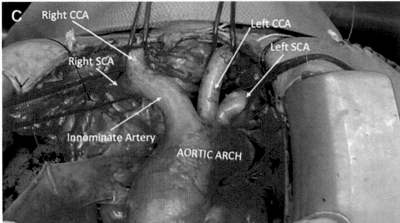

Fig. 2. (*A*) The left innominate vein may be ligated and divided to allow for greater exposure to the aortic arch and proximal innominate artery. (*B*) Dissection and division of the left innominate vein. (*C*) Improved exposure of the aortic arch and its branches after division of the left innominate vein. CCA, common carotid artery; SCA, subclavian artery. (*From* Demetriades D, Chong V, Varga S. Thoracic Vessels. In: Demetriades D, Inaba K, Velmahos G, eds. Atlas of Surgical Techniques in Trauma. 2nd ed. Cambridge: Cambridge University Press; 2020:118-129; with permission.)

compared to prosthetic grafts. For proximal injuries, another option is to perform an external carotid artery transposition to the distal internal carotid artery (**Fig. 3**). Patients presenting with injuries at the base of the skull often require carotid artery ligation which is associated with a 45% risk of mortality.[17,18]

Endovascular. In the modern era, endovascular interventions have become more popular for the treatment of penetrating carotid injuries particularly the more challenging Zones 1 and 3 injuries. Endovascular techniques can be utilized to obtain proximal balloon control for open repair as well as treat pseudoaneurysms, dissections, and arterial venous fistulas.[19] For over 25 years, case reports of endovascular repair have been described including Parodi's description of covered stent repair.[20] If a repair is performed with covered stents, these patients should be followed closely

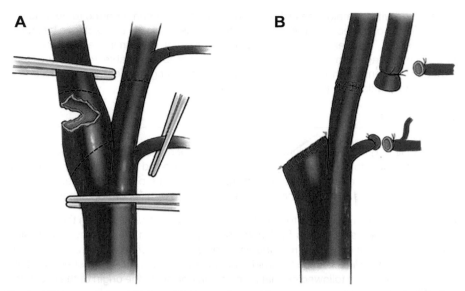

Fig. 3. (*A*) Internal carotid injury. (*B*) External carotid artery transposition to the internal carotid artery. (*From* K.L. Mattox, E.E. Moore, D.V. Feliciano. Trauma. (7th ed.), McGraw-Hill Medical, New York (2013), pp. 471-472; with permission.)

due to the thrombotic nature of covered stents in this area and often it is considered a temporizing procedure until the patient is stable for an open repair (**Fig. 4**).

Cervical venous injuries

Venous injuries are caused almost exclusively by penetrating trauma and internal jugular vein injuries represent 20% of all injuries to the neck.[21] These injuries differ from arterial injuries as they represent injuries to a low-pressure system that can

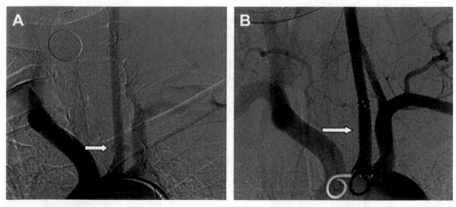

Fig. 4. Treatment of a false aneurysm of the proximal left carotid artery. (*A*) Selective common arteriogram demonstrating the false aneurysm (*arrow*); (*B*) Completion arteriogram showing exclusion of the false aneurysm and stent (*arrow*). (*From* du Toit DF, Coolen D, Lambrechts A, de V Odendaal J, Warren BL. The endovascular management of penetrating carotid artery injuries: long-term follow-up. Eur J Vasc Endovasc Surg. 2009 Sep;38(3):267-72; with permission.)

tamponade with no major hemorrhage and mortality has been reported to be as low as 2.6%.[22,23] As opposed to arterial injuries, the venous injuries in the neck can be ligated with impunity. Madsen and colleagues reported that performing a selective non-operative management for cervical venous injuries is applicable to a well-defined subset of patients with thrombosed isolated penetrating cervical venous trauma to the internal jugular vein (IJV) identified on CTA.[22]

Thoracic Injuries

Great vessels

About 90% of great vessel injuries are caused by penetrating trauma.[2] The mortality for penetrating thoracic aortic injuries has been reported to be greater than 90% and for subclavian artery injuries greater than 65%.[24] The premise of treating injuries to the great vessels is understanding the exposures to obtain control of these vessels.

Exposures. Surgical exposure to the ascending aorta and branches with the exception of the left subclavian artery is facilitated through a median sternotomy. To obtain a complete proximal exposure from the ascending aortic arch, the pericardium should be opened in a vertical fashion to avoid phrenic nerve injury. After the ascending aorta is localized, it can be followed cephalad to obtain control of the origin of the great vessels (**Fig. 5**).

Injuries to the proximal descending aorta should be exposed via a left 4th or 5th intercostal space posterolateral thoracotomy (**Fig. 6**). After obtaining access to the pleural cavity, the left lung is retracted inferiorly and blunt dissection performed medially and cephalad to identify the distal aortic arch and the origin of the left subclavian artery.

Exposure of the left subclavian artery is one of the most challenging exposures in a trauma setting. When an injury to the proximal left subclavian artery is suspected, a left anterior 3rd or 4th intercostal space thoracotomy should be performed. After obtaining

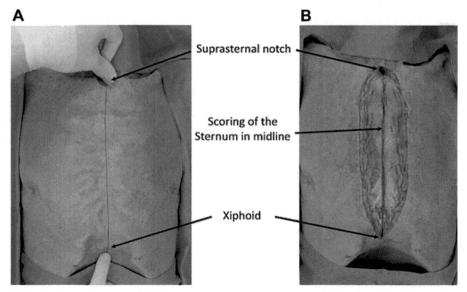

A   **B**

Suprasternal notch

Scoring of the
Sternum in midline

Xiphoid

Fig. 5. Median sternotomy. (*A*) The median sternotomy incision extends from the suprasternal notch to the xiphoid and (*B*) is carried down to the sternum. (*From* Demetrios D, Forestiere M. J., Gelbard R. Chest. In Demetriades D, Inaba K, & Velmahos G, eds, Atlas of Surgical Techniques in Trauma (pp. 95-170). Cambridge: Cambridge University Press; with permission.)

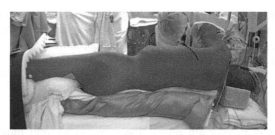

Fig. 6. Intercostal space posterolateral thoracotomy. (*From* Hazim J. Safi and Anthony L. Estrera Direct Surgical Repair of Aneurysms of the Thoracic and Thoracoabdominal Aorta. In: Chaikof, Elliot L. Atlas of Vascular Surgery and Endovascular Therapy, Elsevier, 2014, Pages 216-231; with permission.)

access to the pleural cavity, digital compression should be applied on the left supraclavicular fossa. If proximal control cannot be obtained via this incision, performing a median sternotomy and extending the anterior thoracotomy incision medially can allow for adequate exposure. If a supraclavicular incision is utilized as well, the entire left subclavian artery can be visualized (trapdoor thoracotomy) (**Fig. 7**).

Another advantage of performing a left anterolateral thoracotomy is the incision can also be extended across the sternum and converted into a "clamshell thoracotomy" to provide access to the right pleural space. This incision brings excellent exposure to the ascending aorta, aortic arch, and major aortic branches but at a high morbidity.[25]

Aorta

After performing adequate vascular exposure, injuries to the thoracic aorta can be controlled digitally or with a side-biting vascular clamp. Small injuries can be repaired primarily taking large bites with pledget reinforcement as needed.

Endovascular repair is the treatment of choice for blunt thoracic aortic injuries and is associated with a clear reduction in mortality.[26,27] Several reports have shown the

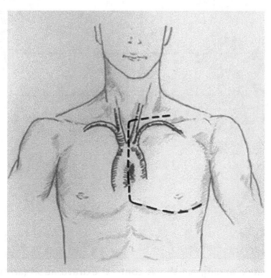

Fig. 7. "Trapdoor" thoracotomy. (*From* Imazeki T, Yamada T, Irie Y, Katayama Y, Kiyama H. Trapdoor thoracotomy as a surgical approach for aortic arch aneurysm. Ann Thorac Surg. 1998 Jul;66(1):272-4; with permission.)

successful treatment of penetrating aortic injuries with endovascular techniques[28–30] (**Fig. 8**) When planning an endovascular repair, a CT angiogram is required for correct stent-graft sizing or intraoperatively intravascular ultrasound can be utilized.[31] Finally, when performing an endovascular treatment, consideration should be taken to avoid covering the left subclavian artery, however, in a life-threatening circumstance, it can be covered with impunity without the need for revascularization.[32]

Innominate (brachiocephalic) artery

When exposing the innominate artery, the innominate vein must be ligated and vascular control can be achieved digitally or with a side-biting clamp. Aberrant anatomy such as a bovine arch anomaly (common origin of the innominate and left common carotid arteries) should be recognized to avoid clamping both carotid arteries.

Small injuries can be repaired primarily or with a patch angioplasty, and major injuries require an interposition graft or a bypass grafting. In the cases where the patient is hemodynamically unstable surgical options include ligating the innominate artery and performing an extra-anatomic bypass including a carotid-carotid, carotid-subclavian bypass.[33]

Several reports have shown successful endovascular treatment of innominate artery injuries using stent grafts, however, in distal innominate injures, these repairs require careful placement of the stent grafts in a "kissing" configuration extending each stent into the right subclavian and common carotid artery to avoid potential coverage of these vessels[34] (**Fig. 9**).

Subclavian artery

Exposure of the proximal left and right subclavian artery has been previously described. Injuries to the second portion of either of the subclavian arteries can be

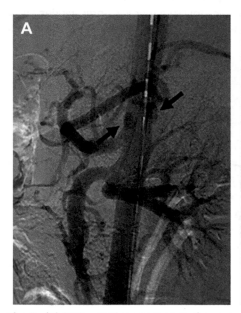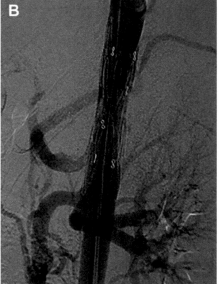

Fig. 8. (*A*) Perioperative angiogram shows contrast extravasation (*arrows*). (*B*) Angiogram shows total exclusion of the penetrating injury without endoleak. (*From* Ding X, Jiang J, Su Q, Hu S. Endovascular stent graft repair of a penetrating aortic injury. Ann Thorac Surg. 2010 Aug;90(2):632-4; with permission.)

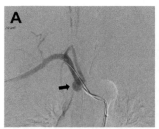
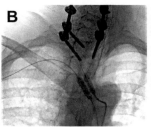
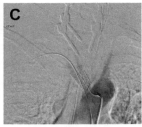

Fig. 9. (*A*) Initial angiogram showing a lesion near the innominate artery bifurcation (*arrow*). (*B*) Innominate artery repair with kissing stent technique. (*C*) Completion angiogram showing total exclusion of the injury. (*Courtesy of* Dr. Singh, N. Professor of Surgery and Associate Chief of the Division of Vascular Surgery. University of Washington, Seattle, WA.)

approached via a supraclavicular incision. If the incision is behind the clavicle and is difficult to obtain adequate exposure, a resection of a segment of the clavicle can be performed. Injuries to the third segment of the subclavian artery can be usually controlled via a supraclavicular approach, however, an infraclavicular incision and a clavicle resection can also be performed (**Fig. 10**).

After obtaining vascular control, the decision should be made to repair or ligate the affected artery. For small injuries, primary repair can be performed. For more extensive injuries, an interposition graft or bypass graft should be done with either a vein or prosthetic grafts. If the patient is hemodynamically unstable, the subclavian artery can be ligated and it is usually well tolerated.[35] With advances in endovascular techniques, there are several reports that describe the endovascular treatment of subclavian arteries injuries.[36–40] Endovascular repair can be achieved by deploying 7 to 8 mm stent grafts. This is reported to be more successful in patients with focal injuries that are able to be crossed with a guidewire[41] (**Fig. 11**).

Abdominal Injuries

Penetrating trauma to the abdomen is classified by the anatomic location of the injuries and separated into four zones (**Fig. 12**). Zone I includes the aortic hiatus and

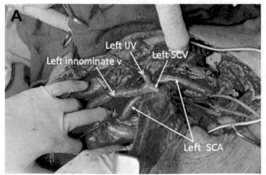
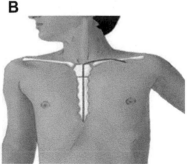

Fig. 10. Satisfactory exposure of the left subclavian artery may require a combination of a median sternotomy with a left clavicular incision. Note the junction of the left internal jugular and left subclavian vein to form the left innominate vein. IJV, internal jugular vein; SCV, subclavian vein. (*From* Demetriades D, Chong V, Varga S. Thoracic Vessels. In: Demetriades D, Inaba K, Velmahos G, eds. Atlas of Surgical Techniques in Trauma. 2nd ed. Cambridge: Cambridge University Press; 2020:118-129; with permission.)

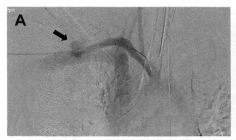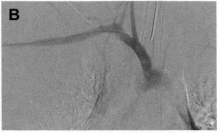

Fig. 11. (*A*) Perioperative angiogram shows contrast extravasation on the right subclavian artery (*arrow*). (*B*) Completion angiogram after treatment with cover stent shows total exclusion of the penetrating injury. (*Courtesy of* Dr. Singh, N. Professor of Surgery and Associate Chief of the Division of Vascular Surgery. University of Washington, Seattle, WA.)

extends down to the sacrum. This area can be further divided into the supramesocolic and inframesocolic. The vascular structures in Zone I include the aorta, inferior vena cava (IVC), and their major branches. Zone II is lateral Zone I and contains the hilar vessels, kidneys, and the paracolic gutter. Zone III includes the pelvic retroperitoneum below the sacrum and includes the iliac vessels and its branches. Finally, Zone IV includes the hepatic artery, portal vein, hepatic veins, and the retro-hepatic IVC. In contrast to blunt abdominal injuries, all penetrating injuries require surgical

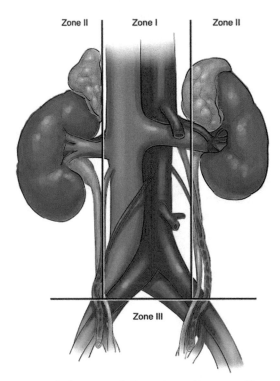

Fig. 12. The three anatomical zones of the retroperitoneum. (*From* Marcus Cleanthis, Michael Jenkins. Abdominal Aortic Trauma, Iliac and Visceral Vessel Injuries. In: Todd E. Rasmussen, Nigel R.M. Tai, Rich's Vascular Trauma (Third Edition), Elsevier, 2016, Pages 113-125; with permission.)

exploration. The exception to this rule is the Zone IV penetrating injuries that are not expanding or pulsatile hematomas or actively bleeding.

The initial approach to patients with penetrating abdominal injuries is a wide operative field with the chest, abdomen, and proximal thighs prepped for potential proximal clamping of the descending thoracic aorta and potential saphenous vein harvest. Penetrating injuries to the abdomen are often associated with bowel and colon injuries and any immediate vascular repair will likely be in a contaminated field, therefore, an autogenous conduit is preferred with tissue coverage utilizing omentum or local or rotational muscle flap.

As a general concept, for Zone I supramesocolic injuries and left Zone II injuries, a left visceral rotation (Mattox maneuver) should be performed and for suspected IVC and for right Zone II injuries, a right visceral rotation (Cattel-Braasch maneuver) should be performed.[42]

Surgical exposure

Zone I injuries. If a Zone I injury is encountered, the approach depends on whether the injury is supramesocolic or inframesocolic. For supramesocolic injuries, a left visceral rotation should be performed (**Fig. 13**). This approach requires transection of the peritoneal reflection (the line of Toldt) of the left colon, dividing the lienosplenic ligament and elevating the left colon, spleen, pancreas, kidneys, and the stomach medially. This exposure allows access to the supraceliac aorta from the aortic hiatus and includes exposure to the origin of the celiac axis, SMA, and the left renal vascular pedicle.[43–45]

For inframesocolic injuries, exposure differs whether it is the infrarenal aorta or the IVC that requires control or repair. Aortic exposure is achieved mobilizing the transverse colon cephalad, mobilizing the small bowel to the right and transecting the ligament of Treitz until the left renal vein is visualized similar to an open infrarenal repair.[43–45]

For IVC exposure, a right medial visceral rotation should be performed (**Fig. 14**). This consists of mobilizing the right colon, and mobilizing the proximal duodenum and pancreatic head (Kocher maneuver). A complete right medial visceral rotation exposes

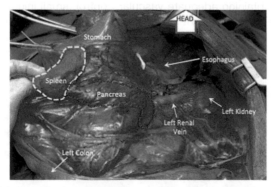

Fig. 13. Left medial visceral rotation has been performed after division of the splenorenal and splenophrenic ligaments. The pancreas and the spleen have been rotated medially. The left kidney remains at its original position in the retroperitoneal. Note the left renal vein crossing anteriorly over the aorta. (*From* Teixeira PG, Magee GA, Rowe VL. Abdominal Aorta and Splachnic Vessels. In: Demetriades D, Inaba K, Velmahos G, eds. Atlas of Surgical Techniques in Trauma. 2nd ed. Cambridge: Cambridge University Press; 2020:268-285; with permission.)

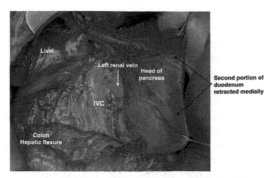

Fig. 14. Kocher maneuver: the duodenum is mobilized medially until the IVC and left renal vein are encountered. (*From* Kwon E, Demetriades D. Duodenum. In: Atlas of Surgical Techniques in Trauma. 1st ed. Cambridge: Cambridge University Press; 2015:189-197; with permission.)

the IVC from the inferior border of the liver to its bifurcation and includes the entry of the left renal vein to the IVC.[42]

Finally, if emergent supraceliac aortic control is required, the gastrohepatic ligament should be divided, the distal esophagus and stomach should be retracted to the left, and the crus of the diaphragm should be divided. A vascular clamp is then placed to control the aorta (**Fig. 15**).

Zone II injuries. Zone II injuries are best approached through a right or left medial visceral rotation as described above.

Zone III injuries. Zone III exposures can be achieved by dissecting the right or left colons attachments and reflecting them medially utilizing a combination of blunt and sharp dissection to locate the iliac vessels.[43–45]

Aorta

Most aortic injuries are caused by penetrating trauma and the mortality has been reported to be over 60%.[46] Exposure of the abdominal aorta has been previously described. After obtaining adequate vascular control, small injuries can be repaired primarily. If there is a significant defect of the aorta, a patch angioplasty can be

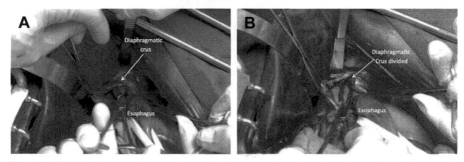

Fig. 15. (*A*) With the esophagus retracted downward, a clamp is advanced into the esophageal hiatus of the diaphragm to facilitate the division of the muscle fibers. (*B*) The diaphragmatic crus is divided at the 2 o'clock position. (*From* Teixeira PG, Magee GA, Rowe VL. Abdominal Aorta and Splanchnic Vessels. In: Demetriades D, Inaba K, Velmahos G, eds. Atlas of Surgical Techniques in Trauma. 2nd ed. Cambridge: Cambridge University Press; 2020:268-285; with permission.)

performed or the injured segment can be resected and the aorta can be mobilized for an end-to-end repair. If these options are not available, the aorta can be repaired with a 12 to 14 mm dacron or polytetrafluoroethylene (PTFE) graft. In the face of contamination, soaking a dacron graft in rifampin (1200 mg of rifampin in 20 mL of saline) and covering the repair with omentum has been utilized as well. Other described techniques involve ligation of the aorta and an extra-anatomic bypass (axillo-bifemoral) to maintain perfusion to the lower extremities.[47]

Endovascular treatment has emerged as an effective and minimally invasive alternative treatment option. The most frequent endovascular techniques include balloon occlusion and stent-graft placements.[48,49] The intra-aortic balloon occlusion of the aorta (IABO) helps to temporize the hemorrhage and allows time for resuscitation and repair. By inflating the balloon in the proximal aorta, one can replace the classic resuscitative thoracotomy and aortic cross-clamping by proving endovascular proximal vascular control prior or during the abdominal exploration.[50]

In the case of potential endovascular treatment, the repair should be considered a temporizing measure as there is often bowel injury as well. Once the hemorrhage is controlled and the contamination cleared, an open direct repair or extra-anatomic repair should be performed.

Inferior vena cava

Penetrating IVC injuries carry a high mortality and one-third of the patients will die before reaching the hospital.[51] Exposure of the IVC is made via a right medial visceral rotation. Exposure of the retro-hepatic IVC is technically more challenging and usually requires extensive mobilization of the liver. Vascular control is often accomplished with sponge sticks above and below the injury or using a side-biting clamp. In patients presenting anterior wall injuries, it is important to remember to look for concomitant posterior wall injury. Partial injuries can be repaired primarily and performing a transverse closure of longitudinal injuries can prevent vessel stenosis. In the cases where primary repair is not possible, a patch angioplasty, end-to-end anastomosis or interposition grafts can be performed. In the setting of concomitant hollow viscus injury, an autogenous graft is preferred, usually from internal jugular vein, or external iliac vein. The saphenous vein can also be utilized; however, it will require the construction of a spiral vein graft that is time-consuming. In the cases where the patient is hemodynamically unstable, a temporary shunt can be placed or the IVC can be ligated.[51] Atriocaval shunts may be a life-saving option, however, the survival in these patients has been reported to be less than 20%[52] (Fig. 16). In general, infrarenal IVC ligation is well tolerated and is not associated with an increased risk of mortality.[53] However, ligation of the suprarenal and retro-hepatic IVC is not well tolerated and carries significant hemodynamic instability.[54]

Innovations in endovascular technology provide an alternative to the management of IVC injuries. Several studies have reported the use of occlusion balloons to obtain vascular control.[55] In addition, stent-graft repair for IVC injuries has been reported in highly selective patients.[56,57]

Celiac artery

Injury to the celiac artery is rare and is mainly associated with penetrating trauma. Exposure and vascular control should be attempted through a supraceliac aortic exposure. All branches from the celiac artery can be ligated with no major consequences.[58] If the hepatic artery is injured, it is preferable to ligate it prior to the origin of the gastroduodenal artery. If this is not possible, a reconstruction should be considered to avoid possible ischemic sequelae.

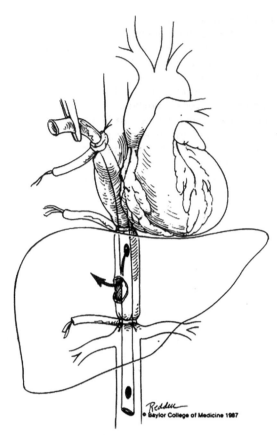

Fig. 16. Atriocaval shunt. (Courtesy of the Baylor College of Medicine Archives.)

Superior mesenteric artery

Injuries to the superior mesenteric artery (SMA) are uncommon and highly lethal. SMA injuries can be classified into four anatomical zones described by Fullen and colleagues.[59] Zone I represents the proximal SMA, Zone II is between the pancreaticoduodenal and middle colic branches of the artery, Zone III is beyond the middle colic branch, and Zone IV is at the level of the enteric branches (**Fig. 17**). All injuries to the SMA should be repaired if possible based on the correlation between mortality and Fullen's classification of 100% for Zone I, 43% for Zone II, and 25% for Zones III and IV.[60]

Exposure of the SMA necessitates a left medial visceral rotation, however, Zone I injuries may also be approached by dissecting the vessel directly through the lesser sac or at the base of the transverse mesocolon[61] (**Fig. 18**). After vascular control has been achieved, for small partial injuries, a primary repair can be performed. In the cases where this is not possible, an interposition graft or bypass graft with saphenous vein or a prosthetic graft should be done. If the patient is unstable, another alternative is to place a temporary arterial shunt.[62] All patients who undergo an SMA repair should have a temporary closure and second-look laparotomy to ensure bowel viability.[63] Successful endovascular treatment of SMA penetrating injuries with covered stents has also been described.[64,65]

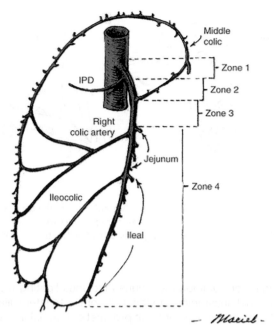

Fig. 17. Fullen's classification. (Fullen, William D. M.d.; Hunt, John M.d.; Altemeier, William A. M.d.. The Clinical Spectrum Of Penetrating Injury To The Superior Mesenteric Arterial Circulation. The Journal Of Trauma: Injury, Infection, And Critical Care 12(8):p 656-664, August 1972.)

Iliac artery

Penetrating trauma to the iliac arteries carries a high mortality. Mattox and colleagues reported a 39% 30-day mortality for patients who presented with iliac artery injuries.[66] Ligation of the internal iliac artery is well tolerated.[67] On the contrary, given the risk of limb ischemia, injuries to the common and external iliac artery require repair or ligation and extra-anatomic bypass.[68]

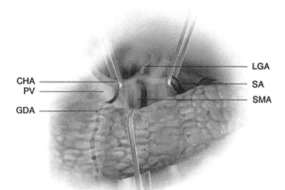

Fig. 18. SMA in the lesser sac above the neck of the pancreas. CHA, common hepatic artery; GDA, gastroduodenal artery; LGA, left gastric artery; PV, portal vein; SA, splenic artery. (*From* Sanjay P, Takaori K, Govil S, Shrikhande SV, Windsor JA. 'Artery-first' approaches to pancreatoduodenectomy. Br J Surg. 2012 Aug;99(8):1027-35; with permission.)

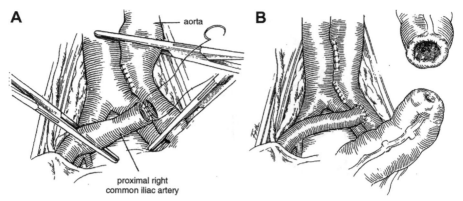

Fig. 19. Iliac artery transposition technique. (*A*), Vascular control with adequate mobilization is obtained, and an end-to-side tension-free anastomosis performed. (*B*) Completed transposition. (*From* Lee JT, Bongard FS. Iliac vessel injuries. Surg Clin North Am. 2002;82(1):21-xix; with permission.)

Another technique for common iliac injuries includes ligating the proximal injured segment and rotational anastomosis to the aorta or contralateral iliac artery (**Fig. 19**). This approach allows for the avoidance of prosthetic material in the face of possible contamination.

In the situation where the external iliac artery is injured, a repair can be performed by ligating the distal ipsilateral internal iliac artery and performing a transposition of the proximal internal iliac to the distal external iliac artery (**Fig. 20**).

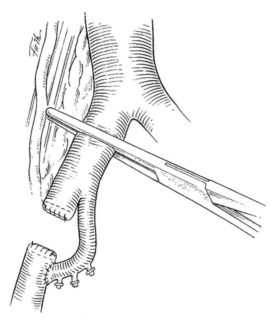

Fig. 20. Ipsilateral hypogastric artery interposition. (*From* Lee JT, Bongard FS. Iliac vessel injuries. Surg Clin North Am. 2002;82(1):21-xix; with permission.)

Endovascular techniques to control bleeding from iliac vessels in association with trauma are well documented and often easily achieved. This can be done with stent-graft placement or internal iliac artery embolization.[69,70] Studies have reported that endovascular repair of iliac arterial injury, irrespective of mechanism, is associated with a significantly lower rate of amputation than open surgery.[71] However, if associated with a contaminated field, the endovascular repair is again considered temporizing with planned open repair or extra-anatomic bypass when the patient's condition has stabilized.

Endovascular. As previously described, REBOA-intra-aortic balloon occlusion can be used to obtain proximal vascular control. For pelvic vascular injuries, the balloon should be inflated in the infrarenal aorta (Zone III), and should be deflated once hemostasis has been achieved.

Current guidelines recommend that the intra-aortic balloon in Zone 1 should only be performed if the anticipated time to start the operation is less than 15 minutes and that in Zone 3 may be tolerated for longer periods, however, the balloon should be deflated as soon as possible.[72] For a trained team, REBOA placement has been reported to be performed in less than 6 minutes and partial balloon inflation at either location may prolong inflation time.[72,73] After vascular control is achieved, the patient should undergo expeditious and definitive endovascular or open treatment. Due to the potential access-vessel complications, aortic dissections, vessel rupture, perforation, and peripheral ischemia, REBOA should only be performed by a trained team with the availability of a specialist who can deal with these complications if they are encountered.[74]

Extremity Vascular Injuries

Vascular injuries account for 6% of all traumatic injuries to extremities, with the femoral artery being the most frequently injured vessel (35%).[75] Extremity vascular injuries are frequently associated with injuries to major veins (62%), nerves (34%), and bones (19%).[76] Combined major artery and vein injury are an indicator of poor limb salvage prognosis.[77,78] Multiple scoring systems have been created to predict limb salvage; however, the Mangled Extremity Severity Score (**Table 1**) is probably the most well-known. These classification systems are used to determine if amputation is likely needed.[79,80]

Patients with extremity vascular injury can be divided into "hard" or "soft" signs of injury as previously described. These findings will dictate if the patient requires an immediate operation or if further study can be done. For diagnosis, CTA has become the gold standard imaging modality and can show signs such as active extravasation of contrast, loss of opacification, pseudoaneurysm, and arteriovenous fistula.[81,82] When approaching a patient with an extremity vascular injury, successful management requires hemorrhage control to prevent mortality, avoid limb loss, and finally restore limb function. The majority of patients will have tourniquets in place if active bleeding is noted at the scene. The tourniquet can be loosened to evaluate for active hemorrhage and re-applied if bleeding is noted. In this scenario, the patient should be taken to the OR immediately.

Operative planning

The patient's extremity should be circumferentially prepped and draped and in the case of lower extremity injuries the contralateral lower extremity as well. For upper extremity injuries the bilateral thighs should be prepped for potential saphenous vein harvest. In the scenario where a tourniquet is controlling hemorrhage in the proximal thigh or upper extremity, it can be replaced with digital pressure over the injury and a sterile tourniquet can be re-applied. If the patient has a concomitant fracture and there is no

Table 1
Mangled extremity severity score

Skeletal/soft-tissue Group			
1	Low-energy	Stab wounds, simple closed fracture, small calliber gunshot wounds	1
2	Medium-energy	Open or multiple level fractures, dislocations, moderate crush injuries	2
3	High-energy	Shotgun blast (close range) high-velocity gunshot wounds, crush injuries	3
4	Very high-energy	Above + gross contamination, soft-tissue avulsion	4
Shock group			
1	Normotensive hemodynamics	BP stable in field and in operation theatre	0
2	Transiently hypotensive	BP unstable in field but responsive to intravenous fluids	1
3	Prolonged hypotension	Systolic BP <90 mm Hg in field and responsive to intravenous fluids only in operation theatre	2
Ischemia group			
1	None	A pulsatile limb without signs of ischemia	0[a]
2	Mild	Pulse reduced or absent but perfusion normal	1[a]
3	Moderate	Pulseless; paraesthesia, diminished capillary refill	2[a]
4	Advanced	Pulseless, cool, paralyzed and numb without capillary refill	3[a]
Age group			
1	<30 y		0
2	>30 - <50 y		1
3	>50 y		2

[a] Points × 2 if ischemia time exceeds 6 hours
Adapted from from Johansen K, Daimes M, Howey T, Helfet DL, Hansen ST. Objective criteria accurately predict amputation following lower extremity trauma. J Trauma. 1990;30:568-73.

active hemorrhage, expeditious external fixation of the fracture should be performed initially so the extremity is at length and it does not compromise the vascular repair. It is important to follow this chronology, given that the use of external fixation will correct the alignment, length, and rotation of the fractured limb to allow the vascular repair to be performed in a controlled environment to protect the completed vascular repair from disruption. In addition to ensuring no tension is on the vascular repair, stabilizing the fracture can help control bleeding from the bone if the patient receives anticoagulation during the procedure.

In a patient with a fracture with active arterial hemorrhage, the injury should be explored, and the bleeding artery controlled. If possible, a shunt should be placed to restore perfusion while the fracture is stabilized to avoid additional ischemic time. Many types of commercial shunts are available and it is crucial that the shunts approximate the diameter of the artery to prevent hemorrhage or thrombosis.[83] These are designed to avoid trauma to the intima of the artery and can be classified as straight and looped shunts. Straight shunts are shorter and useful when operative space is limited and when the gap in or injury to the vessel is short. They lie inside of the injured vessel and are not likely to become compressed with wound dressing material, surgical retractors, or orthopedic fixator devices. These include the Javid (Bard Peripheral

Vascular Inc. Tempe, Arizona, USA) and the Argyle (Kendall Healthcare Products, Mansfield, Mass, USA). Looped shunts are longer and are more effective at bridging longer injuries or segments of missing vessel, and this design may be preferable when the vascular injury crosses an unstable fracture. In these instances, looped shunts have a lower likelihood of being dislodged. These include the Sundt (Integra Neurosciences, Plansboro, NJ, USA) or the Pruitt-Inahara (Horizon Medical, Santa Ana, Calif, USA).

Arterial injuries from stab wounds can often be mobilized, debrided, and repaired in an end-to-end fashion. Ballistic arterial injuries, in our opinion, require an interposition graft as the zone of injury may be greater than what is visible requiring greater mobilization and debridement.

When primary repair cannot be accomplished, a patch, interposition graft, or bypass can be performed with vein or synthetic grafts. Autogenous veins are preferred because of high patency rates and low incidence of secondary graft infection.[84,85] The best conduit for reconstruction is the great saphenous vein (GSV). Traditionally, the contralateral GSV is the conduit of choice given the risk of occult ipsilateral deep venous injury, however, several studies have showed that if no vein is available, and there is no associated venous injury, ipsilateral GSV can be safely used.[86] Prosthetic grafts are not ideal in penetrating trauma as the wound may not be clean or may not have adequate coverage which can lead to infection and potential blowout of the anastomosis. If it is the only option, PTFE grafts have been shown to be effective and more resistant to infections.[87]

In patients who are hemodynamically unstable, a vascular shunt should be placed and it is associated with lower mortality and amputation rates versus ligation[88] (**Fig. 21**).

After a penetrating extremity artery injury and repair, performing a fasciotomy is strongly recommended. The majority of penetrating injuries occurs in young patients with a moderate amount of muscle mass and the edema that occurs with reperfusion will often lead to a compartment syndrome. Numerous studies have shown that early fasciotomy reduces amputation rates.[89,90] It is important to take into consideration that despite the best efforts to perform a vascular reconstruction in a timely manner to achieve limb salvage, functional outcomes will be harder to achieve.[91]

Open exposure
Upper extremity
Axillary and brachial arteries Vascular control of the axillary artery depends on the location of the injury. The affected extremity, the chest, and neck should be prepped to

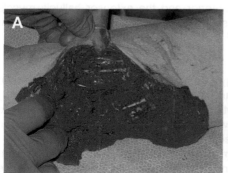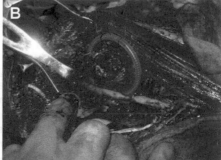

Fig. 21. (*A*) Shunt placed in the brachial artery. (*B*) Repair of Shunted Popliteal Artery. (*Courtesy of* Dr. Singh, N. Professor of Surgery and Associate Chief of the Division of Vascular Surgery. University of Washington, Seattle, WA.)

permit exposure if necessary. If the injury is to the proximal axillary artery, vascular control should be achieved exposing the subclavian artery as described earlier.

For exposure of the axillary artery distal to the first rib, an infra-clavicular incision should be done with extension along the deltopectoral groove. The exposure of the axillary artery requires the dissection between the pectoralis major muscle fibers and the retraction of the underlying pectoralis minor muscle. This incision can be further extended into the proximal arm into the medial bicipital sulcus to obtain additional exposure of the distal axillary and brachial artery. Care should be taken to preserve collateral branches and avoid brachial plexus injury.

When exposing the brachial artery, the incision should be done between the biceps and triceps muscles. This incision can be extended proximally as previously described or distally curving toward the radius in the antecubital fossa to gain access to the brachial artery bifurcation.

Lower extremity

Femoral and popliteal vessels The majority of injuries that involve the proximal common femoral artery are highly lethal as they can result in hemorrhage that is non-compressible. For proximal superficial femoral artery (SFA) and profunda injuries, the exposure is similar for the common femoral artery and involves a vertical incision halfway between the pubic tubercle and the anterior iliac spine below the inguinal ligament. This incision can be extended proximally or distally if needed. When dissecting, care must be taken to avoid injuring the greater saphenous vein.

In penetrating injuries, the thigh is often the location of the injury, and hence, the SFA and above-knee popliteal arteries. In this scenario, if the vessel is completely transected, the injury can be approached directly. In the upper thigh, this exposure is accomplished by rotating the sartorius muscle laterally to expose the SFA and for more distal SFA or above-knee popliteal injuries approaching it via the muscular groove between the sartorius and vastus medialis muscles. The below-knee popliteal artery is approached in the same manner as an elective repair with a medial upper leg incision to enter the popliteal fossa and divide the pes anserine superiorly.

Infra-popliteal vessels. The patency of one of the tibial vessels is sufficient to obtain limb viability and vascular function. The posterior tibial and peroneal vessels can be achieved via the medial incision previously described. In the case of the anterior tibial artery, an approach to its origin can be achieved via the previously described medial incision. These vessels can be explored from the fasciotomy incision. For the lateral incision to decompress the anterior compartment, the anterior tibial artery and deep peroneal nerve are between the tibialis anterior and the extensor hallucis muscle bellies. In general, these vessels can be safely treated with arterial ligation if repair is not feasible or the patient is unstable.[92]

Endovascular

With the advances of stent-graft technology and procedural techniques, endovascular approaches in the management of upper and lower vascular trauma have significantly increased.[93] These techniques can be both diagnostic and therapeutic. Therapeutic options usually include vascular control with a balloon, covered stent repair of an injury, or embolization of a bleeding vessel.[94,95]

In this young patient population in whom these injuries most often occur, the long-term patency of a stent-graft is unknown and long-term surveillance studies should be done. Embolization techniques using different types of materials in smaller vessels have also been described. This has been mainly used for the treatment of pseudoaneurysms and arteriovenous fistulas.[96]

DECLARATION OF CONFLICTING INTERESTS

The authors declared no commercial, or financial conflicts of interest or any funding sources.

REFERENCES

1. DeBakey ME, Simeone FA. Battle injuries of the arteries in World War II: an analysis of 2471 cases. Ann Surg 1946;123:534–79.
2. Hughes CW. Arterial repair during Korean War. Ann Surg 1958;147(4):555–61.
3. Rich NM, Baugh JH, Hughes CW. Acute arterial injuries in Vietnam: 1000 cases. J Trauma 1970;10(5):359–69.
4. Demetriades D, Kimbrell B, Salim A, et al. Trauma deaths in a mature urban trauma system: is "trimodal" distribution a valid concept? J Am Coll Surg 2005; 201:343–8.
5. Advanced trauma life Support: student course manual. 10th edition. Chicago, IL: American College of Surgeons; 2018.
6. Frykberg ER, Dennis JW, Bishop K, et al. The reliability of physical examination in the evaluation of penetrating extremity trauma for vascular injury: results at one year. J Trauma 1991 Apr;31(4):502–11.
7. Johansen K, Lynch K, Paun M, et al. Non-invasive vascular tests reliably exclude occult arterial trauma in injured extremities. J Trauma 1991;31(4):515–9.
8. Feliciano DV, Moore FA, Moore EE, et al. Evaluation and management of peripheral vascular injury. Part 1.
9. Vishwanatha B, Sagayaraj A, Huddar SG, et al. Penetrating neck injuries. Indian J Otolaryngol Head Neck Surg 2007;59:221–4.
10. Saito N, Hito R, Burke PA, et al. Imaging of penetrating injuries of the head and neck: current practice at a level I trauma center in the United States. Keio J Med 2014;63:23–33.
11. Tisherman SA, Bokhari F, Collier B, et al. Clinical practice guideline: penetrating zone II neck trauma. J Trauma 2008;64(5):1392–405.
12. Monson DO, Saletta JD, Freeark RJ. Carotid vertebral trauma. J Trauma 1969; 9:987.
13. Múnera F, Soto JA, Palacio D, et al. Diagnosis of arterial injuries caused by penetrating trauma to the neck: comparison of helical CT angiography and conventional angiography. Radiology 2000;216(2):356–62.
14. Montalvo BM, LeBlang SD, Nunez DB, et al. Color Doppler sonography in penetrating injuries of the neck. AJNR Am J Neuroradiol 1996;17:943–51.
15. Roon AJ, Christensen N. Evaluation and treatment of penetrating cervical injuries. J Trauma 1979;19:391–7.
16. Apffelstaedt JP, Muller R. Results of mandatory exploration for penetrating neck trauma. World J Surg 1994;18:917–9 [discussion: 920].
17. Weaver FA, Yellin AE, Wagner WH, et al. The role of arterial reconstruction in penetrating carotid injuries. Arch Surg 1988;123:1106–11.
18. du Toit D, van Schalkwyk GD, Wadee SA, et al. Neurologic outcome after penetrating extracranial arterial trauma. J Vasc Surg 2003;38:257–62.
19. Moulakakis KG, Mylonas S, Avgerinos E, et al. An update of the role of endovascular repair in blunt carotid artery trauma. Eur J Vasc Endovasc Surg 2010;40(3): 312–9.
20. Parodi JC, Schönholz C, Ferreira LM, et al. Endovascular stent-graft treatment of traumatic arterial lesions. Ann Vasc Surg 1999;13(2):121–9.

21. Nair R, Robbs JV, Muckart DJ. Management of penetrating cervicomediastinal venous trauma. Eur J Vasc Endovasc Surg 2000;19(1):65–9.

22. Madsen AS, Bruce JL, Oosthuizen GV, et al. The Selective Non-operative Management of Penetrating Cervical Venous Trauma is Safe and Effective. World J Surg 2018;42(10):3202–9.

23. Mattox KL, Feliciano DV, Burch J, et al. Five thousand seven hundred sixty cardiovascular injuries in 4459 patients. Epidemiologic evolution 1958 to 1987. Ann Surg 1989;209(6):698–705 [discussion: 706–].

24. Demetriades D. Penetrating injuries to the thoracic great vessels. J Cardiovasc Surg 1997;12(2 Suppl):173–9 [discussion: 179–80].

25. Hoyt DB, Coimbra R, Potenza BM, et al. Anatomic exposures for vascular injuries. Surg Clin North Am 2001;81(6):1299–330, xii.

26. Lee WA, Matsumura JS, Mitchell RS, et al. Endovascular repair of traumatic thoracic aortic injury: clinical practice guidelines of the Society for Vascular Surgery. J Vasc Surg 2011;53:187–92.

27. Murad MH, Rizvi AZ, Malgor R, et al. Comparative effectiveness of the treatments for thoracic aortic transection [corrected]. J Vasc Surg 2011;53:193–9.e1-21.

28. Ding X, Jiang J, Su Q, et al. Endovascular stent graft repair of a penetrating aortic injury. Ann Thorac Surg 2010;90(2):632–4.

29. Feyko JT, Zmijewski P, Lyle C, et al. Transaortic gunshot wound through perivisceral segment successfully managed by placement of thoracic stent graft. J Vasc Surg Cases Innov Tech 2018;4(1):24–6.

30. Fang TD, Peterson DA, Kirilcuk NN, et al. Endovascular management of a gunshot wound to the thoracic aorta. J Trauma 2006;60(1):204–8.

31. Ceja-Rodriguez M, Realyvasquez A, Galante J, et al. Differences in Aortic Diameter Measurements with Intravascular Ultrasound and Computed Tomography After Blunt Traumatic Aortic Injury. Ann Vasc Surg 2018;50:148–53.

32. Stafforini NA, Singh N, Hemingway J, et al. Reevaluating the Need for Routine Coverage of the Left Subclavian Artery in Thoracic Blunt Aortic Injury. Ann Vasc Surg 2021;73:22–6.

33. Okada Y, Narumiya H, Ishii W, et al. Damage control management of innominate artery injury with tracheostomy. Surg Case Rep 2016;2(1):17.

34. Du Toit DF, Odendaal W, Lambrechts A, et al. Surgical and endovascular management of penetrating innominate artery injuries. Eur J Vasc Endovasc Surg 2008;36:56–62.

35. Smith AA, Gupta N. Subclavian artery trauma. In: StatPearls (Internet). Treasure Island (FL): StatPearls Publishing; 2023.

36. Dubose JJ, Rajani R, Gilani R, et al. Endovascular management of axillosubclavian arterial injury: a review of published experience. Injury 2012;43:1785–92.

37. Branco BC, Boutrous ML, DuBose JJ, et al. Outcome comparison between open and endovascular management of axillosubclavian arterial injuries. J Vasc Surg 2016;63:702–9.

38. Castelli P, Caronno R, Piffaretti G, et al. Endovascular repair of traumatic injuries of the subclavian and axillary arteries. Int J Care Injured 2005;36:778–82.

39. Xenos ES, Freeman M, Stevens S, et al. Covered stents for injuries of subclavian and axillary arteries. J Vasc Surg 2003;38:451–4.

40. Du Toit DF, Strauss DC, Blaszczyk M, et al. Endovascular treatment of penetrating thoracic outlet arterial injuries. Eur J Vasc Endovasc Surg 2000;19:489–95.

41. Danetz JS, Cassano AD, Stoner MC, et al. Feasibility of endovascular repair in penetrating axillosubclavian injuries: a retrospective review. J Vasc Surg 2005; 41:246–54.
42. Fildes J, Meredith JW, Hoyt DB, et al. Trauma ACoSCo. ASSET (advanced surgical skills for exposure in trauma): exposure techniques when time matters. Chicago: American College of Surgeons; 2010.
43. Feliciano DV, Burch JM, Graham JM. Abdominal vascular injury. In: Mattox KL, Feliciano DV, Moore EE, editors. Trauma. 4th edition. New York: McGraw-Hill; 1999. p. 783–805.
44. Feliciano DV. Abdominal vessels. In: Ivatury R, Cayten CG, editors. The textbook of penetrating trauma. Baltimore: Williams and Wilkins; 1996. p. 702–16.
45. Mattox KL, McCollum WB, Jordan GL Jr, et al. Management of upper abdominal vascular trauma. Am J Surg 1974;128(6):823–8.
46. Lopez-Viego MA, Snyder WH 3rd, Valentine RJ, et al. Penetrating abdominal aortic trauma: a report of 129 cases. J Vasc Surg 1992;16(3):332–5 [discussion: 335–6].
47. Oderich GS, Bower TC, Hofer J, et al. In situ rifampin-soaked grafts with omental coverage and antibiotic suppression are durable with low reinfection rates in patients with aortic graft enteric erosion or fistula. J Vasc Surg 2011;53(1):99–106, 107.e1-7; [discussion: 106-7].
48. Ghazala CG, Green BR, Williams R, et al. Endovascular management of a penetrating abdominal aortic injury. Ann Vasc Surg 2014;28(7):1790.e9-11.
49. Singh TM, Hung R, Lebowitz E, et al. Endovascular repair of traumatic aortic pseudoaneurysm with associated celiacomesenteric trunk. J Endovasc Ther 2005;12(1):138–41.
50. Gupta BK, Khaneja SC, Flores L, et al. The role of intra-aortic balloon occlusion in penetrating abdominal trauma. J Trauma 1989;29(6):861–5.
51. Sullivan PS, Dente CJ, Patel S, et al. Outcome of ligation of the inferior vena cava in the modern era. Am J Surg 2010;199(4):500–6.
52. Burch JM, Feliciano DV, Mattox KL. The atriocaval shunt. Facts and fiction. Ann Surg 1988;207(5):555–68.
53. Byerly S, Tamariz L, Lee EE, et al. A Systematic Review and Meta-Analysis of Ligation Versus Repair of Inferior Vena Cava Injuries. Ann Vasc Surg 2021;75: 489–96.
54. Mullins RJ, Lucas CE, Ledgerwood AM. The natural history following venous ligation for civilian injuries. J Trauma 1980;20:737–43.
55. Bui TD, Mills JL. Control of inferior vena cava injury using percutaneous balloon catheter occlusion. Vasc Endovascular Surg 2009;43(5):490–3.
56. Castelli P, Caronno R, Piffaretti G, et al. Emergency endovascular repair for traumatic injury of the inferior vena cava. Eur J Cardio Thorac Surg 2005;28(6):906–8.
57. AlMulhim J, AlMutairi B, Qazi S, et al. Retrohepatic IVC injury: A new treatment approach with arterial stent graft. Radiol Case Rep 2020;16(3):560–3.
58. Mehta M, Darling RC 3rd, Taggert JB, et al. Outcomes of planned celiac artery coverage during TEVAR. J Vasc Surg 2010;52(5):1153–8.
59. Fullen WD, Hunt J, Altemeier WA. The clinical spectrum of penetrating injury to the superior mesenteric arterial circulation. J Trauma 1972;12(8):656–64.
60. Asensio JA, Berne JD, Chahwan S, et al. Traumatic injury to the superior mesenteric artery. Am J Surg 1999;178(3):235–9.
61. Lucas AE, Richardson JD, Flint LM, et al. Traumatic injury of the proximal superior mesenteric artery. Ann Surg 1981;193(1):30–4.

62. Mullins RJ, Huckfeldt R, Trunkey DD. Abdominal vascular injuries. Surg Clin North Am 1996;76(4):813–32.

63. Levy PJ, Krausz MM, Manny J. Acute mesenteric ischemia: improved results–a retrospective analysis of ninety-two patients. Surgery 1990;107:372–80.

64. Kim SK, Lee J, Duncan JR, et al. Endovascular treatment of superior mesenteric artery pseudoaneurysms using covered stents in six patients. AJR Am J Roentgenol 2014;203:432–8.

65. Zhao Y, Xie B, Liu Q, et al. Endovascular Treatment of Post-traumatic Superior Mesenteric Arteriovenous Fistula: A Case Report. Ann Vasc Surg 2018;50:297.e9-13.

66. Mattox KL, Rea J, Ennix CL, et al. Penetrating injuries to the iliac arteries. Am J Surg 1978;136(6):663–7.

67. Chitragari G, Schlosser FJ, Ochoa Chaar CI, et al. Consequences of hypogastric artery ligation, embolization, or coverage. J Vasc Surg 2015;62(5):1340–7.e1.

68. Burdick TR, Hoffer EK, Kooy T, et al. Which arteries are expendable? The practice and pitfalls of embolization throughout the body. Semin Intervent Radiol 2008;25: 191–203.

69. Biagioni RB, Burihan MC, Nasser F, et al. Endovascular treatment of penetrating arterial trauma with stent grafts. Vasa 2018;47(2):125–30.

70. Weir A, Kennedy P, Joyce S, et al. Endovascular management of pelvic trauma. Ann Transl Med 2021;9(14):1196.

71. Abdou H, Kundi R, DuBose JJ, et al. Repair of the Iliac Arterial Injury in Trauma: An Endovascular Operation? J Surg Res 2021;268:347–53.

72. Brenner M, Bulger EM, Perina DG, et al. Joint statement from the American College of Surgeons Committee on Trauma (ACS COT) and the American College of Emergency Physicians (ACEP) regarding the clinical use of Resuscitative Endovascular Balloon Occlusion of the Aorta (REBOA). Trauma Surg Acute Care Open 2018;3(1):e000154.

73. Russo RM, White JM, Baer DG. Partial Resuscitative Endovascular Balloon Occlusion of the Aorta: A Systematic Review of the Preclinical and Clinical Literature. J Surg Res 2021;262:101–14.

74. Osborn LA, Brenner ML, Prater SJ, et al. Resuscitative endovascular balloon occlusion of the aorta: current evidence. Open Access Emerg Med 2019;11:29–38.

75. Sise M.J., Shackford S.R., Peripheral vascular injury. In: Mattox, Moore, Feliciano, editors. Trauma.7th edition. 2014. McGraw Hill; New York, pp. 816–849.

76. Nanobashvili J, Kopadze T, Tvaladze M, et al. War injuries of major extremity arteries. World J Surg 2003;27(2):134–9.

77. Hafez HM, Woolgar J, Robbs JV. Lower extremity arterial injury: results of 550 cases and review of risk factors associated with limb loss. J Vasc Surg 2001; 33:1212–9.

78. Perkins ZB, Yet B, Glasgow S, et al. Meta-analysis of prognostic factors for amputation following surgical repair of lower extremity vascular trauma. Br J Surg 2015; 102:436–50.

79. Johansen K, Daines M, Howey T, et al. Objective criteria accurately predict amputation following lower extremity trauma. J Trauma 1990;30(5):568–72 [discussion: 572–3].

80. Loja MN, Sammann A, DuBose J, et al, AAST PROOVIT Study Group. The mangled extremity score and amputation: Time for a revision. J Trauma Acute Care Surg 2017;82(3):518–23.

81. Inaba K, Potzman J, Munera F, et al. Multi-slice CT angiography for arterial evaluation in the injured lower extremity. J Trauma 2006;60:502–6.

82. Peng PD, Spain DA, Tataria M, et al. CT angiography effectively evaluates extremity vascular trauma. Am Surg 2008;74(2):103–7.

83. Hornez E, Boddaert G, Ngabou UD, et al. Temporary vascular shunt for damage control of extremity vascular injury: A toolbox for trauma surgeons. J Visc Surg 2015;152(6):363–8.

84. Rich NM, Hughes CW. The fate of prosthetic material used to repair vascular injuries in contaminated wounds. J Trauma 1972;12(6):459–67.

85. Faries PL, Logerfo FW, Arora S, et al. A comparative study of alternative conduits for lower extremity revascularization: all-autogenous conduit versus prosthetic grafts. J Vasc Surg 2000;32(6):1080–90.

86. Reddy NP, Rowe VL. Is It Really Mandatory to Harvest the Contralateral Saphenous Vein for Use in Repair of Traumatic Injuries? Vasc Endovascular Surg 2018;52(7):548–9.

87. Feliciano DV, Mattox KL, Graham JM, et al. Five-year experience with PTFE grafts in vascular wounds. J Trauma 1985;25(1):71–82.

88. Ball CG, Feliciano DV. Damage control techniques for common and external iliac artery injuries: have temporary intravascular shunts replaced the need for ligation? J Trauma 2010;68(5):1117–20.

89. Farber A, Tan TW, Hamburg NM, et al. Early fasciotomy in patients with extremity vascular injury is associated with decreased risk of adverse limb outcomes: a review of the National Trauma Data Bank. Injury 2012;43(9):1486–91.

90. Feliciano DV, Moore EE, West MA, et al. Western trauma association critical decisions in trauma: evaluation and management of peripheral vascular injury, part II. J Trauma Acute Care Surg 2013;75(3):391–7.

91. Hurd JR, Emanuels DF, Aarabi S, et al. Limb Salvage Does Not Predict Functional Limb Outcome after Revascularization for Traumatic Acute Limb Ischemia. Ann Vasc Surg 2020;66:220–4.

92. Ballard JL, Bunt TJ, Malone JM. Management of small artery vascular trauma. Am J Surg 1992;164(4):316–9.

93. Branco BC, DuBose JJ, Zhan LX, et al. Trends and outcomes of endovascular therapy in the management of civilian vascular injuries. J Vasc Surg 2014;60:1297–307.

94. Doody O, Given MF, Lyon SM. Extremities—indications and techniques for treatment of extremity vascular injuries. InJ. Int J Care Injured 2008;39:1295–303.

95. White R, Krajcer Z, Johnson M, et al. Results of a multicenter trial for the treatment of traumatic vascular injury with a covered stent. J Trauma 2006;60(6):1189–95 [discussion: 1195–6].

96. Mavili E, Donmez H, Ozcan N, et al. Endovascular treatment of lower limb penetrating arterial traumas. Cardiovasc Intervent Radiol 2007;30:1124–9.

Moving?

Make sure your subscription moves with you!

To notify us of your new address, find your **Clinics Account Number** (located on your mailing label above your name), and contact customer service at:

Email: journalscustomerservice-usa@elsevier.com

800-654-2452 (subscribers in the U.S. & Canada)
314-447-8871 (subscribers outside of the U.S. & Canada)

Fax number: 314-447-8029

Elsevier Health Sciences Division
Subscription Customer Service
3251 Riverport Lane
Maryland Heights, MO 63043

*To ensure uninterrupted delivery of your subscription, please notify us at least 4 weeks in advance of move.

9780323939355